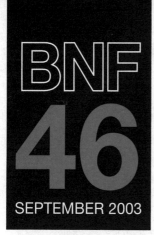

BNF
46
SEPTEMBER 2003

BNF.org

BRITISH
NATIONAL
FORMULARY

•

British Medical Association

Royal Pharmaceutical Society
of Great Britain

Published by the British Medical Association
Tavistock Square, London WC1H 9JP, UK
and the **Royal Pharmaceutical Society of Great Britain**
1 Lambeth High Street, London, SE1 7JN, UK
© 2003 British Medical Association and the Royal Pharmaceutical Society of Great Britain

ISBN: 0 85369 556 3 (Royal Pharmaceutical Society of Great Britain)

ISBN: 0 7279 1789 7 (British Medical Association)

ISSN: 0260-535X

Printed in Great Britain by William Clowes, Beccles, Suffolk

A catalogue record for this book is available from the British Library.

Copies may be obtained through any bookseller or direct from:

Pharmaceutical Press
  PO Box 151
  Wallingford
  Oxon OX10 8QU
  UK
  Tel: +44 (0) 1491 829 272
  Fax: +44 (0) 1491 829 292
  E-mail: rpsgb@cabi.org
  www.pharmpress.com

BMJ Bookshop
  PO Box 295
  London WC1H 9TE
  UK
  Tel: +44 (0) 20 7383 6244
  Fax: +44 (0) 20 7383 6455
  E-mail: orders@bmjbookshop.com
  www.bmjbookshop.com

The Pharmaceutical Press also supplies the BNF in digital formats suitable for standalone use or for small networks, for use over an intranet and for use on a personal digital assistant (PDA).

NHS Responseline
General practitioners and community pharmacies in **England** can telephone the NHS Responseline for enquiries concerning the direct mailing of the *British National Formulary*
Tel: 08701 555 455

For a list of name changes required by Directive 92/27/EEC, see p. x

Contents

Preface

The BNF is a joint publication of the British Medical Association and the Royal Pharmaceutical Society of Great Britain. It is published under the authority of a Joint Formulary Committee which comprises representatives of the two professional bodies and of the UK Health Departments. The BNF aims to provide doctors, pharmacists and other healthcare professionals with sound up-to-date information about the use of medicines.

The BNF includes key information on the selection, prescribing, dispensing and administration of medicines. Drugs that are generally prescribed in the UK are covered and those that are considered less suitable for prescribing are clearly identified. Little or no information is included on medicines that are promoted for purchase by the public.

Basic information about drugs is drawn from the manufacturers' product literature, from medical and pharmaceutical literature, from regulatory and professional authorities, and from the data used for pricing prescriptions. Advice on the therapeutic use of medicines and on the choice of drugs is constructed from clinical literature and reflects, wherever possible, an evaluation of the evidence. The advice also takes account of authoritative national guidelines. In addition, the Joint Formulary Committee receives expert clinical advice on all therapeutic areas, particularly those that are not yet supported by good evidence; this ensures that the BNF's recommendations are relevant to practice. Many individuals and organisations contribute towards the preparation of each edition of the BNF.

The BNF is designed as a digest for rapid reference and it may not always include all the information necessary for prescribing and dispensing. Also, less detail is given on areas such as obstetrics, malignant disease, and anaesthesia since it is expected that those undertaking treatment will have specialist knowledge and access to specialist literature. The BNF is intended to be interpreted in light of professional knowledge and it should be supplemented as necessary by specialised publications and by reference to the manufacturers' product literature. Information is also available from local medicines information services (see inside front cover).

Biannual publication allows the BNF to reflect promptly changes in product availability as well as emerging safety concerns and shifts in clinical practice. The more important changes for this edition are listed on p. viii.

The BNF is now available on the internet (http://BNF.org); the site also includes additional information of relevance to healthcare professionals dealing with medicines. Other digital versions of the BNF—including intranet versions—are produced in parallel with the paper version.

The BNF welcomes comments from healthcare professionals; such comments help to ensure that the BNF remains relevant to practice. Comments and constructive criticism should be sent to:
Executive Editor, British National Formulary,
c/o Royal Pharmaceutical Society of Great Britain,
1 Lambeth High Street, London SE1 7JN.
Email: editor@bnf.org

Acknowledgements

The Joint Formulary Committee is grateful to individuals and organisations that have provided advice and information to the BNF.

The principal contributors for this edition were:

I.H. Ahmed-Jushuf, J.M. Aitken, S.P. Allison, D.G. Arkell, M. Badminton, T.P. Baglin, P.R.J. Barnes, R.H. Behrens, D. Bowsher, M.J. Brodie, R.J. Buckley, I.F. Burgess, D.J. Burn, A.J. Camm, D.A. Chamberlain, C.E. Clarke, C. Diamond, R. Dinwiddie, P.N. Durrington, A.J. Duxbury, T.S.J. Elliott, B.G. Gazzard, A.H. Ghodse, N.J.L. Gittoes, P.J. Goadsby, E.C. Gordon-Smith, I.A. Greer, J. Guillebaud, C.H. Hawkes, C.J. Hawkey, S.H.D. Jackson, J.R. Kirwan, P.G. Kopelman, M.J.S. Langman, T.H. Lee, L. Luzzatto, K.E.L. McColl, G.M. Mead, E. Miller, J.M. Neuberger, J. Nooney, D. Nutt, D.J. Oliver, L.P. Ormerod, P.A. Poole-Wilson, P.A. Routledge, D.J. Rowbotham, P.C. Rubin, R.S. Sawers, R.C. Spencer, I. Stockley, A.E. Tattersfield, H. Thomas, S. Thomas, G.R. Thompson, D.G. Waller, D.A. Warrell, A. Wilcock.

Members of the British Association of Dermatologists Therapy Guidelines and Audit Subcommittee, N.H. Cox, A.S. Highet, M.J.D. Goodfield, R.H. Meyrick-Thomas, A.D. Ormerod, J.K.L. Schofield, C.H. Smith, J.C. Sterling, and D.E. Senner (Secretariat) have provided valuable advice.

The Joint British Societies' Coronary Risk Prediction Charts have been reproduced with the kind permission of P.N. Durrington who has also provided the BNF with access to the computer program for assessing coronary and stroke risk.

Correspondents in the pharmaceutical industry have provided information on new products and commented on products in the BNF. The Prescription Pricing Authority has supplied the prices of products in the BNF.

Numerous doctors, pharmacists, nurses and others have sent comments and suggestions.

The BNF has valuable access to the *Martindale* data banks by courtesy of S. Sweetman and staff.

C.L. Iskander and R.K. Malde provided considerable assistance during the production of this edition of the BNF.

Additional checks on the BNF data were undertaken by A. Breewood, S. Coleman, M.J. Gilmour, E. Laughton, N.J. Morris and E. Rees Evans.

E.I. Connor and K.A. Parsons have assisted with the development of the electronic BNF and publishing software. Xpage and CSW Informatics Ltd have provided technical assistance with the editorial database and typesetting software.

Joint Formulary Committee 2002–2003

Chairman
Martin J. Kendall
MB, ChB, MD, FRCP

Deputy Chairman
Nicholas L. Wood
BPharm, FRPharmS

Committee Members
Peter R. Arlett
BSc, MB BS, MRCP

Alison Blenkinsopp
PhD, BPharm, FRPharmS

Peter Clappison
MB, ChB, MRCGP

Michael J. Goodman
BMBCh, BA, MA, DPhil, MRCP, FRCP

Margaret L. Hewetson
BPharm, DipHospPharm, MRPharmS

Frank P. Marsh
MA, MB, BChir, FRCP

Roopendra K. Prasad
MB BS, MS, FRCS, FRCGP

Jane Richards
OBE, MB BS, MRCS, LRCP, FRCGP, D(Obst) RCOG, DCH

James Smith
BPharm, PhD, FRPharmS, MCPP, MIInfSc

Joint Secretaries
Robert B.K. Broughton
OBE, OStJ, MB, BCh, DMRD, MHSM

Philip E. Green
BSc, MSc, LLM, MRPharmS

Executive Secretary
Lynn Clifton

Editorial Staff

Executive Editor
Dinesh K. Mehta
BPharm, MSc, FRPharmS

Senior Assistant Editor
John Martin
BPharm, PhD, MRPharmS

Assistant Editors
Bryony Jordan
BSc, DipPharmPract, MRPharmS

Colin R. Macfarlane
BPharm, MSc, MRPharmS

Rachel S. M. Ryan
BPharm, MRPharmS

Shama M. S. Wagle
BPharm, DipPharmPract, MRPharmS

Staff Editors
Fauziah T. Hashmi
BSc, MSc, MRPharmS

Sangeeta Kakar
BSc, MRPharmS

Maria Kouimtzi
BPharm, PhD, MRPharmS

Dawud Masieh
BPharm, MRPharmS

Vinaya K. Sharma
BPharm, MSc, MRPharmS

Rob Ticehurst
BSc, MRPharmS

Editorial Assistant
Gerard P. Gallagher

Head of Publishing Services
John Wilson

Director of Publications
Charles Fry

How to use the BNF

Notes on conditions, drugs and preparations

The main text consists of classified notes on clinical conditions, drugs and preparations. These notes are divided into 15 chapters, each of which is related to a particular system of the body or to an aspect of medical care. Each chapter is then divided into sections which begin with appropriate *notes for prescribers*. These notes are intended to provide information to doctors, pharmacists, nurses, and other healthcare professionals to facilitate the selection of suitable treatment. The notes are followed by details of relevant drugs and preparations.

Guidance on prescribing

This part includes information on prescription writing, controlled drugs and dependence, prescribing for children and the elderly, and prescribing in palliative care. Advice is given on the reporting of adverse reactions.

DRUG NAME ◢◣●
Indications: details of uses and indications
Cautions: details of precautions required (with cross-references to appropriate Appendixes) and also any monitoring required
COUNSELLING. Verbal explanation to the patient of specific details of the drug treatment (e.g. posture when taking a medicine)
Contra-indications: details of any contra-indications to use of drug
Side-effects: details of common and more serious side-effects
Dose: dose and frequency of administration (max. dose); CHILD and ELDERLY details of dose for specific age group
By alternative route, dose and frequency

* **Approved Name** (Non-proprietary) PoM●
Pharmaceutical form, colour, coating, active ingredient and amount in dosage form, net price, pack size = basic NHS price. Label: (as in Appendix 9)
Proprietary Name® (Manufacturer) PoM
NHS●
Pharmaceutical form, sugar-free, active ingredient mg/mL, net price, pack size = basic NHS price. Label: (as in Appendix 9)
Excipients: includes clinically important excipients or electrolytes
* exceptions to the prescribing status indicated by a footnote.
Note. Specific notes about the product e.g. handling

Preparations

Preparations usually follow immediately after the drug which is their main ingredient.

Preparations are included under a non-proprietary title, if they are marketed under such a title, if they are not otherwise prescribable under the NHS, or if they may be prepared extemporaneously.

If proprietary preparations are of a distinctive colour this is stated.

In the case of compound preparations the indications, cautions, contra-indications, side-effects, and interactions of all constituents should be taken into account for prescribing.

Emergency treatment of poisoning

This chapter provides information on the management of acute poisoning when first seen in the home, although aspects of hospital-based treatment are mentioned.

Appendixes and indexes

The appendixes include information on interactions, liver disease, renal impairment, pregnancy, breast-feeding, intravenous additives, borderline substances, wound management products, and cautionary and advisory labels for dispensed medicines. They are designed for use in association with the main body of the text.

The Dental Practitioners' List and the Nurse Prescribers' List are also included in this section. The indexes consist of the Index of Manufacturers and the Main Index.

Drugs

Drugs appear under pharmacopoeial or other non-proprietary titles. When there is an *appropriate current monograph* (Medicines Act 1968, Section 65) preference is given to a name at the head of that monograph; otherwise a British Approved Name (BAN), if available, is used (see also p. x).

The symbol ◢◣ is used to denote those preparations that are considered by the Joint Formulary Committee to be less suitable for prescribing. Although such preparations may not be considered as drugs of first choice, their use may be justifiable in certain circumstances.

Prescription-only medicines PoM

This symbol has been placed against those preparations that are available only on medical or dental prescription. For more detailed information see *Medicines, Ethics and Practice*, No. 27, London, Pharmaceutical Press, 2003 (and subsequent editions as available).

The symbol CD indicates that the preparation is subject to the prescription requirements of the Misuse of Drugs Act. For regulations governing prescriptions for such preparations see pages 7–9.

Preparations not available for NHS prescription NHS

This symbol has been placed against those preparations included in the BNF that are not prescribable under the NHS. Those prescribable only for specific disorders have a footnote specifying the condition(s) for which the preparation remains available. Some preparations which are not *prescribable* by brand name under the NHS may nevertheless be *dispensed* using the brand name providing that the prescription shows an appropriate non-proprietary name.

Prices

Prices have been calculated from the basic cost used in pricing NHS prescriptions dispensed in May 2003 or later, see p. vii for further details.

Patient Packs

On January 1 1994, Directive 92/27/EEC came into force, giving the requirements for the labelling of medicines and outlining the format and content of patient information leaflets to be supplied with every medicine. The directive also requires the use of Recommended International Non-proprietary Names for drugs (see p. x).

All medicines have approved labelling and patient information leaflets; anyone who supplies a medicine is responsible for providing the relevant information to the patient (see also Appendix 9).

Many medicines are available in manufacturers' original packs complete with patient information leaflets. Where patient packs are available, the BNF shows the number of dose units in the packs. In particular clinical circumstances, where patient packs need to be split or medicines are provided in bulk dispensing packs, manufacturers will provide additional supplies of patient information leaflets on request.

During the revision of each edition of the BNF careful note is taken of the information that appears on the patient information leaflets. Where it is considered appropriate to alert a prescriber to some specific limitation appearing on the patient information leaflet (for example, in relation to pregnancy) this advice now appears in the BNF.

The patient information leaflet also includes details of all inactive ingredients in the medicine. A list of common E numbers and the inactive ingredients to which they correspond is now therefore included in the BNF (see inside back cover).

PACT and SPA

PACT (Prescribing Analyses and Cost) and SPA (Scottish Prescribing Analysis) provide prescribers with information about their prescribing.

The *PACT Standard Report*, or in Scotland SPA *Level 1 Report*, is sent to all general practitioners on a quarterly basis. It contains an analysis of the practitioner's prescribing over the last 3 months, and for a given topic of prescribing, it compares the individual practice with the Health Authority equivalents.

The *PACT Catalogue*, or in Scotland SPA *Level 2 Report*, provides a full inventory of the prescriptions issued by a prescriber. The PACT catalogue is available on request for periods between 1 and 24 months. To allow the prescriber to target specific areas of prescribing, a Catalogue may be requested to cover individual preparations, BNF sections, or combinations of BNF chapters.

PACT is also available electronically. This system gives users on-line access through NHSnet to the 3 years' prescribing data held on the Prescription Pricing Authority's database.

Prices in the BNF

Basic **net prices** are given in the BNF to provide an indication of relative cost. Where there is a choice of suitable preparations for a particular disease or condition the relative cost may be used in making a selection. Cost-effective prescribing must, however, take into account other factors (such as dose frequency and duration of treatment) that affect the total cost. The use of more expensive drugs is justified if it will result in better treatment of the patient or a reduction of the length of an illness or the time spent in hospital.

Prices have generally been calculated from the net cost used in pricing NHS prescriptions dispensed in May 2003, but where available later prices have been included; unless an original pack is available these prices are based on the largest pack size of the preparation in use in community pharmacies. The price for an extemporaneously prepared preparation has been omitted where the net cost of the ingredients used to make it would give a misleadingly low impression of the final price. In Appendix 8 prices stated are per dressing or bandage.

The unit of 20 is still sometimes used as a basis for comparison, but where suitable original packs or patient packs are available these are priced instead.

Gross prices vary as follows:

1. Costs to the NHS are greater than the net prices quoted and include professional fees and overhead allowances;
2. Private prescription charges are calculated on a separate basis;
3. Over-the-counter sales are at retail price, as opposed to basic net price, and include VAT.

BNF prices are NOT, therefore, suitable for quoting to patients seeking private prescriptions or contemplating over-the-counter purchases.

A fuller explanation of costs to the NHS may be obtained from the Drug Tariff.

It should be noted that separate Drug Tariffs are applicable to England and Wales, Scotland, and Northern Ireland. Prices in the different tariffs may vary.

Changes for this edition

Significant changes

The BNF is revised twice yearly and numerous changes are made between issues. All copies of BNF No. 45 (March 2003) should therefore be withdrawn and replaced by BNF No. 46 (September 2003). Significant changes have been made in the following sections for BNF No. 46:

Combined use of aspirin and clopidogrel [updated advice], section 2.9

Hypothyroidism and lipid-regulating drugs [new text], section 2.12

Statins [revised text], section 2.12

Drugs for asthma in breast-feeding [updated advice], section 3.1

Cromoglicate and related therapy [updated advice], section 3.3.1

Drugs used in Parkinsonism [revised text], section 4.9

Dopaminergic drugs used in Parkinsonism [revised text], section 4.9.1

Antimuscarinic drugs used in Parkinsonism [revised text], section 4.9.2

Paroxetine not recommended for depression in those under 18 years [CSM advice], section 4.3.3

Antibacterial treatment of incubating syphilis [new text], Table 1, section 5.1

Antibacterial treatment of uncomplicated gonorrhoea [revised text], Table 1, section 5.1

Antibacterial treatment of osteomyelitis and septic arthritis [revised text], Table 1, section 5.1

Antibacterial treatment of septicaemia related to vascular catheter [revised text], Table 1, section 5.1

Antibacterial treatment of otitis media [revised text], Table 1, section 5.1

Antibacterial treatment of throat infections [revised text], Table 1, section 5.1

Management of anthrax [revised text], section 5.1.12

Capecitabine and tegafur with uracil for metastatic colorectal cancer [NICE guidance], section 8.1.3

Capecitabine for locally advanced or metastatic breast cancer [NICE guidance], section 8.1.3

Use of irradiated blood products with cladribine and fludarabine [new text], section 8.1.3

Control of microbial contamination of eye preparations [updated advice], section 11.2

Topical pimecrolimus and tacrolimus for atopic eczema [updated advice], section 13.5.3

Meningococcal vaccine for travellers [updated advice], section 14.4

Nephrotoxicity associated with interaction between sevoflurane and carbon dioxide absorbents [new text], section 15.1.2

Dose changes

Changes in dose statements introduced into BNF No. 46:

Amoxicillin [anthrax], p. 261
Caspofungin, p. 295
Ceftazidime, p. 268
Celecoxib, p. 482
Chlorambucil, p. 411
Clozapine, p. 180
Erythromycin [pertussis prevention], p. 275
Etodolac, p. 484
Etomidate-Lipuro®, p. 603
Hypnomidate®, p. 603
Melphalan, p. 412
Prednisolone [daily dose for myasthenia gravis], p. 500
Procaine Benzylpenicillin [for syphilis], p. 255
Tranexamic Acid, p. 122
Viazem XL®, p. 103

Classification changes

Classification changes have been made in the following sections for BNF No. 46:

Section 2.12 Ezetimibe [new subsection]

Section 6.4.1.1 Women with uterus [subsection no longer exists]

Section 6.4.1.1 Women without a uterus [subsection no longer exists]

Section 6.7.1 Bromocriptine and other dopaminergic drugs [title change]

Section 7.3.1 Combined hormonal contraceptives [title change]

Section 7.4.5 Phosphodiesterase type-5 inhibitors [subtitle change]

Section 14.4 Measles, Mumps and Rubella (MMR) vaccine [subtitle change]

New names

Name changes introduced into BNF No. 46 (see also p. x):

Asacol® *MR* [formerly *Asacol*®], p. 48
Actrapid [formerly *Human Actrapid*®], p. 330
Insulatard® [formerly *Human Insulatard*®], p. 331
Lyrinel® *XL* [formerly *Ditropan*® *XL*], p. 401
Mixtard® *10* [formerly *Human Mixtard*® *10*], p. 332
Mixtard® *20* [formerly *Human Mixtard*® *20*], p. 332
Mixtard® *30* [formerly *Human Mixtard*® *30*], p. 332
Mixtard® *40* [formerly *Human Mixtard*® *40*], p. 333
Mixtard® *50* [formerly *Human Mixtard*® *50*], p. 333
Monotard® [formerly *Human Monotard*®], p. 331
Ultratard® [formerly *Human Ultratard*®], p. 331
Velosulin® [formerly *Human Velosulin*®], p. 330

Discontinued preparations

Preparations discontinued during the compilation of BNF No. 46:

Acnecide®
Aerolin® *Autohaler*
Alcoderm®
Aserbine® cream
Becloforte® dry powder for inhalation
Bocasan®
Cogentin® tablets
Duovent® aerosol inhalation and *Autohaler*
Efalith®
Eryacne®
Exosurf Neonatal®
Hexopal® suspension
Ionax Scrub®
Ionil T®
Minims® Homatropine Hydrobromide
Minims® Neomycin Sulphate
Mistamine®
Multibionta®
Mysoline®
Orovite Comploment B₆®
Palfium®
Pnu-Imune®
PostMI® *75EC*
Sterac® sodium chloride
Sterexidine®
Tagamet® effervescent
Tampovagan®
Tenben®
Ticlid®
Trifyba®
Vivotif®
Vitamin Tablets (with Calcium and Iodine) for Nursing Mothers
Xefo®
Zinamide®

New preparations included in this edition

Preparations included in the relevant sections of BNF No. 46:

Avelox® p. 291
Bextra® p. 488
Carbaglu® p. 476
Crestor® p. 128
diabact UBT® p. 37
Evra® p. 392
Ezetrol® p. 125
FemTab® p. 356
FemTab® Continuous p. 354
FemTab® Sequi p. 354
Gammaderm® p. 539
Hepsera® p. 310
Levitra® p. 406
Mastaflu® p. 589
Metrosa® p. 568
Migard® p. 222
Movicol-Half® p. 55
Neulasta® p. 450
Olmetec® p. 96
Opatanol® p. 512
Promixin® p. 280
Rapolyte® p. 452
Risperdal Quicklet® p. 182
Testogel® p. 361
Voltarol® *Ophtha Multidose* p. 520
WinRho SDF® p. 599
Zoton FasTab® p. 43

Name changes

Directive 92/27/EEC requires use of the Recommended International Non-proprietary Name (rINN) for medicinal substances. In most cases the British Approved Name (BAN) and rINN were identical. Where the two differed, the BAN was modified to accord with the rINN.

The following list shows those substances for which the former BAN has been modified to accord with the rINN. The MHRA has proposed a timetable for effecting the change from former BANs to the new names. Former BANs have been retained as synonyms in the BNF.

For substances which were considered to pose the highest risk to public health, a system of showing the new name as well as the former name ('dual-labelling') was advocated and this edition of the BNF shows both names at the head of the drug entries. However, with the exception of adrenaline and noradrenaline, the British Pharmacopoeia (BP 2003) has discontinued the practice of dual-labelling and BNF 47 (March 2004) will show the former names as synonyms.

ADRENALINE AND NORADRENALINE. Adrenaline and noradrenaline are the terms used in the titles of monographs in the European Pharmacopoeia and are thus the official names in the member states. For these substances, BP 2003 shows the European Pharmacopoeia names and the rINNs at the head of the monographs; the BNF has adopted a similar style.

Former BAN	New BAN
adrenaline	*see above*
amethocaine	tetracaine
aminacrine	aminoacridine
amoxycillin	amoxicillin
amphetamine	amfetamine
amylobarbitone	amobarbital
amylobarbitone sodium	amobarbital sodium
beclomethasone	beclometasone
bendrofluazide	bendroflumethiazide
benorylate	benorilate
benzhexol	trihexyphenidyl
benzphetamine	benzfetamine
benztropine	benzatropine
busulphan	busulfan
butobarbitone	butobarbital
carticaine	articane
cephalexin	cefalexin
cephamandole nafate	cefamandole nafate
cephazolin	cefazolin
cephradine	cefradine
chloral betaine	cloral betaine
chlorbutol	chlorobutanol
chlormethiazole	clomethiazole
chlorpheniramine	chlorphenamine
chlorthalidone	chlortalidone
cholecalciferol	colecalciferol
cholestyramine	colestyramine
clomiphene	clomifene
colistin sulphomethate sodium	colistimethate sodium
corticotrophin	corticotropin
cyclosporin	ciclosporin
cysteamine	mercaptamine
danthron	dantron
desoxymethasone	desoximetasone
dexamphetamine	dexamfetamine
dibromopropamidine	dibrompropamidine
dicyclomine	dicycloverine

Former BAN	New BAN
dienoestrol	dienestrol
dimethicone(s)	dimeticone
dimethyl sulphoxide	dimethyl sulfoxide
dothiepin	dosulepin
doxycycline hydrochloride (hemihydrate hemiethanolate)	doxycycline hyclate
eformoterol	formoterol
ethacrynic acid	etacrynic acid
ethamsylate	etamsylate
ethinyloestradiol	ethinylestradiol
ethynodiol	etynodiol
flumethasone	flumetasone
flupenthixol	flupentixol
flurandrenolone	fludroxycortide
frusemide	furosemide
gestronol	gestonorone
guaiphenesin	guaifenesin
hexachlorophane	hexachlorophene
hexamine hippurate	methenamine hippurate
hydroxyurea	hydroxycarbamide
indomethacin	indometacin
lignocaine	lidocaine
lysuride	lisuride
methotrimeprazine	levomepromazine
methyl cysteine	mecysteine
methylene blue	methylthioninium chloride
methylphenobarbitone	methylphenobarbital
mitozantrone	mitoxantrone
mustine	chlormethine
nicoumalone	acenocoumarol
noradrenaline	*see above*
oestradiol	estradiol
oestriol	estriol
oestrone	estrone
oxethazaine	oxetacaine
oxpentifylline	pentoxifylline
pentaerythritol tetranitrate	pentaerithrityl tetranitrate
phenobarbitone	phenobarbital
pipothiazine	pipotiazine
polyhexanide	polihexanide
potassium clorazepate	dipotassium clorazepate
pramoxine	pramocaine
procaine penicillin	procaine benzylpenicillin
prothionamide	protionamide
quinalbarbitone	secobarbital
riboflavine	riboflavin
salcatonin	calcitonin (salmon)
sodium calciumedetate	sodium calcium edetate
sodium cromoglycate	sodium cromoglicate
sodium ironedetate	sodium feredetate
sodium picosulphate	sodium picosulfate
sorbitan monostearate	sorbitan stearate
stibocaptate	sodium stibocaptate
stilboestrol	diethylstilbestrol
sulphacetamide	sulfacetamide
sulphadiazine	sulfadiazine
sulphadimidine	sulfadimidine
sulphamethoxazole	sulfamethoxazole
sulphapyridine	sulfapyridine
sulphasalazine	sulfasalazine
sulphathiazole	sulfathiazole
sulphinpyrazone	sulfinpyrazone
tetracosactrin	tetracosactide
thiabendazole	tiabendazole
thioguanine	tioguanine
thiopentone	thiopental
thymoxamine	moxisylyte
thyroxine sodium	levothyroxine sodium
tribavirin	ribavirin
trimeprazine	alimemazine
urofollitrophin	urofollitropin

Guidance on prescribing

General guidance

Medicines should be prescribed only when they are necessary, and in all cases the benefit of administering the medicine should be considered in relation to the risk involved. This is particularly important during pregnancy where the risk to both mother and fetus must be considered (for further details see Prescribing in Pregnancy, Appendix 4).

It is important to discuss treatment options carefully with the patient to ensure that the patient is content to take the medicine as prescribed (see also Taking Medicines to Best Effect, below). In particular, the patient should be helped to distinguish the side-effects of prescribed drugs from the effects of the medical disorder. Where the beneficial effects of the medicine are likely to be delayed, the patient should be advised of this.

TAKING MEDICINES TO BEST EFFECT. Difficulties in compliance with drug treatment occur regardless of age. Factors contributing to poor compliance with prescribed medicines include:

- Prescription not collected or not dispensed
- Purpose of medicine not clear
- Perceived lack of efficacy
- Real or perceived side-effects
- Instructions for administration not clear
- Physical difficulty in taking medicines (e.g. with swallowing the medicine, with handling small tablets, or with opening medicine containers)
- Unattractive formulation (e.g. unpleasant taste)
- Complicated regimen

The prescriber and the patient should agree on the health outcomes that the patient desires and on the strategy for achieving them ('concordance'). Further information on concordance is available on the Internet (www.medicines-partnership.org).

Taking the time to explain to the patient (and relatives) the rationale and the potential adverse effects of treatment may improve compliance. Reinforcement and elaboration of the physician's instructions by the pharmacist also helps. Advising the patient of the possibility of alternative treatments may encourage the patient to seek advice rather than merely abandon unacceptable treatment.

Simplifying the drug regimen may help; the need for frequent administration may reduce compliance although there appears to be little difference in compliance between once-daily and twice-daily administration. Combination products reduce the number of drugs taken but this may be at the expense of the ability to titrate individual doses.

COMPLEMENTARY MEDICINE. An increasing amount of information on complementary ('alternative') medicine is becoming available. However, the scope of the BNF's advice is restricted to the discussion of conventional medicines but reference will be made to complementary treatments if they affect conventional therapy (e.g. interactions with St John's wort—see Appendix 1). Further information on herbal medicines is available on the Internet (www.mhra.gov.uk/ourwork/licensingmeds/herbalmeds/herbalsafety.htm).

ABBREVIATION OF TITLES. In general, titles of drugs and preparations should be written *in full*. Unofficial abbreviations should not be used as they may be misinterpreted; obsolete titles, such as Mist. Expect. should not be used.

NON-PROPRIETARY TITLES. Where non-proprietary ('generic') titles are given, they should be used in prescribing. This will enable any suitable product to be dispensed, thereby saving delay to the patient and sometimes expense to the health service. The only exception is where bioavailability problems are so important that the patient should always receive the same brand; in such cases, the brand name or the manufacturer should be stated. Non-proprietary titles should **not** be invented for the purposes of prescribing generically since this can lead to confusion, particularly in the case of compound and modified-release preparations.

Titles used as headings for monographs may be used freely in the United Kingdom but in other countries may be subject to restriction.

Many of the non-proprietary titles used in this book are titles of monographs in the European Pharmacopoeia, British Pharmacopoeia or British Pharmaceutical Codex 1973. In such cases the preparations must comply with the standard (if any) in the appropriate publication, as required by the Medicines Act (Section 65).

PROPRIETARY TITLES. Names followed by the symbol® are or have been used as proprietary names in the United Kingdom. These names may in general be applied only to products supplied by the owners of the trade marks.

MARKETING AUTHORISATION AND BNF ADVICE. The doses stated in the BNF are intended for general guidance and represent, unless otherwise stated, the usual range of doses that are generally regarded as being suitable for adults. In general the *doses, indications, cautions, contra-indications and side-effects* in the BNF reflect those in the manufacturers' data sheets or Summaries of Product Characteristics (SPCs) which, in turn, reflect those in the corresponding Marketing Authorisations (formerly known as Product Licences). Where an unlicensed drug is included in the BNF, this is indicated in brackets after the entry. Where a use (or route) is recommended outside the licensed indication ('off-label' use) of an available product, this too is indicated. When a preparation is available from more than one manufacturer, the BNF reflects advice that is the most clinically relevant regardless of any variation in the marketing authorisations.

> It has been noted (*Drug and Therapeutics Bulletin* 1992; **30:** 97–9) that prescribing of licensed medicines outside the recommendations of the Marketing Authorisation alters (and probably increases) the doctor's professional responsibility.

ORAL SYRINGES. An **oral syringe** is supplied when oral liquid medicines are prescribed in doses other than multiples of 5 mL. The oral syringe is marked in 0.5-mL divisions from 1 to 5 mL to measure doses of less than 5 mL. It is provided with an adaptor and an instruction leaflet. The *5-mL spoon* is used for doses of 5 mL (or multiples thereof).

STRENGTHS AND QUANTITIES. The strength or quantity to be contained in capsules, lozenges, tablets, etc. should be stated by the prescriber.

If a pharmacist receives an incomplete prescription for a systemically administered preparation[1] and considers it would not be appropriate for the patient to return to the doctor, the following procedures will apply:

(a) an attempt must always be made to contact the prescriber to ascertain the intention;

(b) if the attempt is successful the pharmacist must, where practicable, subsequently arrange for details of quantity, strength where applicable, and dosage to be inserted by the prescriber on the incomplete form;

(c) where, although the prescriber has been contacted, it has not proved possible to obtain the written intention regarding an incomplete prescription, the pharmacist may endorse the form 'p.c.' (prescriber contacted) and add details of the quantity and strength where applicable of the preparation supplied, and of the dose indicated. The endorsement should be initialled and dated by the pharmacist;

(d) where the prescriber cannot be contacted and the pharmacist has sufficient information to make a professional judgment the preparation may be dispensed. If the quantity is missing the pharmacist may supply sufficient to complete up to 5 days' treatment; except that where a combination pack (i.e. a proprietary pack containing more than one medicinal product) or oral contraceptive is prescribed by name only, the smallest pack shall be dispensed. In all cases the prescription must be endorsed 'p.n.c.' (prescriber not contacted) the quantity, the dose, and the strength (where applicable) of the preparation supplied must be indicated, and the endorsement must be initialled and dated;

(e) if the pharmacist has any doubt about exercising discretion, an incomplete prescription must be referred back to the prescriber.

EXCIPIENTS. Oral liquid preparations that do not contain *fructose, glucose* or *sucrose* are described as 'sugar-free' in the BNF. Preparations containing hydrogenated glucose syrup, mannitol, maltitol, sorbitol or xylitol are also marked 'sugar-free' since there is evidence that they do not cause dental caries. Patients receiving medicines containing cariogenic sugars should be advised of appropriate dental hygiene measures to prevent caries.

Where information on the presence of *aspartame, gluten, tartrazine, arachis (peanut) oil* or *sesame oil* is available, this is indicated in the BNF against the relevant preparation.

Information is provided on *selected excipients* in skin preparations (see section 13.1.3) and on *selected preservatives* and *excipients* in eye drops and injections. Pressurised metered aerosols containing *chlorofluorocarbons* (CFCs) have also been identified throughout the BNF (see section 3.1.1.1).

The presence of *benzyl alcohol* and *polyoxyl castor oil* (polyethoxylated castor oil) in injections is indicated in the BNF. Benzyl alcohol has been associated with a fatal toxic syndrome in premature infants, and parenteral preparations containing the preservative should not be used in neonates. Polyoxyl castor oils, used as vehicles in intravenous injections, have been associated with severe anaphylactoid reactions.

> In the absence of information on excipients in the BNF and in the product literature, contact the manufacturer (see Index of Manufacturers) if it is essential to check details.

EXTEMPORANEOUS PREPARATION. A product should be dispensed extemporaneously only when no product with a marketing authorisation is available.

The BP direction that a preparation must be *freshly prepared* indicates that it must be made not more than 24 hours before it is issued for use. The direction that a preparation should be *recently prepared* indicates that deterioration is likely if the preparation is stored for longer than about 4 weeks at 15–25° C.

The term **water** used without qualification means either potable water freshly drawn direct from the public supply and suitable for drinking or freshly boiled and cooled purified water. The latter should be used if the public supply is from a local storage tank or if the potable water is unsuitable for a particular preparation (Water for injections, section 9.2.2).

DRUGS AND DRIVING. Prescribers should advise patients if treatment is likely to affect their ability to drive motor vehicles. This applies especially to drugs with sedative effects; patients should be warned that these effects are increased by alcohol. General information about a patient's fitness to drive is available from the Driver and Vehicle Licensing Agency at www.dvla.gov.uk/dvla.htm (see also Appendix 9).

PATENTS. In the BNF certain drugs have been included notwithstanding the existence of actual or potential patent rights. In so far as such substances are protected by Letters Patent, their inclusion in this Formulary neither conveys, nor implies, licence to manufacture.

HEALTH AND SAFETY. When handling chemical or biological materials particular attention should be given to the possibility of allergy, fire, explosion, radiation, or poisoning. Substances, including corticosteroids, some antimicrobials, phenothiazines, and many cytotoxics, are irritant or very potent and should be handled with caution. Contact with the skin and inhalation of dust should be avoided.

SAFETY IN THE HOME. Patients must be warned to keep all medicines out of the reach of children. All solid dose and all oral and external liquid prepara-

---

1. With the exception of temazepam, an incomplete prescription is **not** acceptable for controlled drugs in schedules 2 and 3 of the Misuse of Drugs Regulations 2001

tions must be dispensed in a reclosable *child-resistant container* unless:

- the medicine is in an original pack or patient pack such as to make this inadvisable;
- the patient will have difficulty in opening a child-resistant container;
- a specific request is made that the product shall not be dispensed in a child-resistant container;
- no suitable child-resistant container exists for a particular liquid preparation.

All patients should be advised to dispose of *unwanted medicines* by returning them to a supplier for destruction.

NAME OF MEDICINE. The name of the medicine should appear on the label unless the prescriber indicates otherwise.

1. Subject to the conditions of paragraphs 4 and 6 below, the name of the prescribed medicine is stated on the label unless the prescriber deletes the letters 'NP' which appear on NHS prescription forms.
2. The strength is also stated on the label in the case of tablets, capsules, and similar preparations that are available in different strengths.
3. If it is the wish of the prescriber that a description such as 'The Sedative Tablets' should appear on the label, the prescriber should write the desired description on the prescription form.
4. The arrangement will extend to approved names, proprietary names or titles given in the BP, BPC, BNF, DPF, or NPF. The arrangement does not apply when a prescription is written so that several ingredients are given.
5. The name written on the label is that used by the prescriber on the prescription.
6. If more than one item is prescribed on one form and the prescriber does not delete the letters 'NP', each dispensed medicine is named on the label, subject to the conditions given above in paragraph 4. If the prescriber wants only selected items on such a prescription to be so labelled this should be indicated by deleting the letters 'NP' on the form and writing 'NP' alongside the medicines to be labelled.
7. When a prescription is written other than on an NHS prescription form the name of the prescribed preparation will be stated on the label of the dispensed medicine unless the prescriber indicates otherwise.
8. The Council of the Royal Pharmaceutical Society advises that the labels of dispensed medicines should indicate the total quantity of the product dispensed in the container to which the label refers. This requirement applies equally to solid, liquid, internal, and external preparations. If a product is dispensed in more than one container, the reference should be to the amount in each container.

Non-proprietary names of **compound preparations** which appear in the BNF are those that have been compiled by the British Pharmacopoeia Commission or another recognised body; whenever possible they reflect the names of the active ingredients.

Prescribers should avoid creating their own compound names for the purposes of generic prescribing; such names do not have an approved definition and can be misinterpreted.

Special care should be taken to avoid errors when prescribing compound preparations; in particular the hyphen in the prefix 'co-' should be retained.

Special care should also be taken to avoid creating generic names for **modified-release** preparations where the use of these names could lead to confusion between formulations with different lengths of action.

SECURITY AND VALIDITY OF PRESCRIPTIONS. The Councils of the British Medical Association and the Royal Pharmaceutical Society have issued a joint statement on the security and validity of prescriptions.

In particular, prescription forms should:

- not be left unattended at reception desks;
- not be left in a car where they may be visible; and
- when not in use, be kept in a locked drawer within the surgery and at home.

Where there is any doubt about the authenticity of a prescription, the pharmacist should contact the prescriber. If this is done by telephone, the number should be obtained from the directory rather than relying on the information on the prescription form, which may be false.

PATIENT GROUP DIRECTION (PGD). In most cases, the most appropriate clinical care will be provided on an individual basis by a prescriber to a specific individual patient. However, a Patient Group Direction for supply and administration of medicines by other healthcare professionals can be used where it would benefit patient care without compromising safety.

A Patient Group Direction is a written direction relating to supply and administration (or administration only) of a prescription-only medicine by certain classes of healthcare professionals; the Direction is signed by a doctor (or dentist), and by a pharmacist. Further information is available in Health Service Circular (HSC 2000/026) on Patient Group Directions [England only].

Prescription writing

Shared care. In its guidelines on responsibility for prescribing between hospitals and general practitioners, the Department of Health has advised that legal responsibility for prescribing lies with the doctor who signs the prescription.

Prescriptions[1] should be written legibly in ink or otherwise so as to be indelible[2], should be dated, should state the full name and address of the patient, and should be signed in ink by the prescriber[3]. The age and the date of birth of the patient should preferably be stated, and it is a legal requirement in the case of prescription-only medicines to state the age for children under 12 years.

The following should be noted:

(a) The unnecessary use of decimal points should be avoided, e.g. 3 mg, not 3.0 mg.

Quantities of 1 gram or more should be written as 1 g etc.

Quantities less than 1 gram should be written in milligrams, e.g. 500 mg, not 0.5 g.

Quantities less than 1 mg should be written in micrograms, e.g. 100 micrograms, not 0.1 mg.

When decimals are unavoidable a zero should be written in front of the decimal point where there is no other figure, e.g. 0.5 mL, not .5 mL.

Use of the decimal point is acceptable to express a range, e.g. 0.5 to 1 g.

(b) 'Micrograms' and 'nanograms' should **not** be abbreviated. Similarly 'units' should **not** be abbreviated.

(c) The term 'millilitre' (ml or mL)[4] is used in medicine and pharmacy, and cubic centimetre, c.c., or cm[3] should not be used.

(d) Dose and dose frequency should be stated; in the case of preparations to be taken 'as required' a **minimum dose interval** should be specified.

When doses other than multiples of 5 mL are prescribed for *oral liquid preparations* the dose-volume will be provided by means of an **oral syringe**, see p. 2 (except for preparations intended to be measured with a pipette).

Suitable quantities:

Elixirs, Linctuses, and Paediatric Mixtures (5-mL dose), 50, 100, or 150 mL

Adult Mixtures (10-mL dose), 200 or 300 mL

Ear Drops, Eye drops, and Nasal Drops, 10 mL (or the manufacturer's pack)

Eye Lotions, Gargles, and Mouthwashes, 200 mL

(e) For suitable quantities of dermatological preparations, see section 13.1.2.

(f) The names of drugs and preparations should be written clearly and **not** abbreviated, using approved titles **only** (see also advice in box on p. 3 to **avoid** creating generic titles for modified-release preparations).

(g) The symbol 'NP' on NHS forms should be deleted if it is required that the name of the preparation should not appear on the label. For full details see p. 3.

(h) The quantity to be supplied may be stated by indicating the number of days of treatment required in the box provided on NHS forms. In most cases the exact amount will be supplied. This does not apply to items directed to be used as required—if the dose and frequency are not given the quantity to be supplied needs to be stated.

When several items are ordered on one form the box can be marked with the number of days of treatment provided the quantity is added for any item for which the amount cannot be calculated.

(i) Although directions should preferably be in **English without abbreviation**, it is recognised that some Latin abbreviations are used (for details see Inside Back Cover).

(j) A prescription for a preparation that has been withdrawn or needs to be specially imported for a named patient should be handwritten. The name of the preparation should be endorsed with the prescriber's signature and the letters 'WD' (withdrawn or specially-imported drug); there may be considerable delay in obtaining a withdrawn medicine.

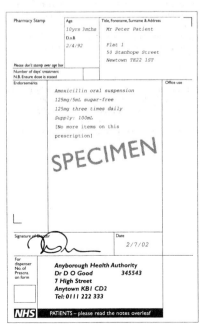

1. The above recommendations are acceptable for **prescription-only medicines** (PoM). For items marked CD see also Controlled Drugs and Drug Dependence p. 7.

2. It is permissible to issue carbon copies of NHS prescriptions as long as they are signed in ink.

3. Computer-generated facsimile signatures do not meet the legal requirement.

4. The use of capital 'L' in mL is a printing convention throughout the BNF; both 'mL' and 'ml' are recognised SI abbreviations.

Computer-issued prescriptions

For computer-issued prescriptions the following recommendations of the Joint Computing Group of the General Practitioners Committee and the Royal College of General Practitioners should also be noted:

1. The computer must print out the date,[1] the patient's surname, one forename, other initials, and address, and may also print out the patient's title and date of birth. The age of children under 12 years and of adults over 60 years must be printed in the box available; the age of children under 5 years should be printed in years and months. A facility may also exist to print out the age of patients between 12 and 60 years.

2. The doctor's name must be printed at the bottom of the prescription form; this will be the name of the doctor responsible for the prescription (who will normally sign it). The doctor's surgery address, reference number, and Health Authority (HA)[2] are also necessary. In addition, the surgery telephone number should be printed.

3. When prescriptions are to be signed by general practitioner registrars, assistants, locums, or deputising doctors, the name of the doctor printed at the bottom of the form must still be that of the responsible principal.

4. Names of medicines must come from a dictionary held in the computer memory, to provide a check on the spelling and to ensure that the name is written in full. The computer can be programmed to recognise both the non-proprietary and the proprietary name of a particular drug and to print out the preferred choice, but must not print out both names. For medicines not in the dictionary, separate checks are required—the user must be warned that no check was possible and the entire prescription must be entered in the lexicon.

5. The dictionary may contain information on the usual doses, formulations, and pack sizes to produce standard predetermined prescriptions for common preparations, and to provide a check on the validity of an individual prescription on entry.

6. The prescription must be printed in English without abbreviation; information may be entered or stored in abbreviated form. The dose must be in numbers, the frequency in words, and the quantity in numbers in brackets, thus: 40 mg four times daily (112). It must also be possible to prescribe by indicating the length of treatment required, see (h) above.

7. The BNF recommendations should be followed as in (a), (b), (c), (d), and (e) above.

8. Checks may be incorporated to ensure that all the information required for dispensing a particular drug has been filled in. For instructions such as 'as directed' and 'when required', the maximum daily dose should normally be specified.

9. Numbers and codes used in the system for organising and retrieving data must never appear on the form.

10. Supplementary warnings or advice should be written in full, should not interfere with the clarity of the prescription itself, and should be in line with any warnings or advice in the BNF; numerical codes should not be used.

11. A mechanism (such as printing a series of non-specific characters) should be incorporated to cancel out unused space, or wording such as 'no more items on this prescription' may be added after the last item. Otherwise the doctor should delete the space manually.

12. To avoid forgery the computer may print on the form the number of items to be dispensed (somewhere separate from the box for the pharmacist). The number of items per form need be limited only by the ability of the printer to produce clear and well-demarcated instructions with sufficient space for each item and a spacer line before each fresh item.

13. Handwritten alterations should only be made in exceptional circumstances—it is preferable to print out a new prescription. Any alterations must be made in the doctor's own handwriting and countersigned; computer records should be updated to fully reflect any alteration. Prescriptions for drugs used for contraceptive purposes (but which are not promoted as contraceptives) may need to be marked in handwriting with the symbol ♀ (or endorsed in another way to indicate that the item is prescribed for contraceptive purposes).

14. Prescriptions for controlled drugs must not be printed from the computer. Blank forms may be computer-printed with the doctor's name, surgery address and telephone number, reference number and Health Authority (HA)[2]; the remaining details must be handwritten.[3]

15. The strip of paper on the side of the FP10[4](Comp) may be used for various purposes but care should be taken to avoid including confidential information. It may be advisable for the patient's name to appear at the top, but this should be preceded by 'confidential'.

16. In rural dispensing practices prescription requests (or details of medicines dispensed) will normally be entered in one surgery. The prescriptions (or dispensed medicines) may then need to be delivered to another surgery or location; if possible the computer should hold up to 10 alternatives.

17. Prescription forms that are reprinted or issued as a duplicate should be labelled clearly as such.

---

1. The exemption for own handwriting regulations for phenobarbital does not apply to the date; a computer-generated date need not be deleted but the date must also be added by the prescriber.

2. Health Board in Scotland.

3. Except in the case of phenobarbital (but see also footnote 1) or where the prescriber has been exempted from handwriting requirements, for details see Controlled Drugs and Drug Dependence p. 7

4. GP10 in Scotland

Emergency supply of medicines

For details of emergency supply at the request of a doctor, see *Medicines, Ethics and Practice*, No. 27, London, Pharmaceutical Press, 2003 (and subsequent editions).

Pharmacists are sometimes called upon by members of the public to make an emergency supply of medicines. The Medicines (Products Other Than Veterinary Drugs) (Prescription Only) Order 1983, as amended, allows exemptions from the Prescription Only requirements for emergency supply to be made by a person lawfully conducting a retail pharmacy business provided:

(a) that the pharmacist has interviewed the person requesting the prescription-only medicine and is satisfied:
  (i) that there is immediate need for the prescription-only medicine and that it is impracticable in the circumstances to obtain a prescription without undue delay;
  (ii) that treatment with the prescription-only medicine has on a previous occasion been prescribed by a doctor[1] for the person requesting it;
  (iii) as to the dose which it would be appropriate for the person to take;
(b) that no greater quantity shall be supplied than will provide 5 days' treatment except when the prescription-only medicine is:
  (i) insulin, an ointment or, cream, or a preparation for the relief of asthma in an aerosol dispenser when the smallest pack can be supplied;
  (ii) an oral contraceptive when a full cycle may be supplied;
  (iii) an antibiotic in liquid form for oral administration when the smallest quantity that will provide a full course of treatment can be supplied;
(c) that an entry shall be made in the prescription book stating:
  (i) the date of supply;
  (ii) the name, quantity and, where appropriate, the pharmaceutical form and strength;
  (iii) the name and address of the patient;
  (iv) the nature of the emergency;
(d) that the container or package must be labelled to show:
  (i) the date of supply;
  (ii) the name, quantity and, where appropriate, the pharmaceutical form and strength;
  (iii) the name of the patient;
  (iv) the name and address of the pharmacy;
  (v) the words 'Emergency supply'.
(e) that the prescription-only medicine is not a substance specifically excluded from the emergency supply provision, and does not contain a Controlled Drug specified in schedules 1, 2, or 3 to the Misuse of Drugs Regulations 1985 except for phenobarbital or phenobarbital sodium for the treatment of epilepsy: for details see *Medicines, Ethics and Practice*, No. 27, London, Pharmaceutical Press, 2003 (and subsequent editions as available).

Royal Pharmaceutical Society's Guidelines

1. The pharmacist should consider the medical consequences of *not* supplying.
2. If the patient is not known to the pharmacist, the patient's identity should be established by way of appropriate documentation.
3. It may occasionally be desirable to contact the prescriber, e.g. when the medicine requested has a potential for misuse or the prescriber is not known to the pharmacist.
4. Care should be taken to ask whether the patient's doctor has stopped the treatment, or whether the patient is taking any other medication.
5. Except for conditions which may occur infrequently (e.g. hay fever, asthma attack or migraine), a supply should not be made if the item requested was last prescribed more than 6 months ago.
6. Consideration should be given to supplying less than 5 days' quantity if this is justified.
7. Where a prescription is to be provided later, a record of emergency supply as required by law must still be made. It is good practice to add to the record the date on which the prescription is received. Payment for the medicine supplied is not a legal requirement, but may help to minimise the abuse of the emergency supply exemption. If an NHS prescription is to be provided, a refundable charge may be made.

---

1. The doctor must be a UK-registered doctor.

Controlled drugs and drug dependence

PRESCRIPTIONS. Preparations which are subject to the prescription requirements of the Misuse of Drugs Regulations 2001, i.e. preparations specified in schedules 2 and 3, are distinguished throughout the BNF by the symbol CD (Controlled Drugs). The principal legal requirements relating to medical prescriptions are listed below.

Prescriptions ordering Controlled Drugs subject to prescription requirements must be *signed* and *dated*[1] by the prescriber and specify the prescriber's *address*. The prescription must always state *in the prescriber's own handwriting*[2] in ink or otherwise so as to be indelible:

- The name and address of the patient;
- In the case of a preparation, the form[3] and where appropriate the strength[4] of the preparation;
- The total quantity of the preparation, or the number of dose units, *in both words and figures;*[5]
- The dose;[6]
- The words 'for dental treatment only' if issued by a dentist.

A prescription may order a Controlled Drug to be dispensed by instalments; the amount of the instalments and the intervals to be observed must be specified.[7,8] Prescriptions ordering 'repeats' on the same form are **not** permitted. A prescription is valid for 13 weeks from the date stated thereon.

It is an offence for a prescriber to issue an incomplete prescription and a pharmacist is **not** allowed to dispense a Controlled Drug unless all

the information required by law is given on the prescription. Failure to comply with the regulations concerning the writing of prescriptions will result in inconvenience to patients and delay in supplying the necessary medicine.

DEPENDENCE AND MISUSE. The most serious drugs of addiction are **cocaine, diamorphine** (heroin), **morphine**, and the **synthetic opioids**. For arrangements for prescribing of diamorphine, dipipanone or cocaine for addicts, see p. 9.

Despite marked reduction in the prescribing of **amphetamines** there is concern that abuse of illicit amfetamine and related compounds is widespread.

Owing to problems of abuse, **flunitrazepam** and **temazepam** are subject to additional controlled drug requirements (but temazepam remains exempt from the additional prescribing requirements).

The principal **barbiturates** are now Controlled Drugs, but phenobarbital (phenobarbitone) and phenobarbital sodium (phenobarbitone sodium) or a preparation containing either of these are exempt from the handwriting requirement but must fulfil all other controlled drug prescription requirements (**important:** the own handwriting exemption does **not** apply to the date; a computer-generated date need not be deleted but the date must also be added by the prescriber). Moreover, for the treatment of epilepsy phenobarbital and phenobarbital sodium are available under the emergency supply regulations (p. 6).

Cannabis (Indian hemp) has no approved medicinal use and cannot be prescribed by doctors. Its use is illegal but has become widespread. Cannabis is a mild hallucinogen seldom accompanied by a desire

---

1. A computer-generated date is **not** acceptable; however, the prescriber may use a date stamp.

2. Does not apply to prescriptions for temazepam. Otherwise applies unless the prescriber has been specifically exempted from this requirement or unless the prescription contains no controlled drug other than phenobarbital or phenobarbital sodium or a preparation containing either of these; the exemption does **not** apply to the date—a computer-generated date need not be deleted but the date must also be added by the prescriber.

3. The dosage form (e.g. tablets) must be included on a Controlled Drugs prescription irrespective of whether it is implicit in the proprietary name (e.g. *MST Continus*) or of whether only one form is available.

4. When more than one strength of a preparation exists the strength required must be specified.

5. Does not apply to prescriptions for temazepam.

6. The instruction 'one as directed' constitutes a dose but 'as directed' does not.

7. A total of 14 days' treatment by instalment of any drug listed in Schedule 2 of the Misuse of Drugs Regulations may be prescribed in England and Scotland. In *England*, form FP10MDA-SS (blue) or occasionally form FP10MDA (blue) should be used; in hospital, form FP10HP(AD) is being replaced by form FP10MDA-SS. In *Scotland* forms HBP(A) (hospital-based prescribers) or GP10 (general practitioners) should be used. In *Wales* a total of 14 days treatment by instalment of any drug listed in Schedules 2–5 of the Misuse of Drugs Regulations may be prescribed. In Wales form WP10(MDA) or form WP10HP(AD) for hospital prescribers should be used when available; in the meantime existing stocks of FP10(MDA) or FP10HP(AD) for hospital prescribers should continue to be used.

8. Buprenorphine (schedule 3) may be prescribed by instalment in England on form FP10MDA-SS (or on form FP10MDA)

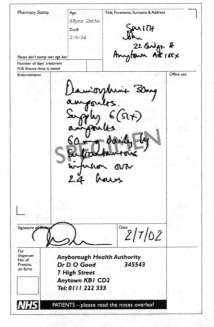

to increase the dose; withdrawal symptoms are unusual. **Lysergide** (lysergic acid diethylamide, LSD) is a much more potent hallucinogen; its use can lead to severe psychotic states in which life may be at risk.

PRESCRIBING DRUGS LIKELY TO CAUSE DEPEND-ENCE OR MISUSE. The prescriber has three main responsibilities:

- To avoid creating dependence by introducing drugs to patients without sufficient reason. In this context, the proper use of the morphine-like drugs is well understood. The dangers of other controlled drugs are less clear because recognition of dependence is not easy and its effects, and those of withdrawal, are less obvious. Perhaps the most notable result of uninhibited prescribing is that a very large number of patients in the country take tablets which do them neither much good nor much harm, but are com-mitted to them indefinitely because they cannot readily be stopped.
- To see that the patient does not gradually increase the dose of a drug, given for good medical reasons, to the point where dependence becomes more likely. This tendency is seen especially with hypnotics and anxiolytics (for CSM advice see section 4.1). The prescriber should keep a close eye on the amount prescribed to prevent patients from accumulating stocks that would enable them to arrange their own dosage or even that of their families and friends. A minimal amount should be prescribed in the first instance, or when seeing a new patient for the first time.
- To avoid being used as an unwitting source of supply for addicts. Methods include visiting more than one doctor, fabricating stories, and forging prescriptions.

Patients under temporary care should be given only small supplies of drugs unless they present an unequivocal letter from their own doctors. Doctors should also remember that their own patients may be doing a collecting round with other doctors, espe-cially in hospitals. It is sensible to decrease dosages steadily or to issue weekly or even daily prescrip-tions for small amounts if it is apparent that depend-ence is occurring.

The stealing and misuse of prescription forms could be minimised by the following precautions:

(a) do not leave unattended if called away from the consulting room or at reception desks; do not leave in a car where they may be visible; when not in use, keep in a locked drawer within the surgery and at home;
(b) draw a diagonal line across the blank part of the form under the prescription;
(c) write the quantity in words and figures when pre-scribing drugs prone to abuse; this is obligatory for controlled drugs (see Prescriptions, above);
(d) alterations are best avoided but if any are made they should be clear and unambiguous; add initials against altered items;
(e) if prescriptions are left for collection they should be left in a safe place in a sealed envelope.

TRAVELLING ABROAD. Prescribed drugs listed in schedules 4 and 5 to the Misuse of Drugs Regula-tions 2001 are not subject to import or export licensing but doctors are advised that patients intending to carry Schedule 2 and 3 drugs abroad may require an export licence. This is dependent upon the amount of drug to be exported and further details may be obtained from the Home Office by telephoning (020) 7273 3806. Applications for licences should be sent to the Home Office, Drugs Branch, Queen Anne's Gate, London SW1H 9AT.

There is no standard application form but applica-tions must be supported by a letter from a doctor giving details of:

- the patient's name and current address;
- the quantities of drugs to be carried;
- the strength and form in which the drugs will be dispensed;
- the dates of travel to and from the United Kingdom.

Ten days should be allowed for processing the application.

Individual doctors who wish to take Controlled Drugs abroad while accompanying patients may similarly be issued with licences. Licences are not normally issued to doctors who wish to take Con-trolled Drugs abroad solely in case a family emer-gency should arise.

These import/export licences for named individuals do not have any legal status outside the UK and are only issued to comply with the Misuse of Drugs Act and facilitate passage through UK Customs and Excise control. For clearance in the country to be visited it would be necessary to approach that country's consulate in the UK.

Misuse of Drugs Act

The Misuse of Drugs Act, 1971 prohibits certain activities in relation to 'Controlled Drugs', in particular their manufacture, supply, and possession. The penalties applicable to offences involving the different drugs are graded broadly according to the *harmfulness attributable to a drug when it is misused* and for this purpose the drugs are defined in the following three classes:

Class A includes: alfentanil, cocaine, dextromoramide, diamorphine (heroin), dipipanone, lysergide (LSD), methadone, methylenedioxymethamfetamine (MDMA, 'ecstasy'), morphine, opium, pethidine, phencyclidine, remifentanil, and class B substances when prepared for injection

Class B includes: oral amphetamines, barbiturates, cannabis, cannabis resin, codeine, ethylmorphine, glu-tethimide, pentazocine, phenmetrazine, and pholcodine

Class C includes: certain drugs related to the amphet-amines such as benzfetamine and chlorphentermine, buprenorphine, diethylpropion, mazindol, mepro-bamate, pemoline, pipradrol, most benzodiazepines, zolpidem, androgenic and anabolic steroids, clenbuterol, chorionic gonadotrophin (HCG), non-human chorionic gonadotrophin, somatotropin, somatrem, and soma-tropin

The Misuse of Drugs Regulations 2001 define the classes of person who are authorised to supply and possess controlled drugs while acting in their professional capacities and lay down the conditions under which these activities may be carried out. In the regulations drugs are divided into five schedules each specifying the requirements governing such activities as import, export, production, supply, possession, prescribing, and record keeping which apply to them.

Schedule 1 includes drugs such as cannabis and lysergide which are not used medicinally. Possession and supply are prohibited except in accordance with Home Office authority.

Schedule 2 includes drugs such as diamorphine (heroin), morphine, remifentanil, pethidine, secobarbital, glutethi-mide, amfetamine, and cocaine and are subject to the full controlled drug requirements relating to prescriptions, safe custody (except for secobarbital), the need to keep registers, etc. (unless exempted in schedule 5).

Schedule 3 includes the barbiturates (except secobarbital, now schedule 2), buprenorphine, diethylpropion, flunitrazepam, mazindol, meprobamate, pentazocine, phentermine, and temazepam. They are subject to the special prescription requirements (except for phenobarbital and temazepam, see p. 7) but not to the safe custody requirements (except for buprenorphine, diethylpropion, flunitrazepam, and temazepam) nor to the need to keep registers (although there are requirements for the retention of invoices for 2 years).

Schedule 4 includes in Part I benzodiazepines (except flunitrazepam and temazepam which are in schedule 3) and zolpidem, which are subject to minimal control. Part II includes androgenic and anabolic steroids, clenbuterol, chorionic gonadotrophin (HCG), non-human chorionic gonadotrophin, somatotropin, somatrem, and somatropin. Controlled drug prescription requirements do not apply and Schedule 4 Controlled Drugs are not subject to safe custody requirements.

Schedule 5 includes those preparations which, because of their strength, are exempt from virtually all Controlled Drug requirements other than retention of invoices for two years.

Notification of drug misusers

Doctors are expected to report on a standard form cases of drug misuse to their regional or national drug misuse database or centre—see below for contact telephone numbers. The National Drugs Treatment Monitoring System was introduced in England in April 2001; regional centres replace the Regional Drug Misuse Databases. A similar system has been introduced in Wales.

A report (notification) to their regional or national drug misuse database or centre should be made when a patient starts treatment for drug misuse. In England and Wales further information is collected in Spring, including whether or not patients are continuing to receive treatment. All types of problem drug misuse should be reported including opioid, benzodiazepine, and CNS stimulant.

The regional or national drug misuse database or centres are now the only national and local source of epidemiological data on people presenting with problem drug misuse; they provide valuable information to those working with drug misusers and those planning services for them. The databases cannot, however be used as a check on multiple prescribing for drug addicts because the data are anonymised.

Enquiries about the regional or national drug misuse database or centres (including requests for supplies of notification forms) can be made by contacting one of the centres listed below:

ENGLAND

Eastern and South East (West)
Tel: (01865) 226 734
Fax: (01865) 226 652

London and South East (East)
Tel: (020) 7972 2214

Mersey and Yorkshire
Tel: (0151) 231 4486
Fax: (0151) 231 4320

North West
Tel: (0161) 772 3782
Fax: (0161) 772 3445

South West
Tel: (0117) 918 6880
Fax: (0117) 918 6883

Trent
Tel: (0116) 225 6360
Fax: (0116) 225 6370

West Midlands
Tel: (0121) 580 4331
Fax: (0121) 525 7980

SCOTLAND
Tel: (0131) 551 8715
Fax: (0131) 551 1392

WALES
Tel: (02920) 502 639
Fax: (02920) 502 504

In **Northern Ireland**, the Misuse of Drugs (Notification of and Supply to Addicts) (Northern Ireland) Regulations 1973 require doctors to send particulars of persons whom they consider to be addicted to certain controlled drugs to the Chief Medical Officer of the Department of Health and Social Services. The Northern Ireland contacts are:

Medical contact:

Dr Ian McMaster
C3 Castle Buildings
Belfast BT4 3PP
Tel: (028) 9052 2421
Fax: (028) 9052 0781

Administrative contact:

Health Promotion Branch
C4.22 Castle Building
Belfast BT4 3PP
Tel: (028) 9052 0532

Prescribing of diamorphine (heroin), dipipanone, and cocaine for addicts

The Misuse of Drugs (Supply to Addicts) Regulations 1997 require that only medical practitioners who hold a special licence issued by the Home Secretary may prescribe, administer or supply diamorphine, dipipanone[1] (*Diconal®*) or cocaine in the treatment of drug addiction; other practitioners must refer any addict who requires these drugs to a treatment centre. Whenever possible the addict will be introduced by a member of staff from the treatment centre to a pharmacist whose agreement has been obtained and whose pharmacy is conveniently sited for the patient. Prescriptions for weekly supplies will be sent to the pharmacy by post and will be dispensed on a daily basis as indicated by the doctor. If any alterations of the arrangements are requested by the addict, the portion of the prescription affected must be represcribed and not merely altered. *General practitioners and other doctors may still prescribe diamorphine, dipipanone, and cocaine for patients (including addicts) for relief of pain due to organic disease or injury without a special licence.* For guidance on prescription writing, see p. 7.

---

1. Dipipanone in *Diconal®* tablets has been much misused by opioid addicts in recent years. Doctors and others should be suspicious of people who ask for the tablets, especially if temporary residents.

Rare paediatric conditions

Information on substances such as *biotin* and *sodium benzoate* used in rare metabolic conditions can be obtained from:

Alder Hey Children's
Hospital
Drug Information Centre
Liverpool L12 2AP
Tel: (0151) 252 5381

Great Ormond Street
Hospital for Children
Pharmacy
Great Ormond St
London WC1N 3JH
Tel: (020) 7405 9200

Dosage in Children

Children's doses in the BNF are stated in the individual drug entries as far as possible, except where paediatric use is not recommended, information is not available, or there are special hazards.

Doses are generally based on body-weight (in kilograms) or the following age ranges:

first month (neonate)
up to 1 year (infant)
1–5 years
6–12 years

Unless the age is specified, the term 'child' in the BNF includes persons aged 12 years and younger.

DOSE CALCULATION. Children's doses may be calculated from adult doses by using age, body-weight, or body-surface area, or by a combination of these factors. The most reliable methods are those based on body-surface area.

Body-weight may be used to calculate doses expressed in mg/kg. Young children may require a higher dose per kilogram than adults because of their higher metabolic rates. Other problems need to be considered. For example, calculation by body-weight in the obese child may result in much higher doses being administered than necessary; in such cases, dose should be calculated from an ideal weight, related to height and age.

Body-surface area (BSA) estimates are more accurate for calculation of paediatric doses than body-weight since many physiological phenomena correlate better to body-surface area. The average body-surface area of a 70-kilogram human is about $1.8\,m^2$. Thus, to calculate the dose for a child the following formula may be used:

Approximate dose for patient =

$$\frac{\text{surface area of patient } (m^2)}{1.8} \times \text{adult dose}$$

More precise body-surface values may be calculated from height and weight by means of a nomogram (e.g. J. Insley, *A Paediatric Vade-Mecum*, 13th Edition, London, Arnold, 1996); see also inside back cover.

Where the dose for children is not stated, prescribers should seek advice from a drug information centre or refer to a current edition of a specialist text on the use of medicines in children.

DOSE FREQUENCY. Antibacterials are generally given at regular intervals throughout the day. Some flexibility should be allowed in children to avoid waking them during the night. For example, the night-time dose may be given at the parent's bed-time.

Where new or potentially toxic drugs are used, the manufacturers' recommended doses should be carefully followed.

Equivalent doses of morphine sulphate by mouth (as oral solution or standard tablets or as modified-release tablets) or of diamorphine hydrochloride by intramuscular injection or by subcutaneous infusion

These equivalences are approximate only and may need to be adjusted according to response

ORAL MORPHINE		PARENTERAL DIAMORPHINE	
Morphine sulphate oral solution or standard tablets	Morphine sulphate modified-release tablets	Diamorphine hydrochloride by intramuscular injection	Diamorphine hydrochloride by subcutaneous infusion
every 4 hours	every 12 hours	every 4 hours	every 24 hours
5 mg	20 mg	2.5 mg	15 mg
10 mg	30 mg	5 mg	20 mg
15 mg	50 mg	5 mg	30 mg
20 mg	60 mg	7.5 mg	45 mg
30 mg	90 mg	10 mg	60 mg
40 mg	120 mg	15 mg	90 mg
60 mg	180 mg	20 mg	120 mg
80 mg	240 mg	30 mg	180 mg
100 mg	300 mg	40 mg	240 mg
130 mg	400 mg	50 mg	300 mg
160 mg	500 mg	60 mg	360 mg
200 mg	600 mg	70 mg	400 mg

If breakthrough pain occurs give a subcutaneous (preferable) or intramuscular injection of diamorphine equivalent to one-sixth of the total 24-hour subcutaneous infusion dose. It is kinder to give an intermittent bolus injection *subcutaneously*—absorption is smoother so that the risk of adverse effects at peak absorption is avoided (an even better method is to use a subcutaneous butterfly needle).
To minimise the risk of infection no individual subcutaneous infusion solution should be used for longer than 24 hours.

Prescribing for the elderly

Old people, especially the very old, require special care and consideration from prescribers. *Medicines for Older People*, a component document of the National Service Framework for Older People,[1] describes how to maximise the benefits of medicines and how to avoid excessive, inappropriate, or inadequate consumption of medicines by older people.

APPROPRIATE PRESCRIBING. Elderly patients often receive multiple drugs for their multiple diseases. This greatly increases the risk of drug interactions as well as adverse reactions, and may affect compliance (see Taking medicines to best effect under General guidance). The balance of benefit and harm of some medicines may be altered in the elderly. Therefore, elderly patients' medicines should be reviewed regularly and medicines which are not of benefit should be stopped. In some cases prophylactic drugs may be inappropriate if they are likely to complicate existing treatment or introduce unnecessary side-effects, especially in elderly patients with poor prognosis or with poor overall health. However, elderly patients should not be denied medicines which may help them, such as anticoagulants or antiplatelet drugs for atrial fibrillation, antihypertensives, statins, and drugs for osteoporosis.

FORM OF MEDICINE. Frail elderly patients may have difficulty swallowing tablets; if left in the mouth, ulceration may develop. They should always be encouraged to take their tablets or capsules with enough fluid, and in some cases it may be helpful to

1. Department of Health. National Service Framework for Older People. London: Department of Health, March 2001

discuss with the patient the possibility of prescribing the drug as a liquid if available.

MANIFESTATIONS OF AGEING. In the very old, manifestations of normal ageing may be mistaken for disease and lead to inappropriate prescribing. In addition, age-related muscle weakness and difficulty in maintaining balance should not be confused with neurological disease. Disorders such as lightheadedness not associated with postural or postprandial hypotension are unlikely to be helped by drugs.

SELF-MEDICATION. Just as in a younger patient self-medication with over-the-counter products or with drugs prescribed for a previous illness (or even for another person) may be an added complication. Discussion with both the patient and relatives as well as a home visit may be needed to establish exactly what is being taken.

SENSITIVITY. The ageing nervous system shows increased *susceptibility* to many commonly used drugs, such as opioid analgesics, benzodiazepines, antipsychotics, and antiparkinsonian drugs, all of which must be used with caution. Similarly, other organs may also be more susceptible to the effects of drugs such as antihypertensives and NSAIDs.

Pharmacokinetics

The most important effect of age is reduction in renal clearance. Many aged patients thus *excrete drugs slowly*, and are *highly susceptible to nephrotoxic drugs*. Acute illness may lead to rapid reduction in renal clearance, especially if accompanied by dehydration. Hence, a patient stabilised on a drug with a narrow margin between the therapeutic and the toxic dose (e.g. digoxin) may rapidly develop adverse effects in the aftermath of a myocardial infarction or a respiratory-tract infection. The metabolism of some drugs may be reduced in the elderly.

Pharmacokinetic changes may markedly increase the tissue concentration of a drug in the elderly, especially in debilitated patients.

Adverse reactions

Adverse reactions often present in the elderly in a vague and non-specific fashion. *Confusion* is often the presenting symptom (caused by almost any of the commonly used drugs). Other common manifestations are *constipation* (with antimuscarinics and many tranquillisers) and postural *hypotension* and *falls* (with diuretics and many psychotropics).

HYPNOTICS. Many hypnotics with long half-lives have serious hangover effects of drowsiness, unsteady gait, and even slurred speech and confusion. Those with short half-lives should be used but they too can present problems (section 4.1.1). Short courses of hypnotics are occasionally useful for helping a patient through an acute illness or some other crisis but every effort must be made to avoid dependence. Benzodiazepines impair balance, which may result in falls.

DIURETICS. Diuretics are overprescribed in old age and should **not** be used on a long-term basis to treat simple gravitational oedema which will usually respond to increased movement, raising the legs, and support stockings. A few days of diuretic treatment may speed the clearing of the oedema but it should rarely need continued drug therapy.

NSAIDs. Bleeding associated with *aspirin* and *other NSAIDs* is more common in the elderly who are more likely to have a fatal or serious outcome. NSAIDs are also a special hazard in patients with cardiac disease or renal impairment which may again place older patients at particular risk.

Owing to the *increased susceptibilty of the elderly* to the *side-effects of NSAIDs* the following recommendations are made:

- for *osteoarthritis, soft-tissue lesions* and *back pain* first try measures such as weight reduction (if obese), warmth, exercise and use of a walking stick;
- for *osteoarthritis, soft-tissue lesions, back pain* and *pain in rheumatoid arthritis*, paracetamol should be used first and can often provide adequate pain relief;
- alternatively, a low-dose NSAID (e.g. ibuprofen up to 1.2 g daily may be given;
- for pain relief when either drug is inadequate, paracetamol in a full dose plus a low-dose NSAID may be given;
- if necessary, the NSAID dose can be increased or an opioid analgesic given with paracetamol;
- do not give two NSAIDs at the same time.

For advice on prophylaxis of NSAID-induced peptic ulcers if continued NSAID treatment is necessary, see section 1.3.

OTHER DRUGS. Other drugs which commonly cause adverse reactions are *antiparkinsonian drugs, antihypertensives, psychotropics,* and *digoxin*. The usual maintenance dose of digoxin in very old patients is 125 micrograms daily (62.5 micrograms in those with renal disease); lower doses are often inadequate but toxicity is common in those given 250 micrograms daily.

Drug-induced blood disorders are much more common in the elderly. Therefore drugs with a tendency to cause bone marrow depression (e.g. *co-trimoxazole, mianserin*) should be avoided unless there is no acceptable alternative.

The elderly generally require a lower maintenance dose of *warfarin* than younger adults; once again, the outcome of bleeding tends to be more serious.

Guidelines

First always question whether a drug is indicated at all.

LIMIT RANGE. It is a sensible policy to prescribe from a limited range of drugs and to be thoroughly familiar with their effects in the elderly.

REDUCE DOSE. Dosage should generally be substantially lower than for younger patients and it is common to start with about 50% of the adult dose. Some drugs (e.g. long-acting antidiabetic drugs such as glibenclamide and chlorpropamide) should be avoided altogether.

REVIEW REGULARLY. Review repeat prescriptions regularly. In many patients it may be possible to stop some drugs, provided that clinical progress is monitored. It may be necessary to reduce the dose of some drugs as renal function declines.

SIMPLIFY REGIMENS. Elderly patients benefit from simple treatment regimens. Only drugs with a clear indication should be prescribed and whenever possible given once or twice daily. In particular, regimens which call for a confusing array of dosage intervals should be avoided.

EXPLAIN CLEARLY. Write full instructions on every prescription (*including* repeat prescriptions) so that containers can be properly labelled with full directions. Avoid imprecisions like 'as directed'. Child-resistant containers may be unsuitable.

REPEATS AND DISPOSAL. Instruct patients what to do when drugs run out, and also how to dispose of any that are no longer necessary. Try to prescribe matching quantities.

If these guidelines are followed most elderly people will cope adequately with their own medicines. If not then it is essential to enrol the help of a third party, usually a relative or a friend.

Drugs and sport

uk sport

Drug-Free Sport
Advice Card

Prohibited Classes of Substances and Prohibited Methods
and Examples of Permitted Substances in Sport

If in doubt - check it out

Examples of Permitted Substances

Anti-allergic	cetirizine dihydrochloride, chlorpheniramine maleate, desloratadine, loratadine, mizolastine, terfenadine
Anti-diarrhoeal	atropine, diphenoxylate, loperamide, and products containing electrolytes
Anti-fungal	clotrimazole, amphotericin, fluconazole, miconazole, nystatin, terbinafine hydrochloride
Anti-viral/Infections	aciclovir, idoxuridine, penciclovir
Antibiotics	all antibiotics are PERMITTED
Asthma	sodium cromoglicate and theophylline, salbutamol, formoterol, terbutaline, salmeterol, beclometasone, fluticasone (are all permitted with prior notification)
Cough/Cold	non-sedative antihistamines, paracetamol, astemizole, terfenadine, steam and menthol inhalations, guaiphenesin, pholcodine, dextromethorphan
Ear/Nose	oral/nasal drops or sprays containing: betamethasone sodium phosphate, beclometasone, dexamethasone, fluticasone, hydrocortisone, docusate sodium, tramazoline hydrochloride
Eye preparations	drops or creams containing: antazoline, betamethasone sodium phosphate, flurometholone, hydrocortisone acetate, sodium cromoglicate, chloramphenicol
Hayfever	non-sedative antihistamines, nasal sprays containing a corticosteroid
Pain/Inflammation	all non-steroidal anti-inflammatories (NSAIDs), codeine, aspirin, ibuprofen, paracetamol dextropropoxyphene
Vomiting/Nausea	cinnarizine, domperidone, metoclopramide, prochlorperazine

WARNING: Medications prescribed by your doctor or purchased over the counter may contain prohibited substances. Inform your doctor and your pharmacist of your need to take permitted substances if you are eligible for testing. Consider giving your doctor and pharmacist a copy of this advice card.

SUPPLEMENTS: Some vitamin, herbal and nutritional supplements may contain prohibited substances. Use of supplements is at your own risk.

NOTE: Listed on this card are examples only of substances prohibited and permitted by the IOC Medical Commission and World Anti-Doping Agency (January 2003). Some sports may apply minor exceptions to this list.

If in doubt check with the medical officer of your governing body or international federation.

USEFUL CONTACTS:

UK Sport Drug Information Database (DID):	www.uksport.gov.uk/did
UK Sport Drug Information Line:	+44 (0)800 528 0004
Drug-Free Sport email address:	drug-free@uksport.gov.uk

Add your own useful numbers:

_____

_____

_____

Version 2 January 2003

Classes of Prohibited Substances and Methods

Prohibited classes and related substances	**Stimulants:** amfetamine, bromantan, caffeine*, cocaine, ephedrines**, fenproporex, methylphenidate, pseudoephedrine***, phenmetrazine, phenylpropanolamine***, salbutamol****, salmeterol****, terbutaline****, formoterol**** and certain beta2agonists**** **Narcotics Analgesics:** morphine, diamorphine (heroin), pethidine, methadone **Anabolic Agents:** androstenedione, bolasterone, clenbuterol, DHEA, methandienone, nandrolone, norbolethone, 19 nor-steroids, stanozolol, testosterone and certain beta2agonists**** **Diuretics:** amiloride, bendrofluazide, furosemide, mannitol (prohibited by intravenous injection), triamterene, hydrochlorothiazide **Peptide Hormones, Mimetics and Analogues** (and all releasing factors): growth hormone, corticotrophins, chorionic gonadotrophin and pituitary and synthetic gonadotrophins are prohibited in males only, erythropoietin (EPO), insulin-like growth factor, insulin (allowed only to treat certified insulin dependent diabetes and with prior written notification to the relevant authority) **Anti-oestrogenic activity:** (Prohibited in males only) aromatase inhibitors, clomiphene, cyclofenil, tamoxifen **Masking Agents:** diuretics (see above), epitestosterone (a urinary concentration greater than 200 ng/ml) probenecid, hydroxyethyl starch

Urinary concentration above the following levels constitutes as a doping offence: * Caffeine 12mcg/ml **Ephedrine and methylephedrine 10mcg/ml ***Phenylpropanolamine and pseudoephedrine 25mcg/ml ****Salbutamol (above 1000 ng/ml), salmeterol, terbutaline, formoterol and certain other beta2agonists are allowed by inhaler only to prevent and/or treat asthma and exercise-induced asthma. Written notification by a respiratory or team physician must be given to the relevant authority prior to competition, for example, the governing body or international federation medical officer. Check the procedure for notifying medication within your sport.

Prohibited Methods	**Enhancement of Oxygen Transfer:** blood doping, administration of blood, red blood cells, and related blood products that enhance the uptake, transport or delivery of oxygen **Pharmacological, Chemical or Physical Manipulation:** substances or methods that alter the validity and integrity of the urine, e.g. catheterisation, diuretics, epitestosterone, urine substitution **Gene Doping:** non-therapeutic use of genes and/or genetic elements that have the capacity to enhance performance
Classes of prohibited substances in certain circumstances	**Alcohol/Cannabinoids:** restricted in certain sports. Refer to national/international federation regulations. N.B. Cannabinoids may be controlled at certain major events. **Local Anaesthetics:** administration restricted to local or intra-articular injection when medically justified***** **Glucocorticosteroids:** systemic use is prohibited when administered orally, rectally, or by intravenous or intramuscular injection **Beta-blockers:** restricted in certain sports. Refer to national/international sports federation regulations. Prohibited substances include, acebutolol, atenolol, carvedilol, oxprenolol, propranolol

*****Written notification should be sent to the relevant authority, for example, your governing body or international federation medical officer.

Beware of products to treat the following conditions that may contain:

Asthma	sympathomimetics e.g. ephedrine, isoprenaline, fenoterol and rimiterol
Cough/Cold	sympathomimetics/stimulants e.g. ephedrine, pseudoephedrine, phenylpropanolamine
Hayfever	ephedrine and pseudoephedrine
Pain/Inflammation	opioids and caffeine
Diarrhoea	opioids e.g. morphine

It is the responsibility of the athlete to check the status of all medications

---

Supplies of this card are available from: UK Sport, Ethics & Anti-Doping, 40 Bernard Street, London WC1N 1ST.

A similar card detailing classes of drugs and doping methods prohibited in football is available from the Football Association.

General Medical Council's advice. Doctors who prescribe or collude in the provision of drugs or treatment with the intention of improperly enhancing an individual's performance in sport would be contravening the GMC's guidance, and such actions would usually raise a question of a doctor's continued registration. This does not preclude the provision of any care or treatment where the doctor's intention is to protect or improve the patient's health.

Emergency treatment of poisoning

These notes are only guidelines and it is strongly recommended that a **poisons information centre** (see below) be consulted in cases where there is doubt about the degree of risk or about appropriate management.

HOSPITAL ADMISSION. All patients who show features of poisoning should generally be admitted to hospital. Patients who have taken poisons with delayed actions should also be admitted, even if they appear well. Delayed-action poisons include aspirin, iron, paracetamol, tricyclic antidepressants, co-phenotrope (diphenoxylate with atropine, *Lomotil*®), and paraquat; the effects of modified-release preparations are also delayed. A note of what is known and what treatment has been given should accompany the patient to hospital.

only a few poisons (such as opioids, paracetamol, and iron) have specific antidotes; few patients require active removal of the poison. In most patients, treatment is directed at managing symptoms as they arise. Nevertheless, knowledge of the type and timing of poisoning can help in anticipating the course of events. All relevant information should be sought from the poisoned individual and from carers or parents. However, such information should be interpreted with care because it may not be complete or entirely reliable. Sometimes symptoms are due to an illness such as appendicitis. Accidents can arise from a number of domestic and industrial products (the contents of which are not generally known). A **poisons information centre** should be consulted where there is doubt about any aspect of suspected poisoning.

TOXBASE

TOXBASE, the primary clinical toxicology database of the National Poisons Information Service, is available on the Internet (www.spib.axl.co.uk/). It provides information about routine diagnosis, treatment and management of patients exposed to drugs, household products, and industrial and agricultural chemicals. **Important:** for specialised information telephone a Poisons Information Centre.

TICTAC

TICTAC is a computer-aided tablet and capsule identification system. It is available to authorised users including Regional Medicines Information Centres (see inside front cover) and Poisons Information Centres.

Poisons information centres (consult day and night)

The following single number for the UK National Poisons Information Service directs the caller to the local poisons information centre:

Tel: (0870) 600 6266

NOTE. Some centres also advise on laboratory analytical services which may be of help in the diagnosis and management of a small number of cases. For advice on snake bites see p. 29.

> The **poisons information centres** (see above) will provide advice on all aspects of poisoning day and night

General care

It is often impossible to establish with certainty the identity of the poison and the size of the dose. Fortunately this is not usually important because

Respiration

Respiration is often impaired in unconscious patients. An obstructed airway requires immediate attention. Pull the tongue forward, remove dentures and oral secretions, hold the jaw forward, insert an oropharyngeal airway if one is available, and turn the patient semiprone. The risk of inhaling vomit is minimised with the patient positioned semiprone and head down.

Most poisons that impair consciousness also depress respiration. Assisted ventilation by mouth-to-mouth or *Ambu-bag* inflation may be needed. Oxygen is not a substitute for adequate ventilation, though it should be given in the highest concentration possible in poisoning with carbon monoxide and irritant gases.

Respiratory stimulants do not help and are **potentially dangerous**.

Blood pressure

Hypotension is common in severe poisoning with central nervous system depressants. A systolic blood pressure of less than 70 mmHg may lead to irreversible brain damage or renal tubular necrosis. The patient should be carried head downwards on a stretcher and nursed in this position in the ambulance. Oxygen should be given to correct hypoxia and an intravenous infusion set up if practicable. Vasopressor drugs should **not** be used.

Fluid depletion without hypotension is common after prolonged coma and after aspirin poisoning due to vomiting, sweating, and hyperpnoea.

Hypertension, often transient, occurs less frequently than hypotension in poisoning; it may be associated with sympathomimetic drugs such as amphetamines, phencyclidine, and cocaine.

Heart

Cardiac conduction defects and arrhythmias may occur in acute poisoning, notably with tricyclic antidepressants. Arrhythmias often respond to correction of underlying hypoxia, acidosis, or other biochemical abnormalities. Ventricular arrhythmias that have been confirmed by emergency ECG and which are causing serious hypotension may require treatment. If the QT interval is prolonged, specialist advice should be sought because the use of some anti-arrhythmic drugs may be inappropriate. Supra-ventricular arrhythmias are seldom life-threatening and drug treatment is best withheld until the patient reaches hospital.

Body temperature

Hypothermia may develop in patients of any age who have been deeply unconscious for some hours particularly following overdose with barbiturates or phenothiazines. It may be missed unless core temperature is measured using a low-reading rectal thermometer or by some other means. Hypothermia is best treated by wrapping the patient (e.g. in a 'space blanket') to conserve body heat. A *mild* source of heat (such as water bottles heated to 42°C) may be used but care must be taken to avoid causing burns.

Hyperthermia can develop in patients taking CNS stimulants; children and the elderly are also at risk when taking drugs with antimuscarinic properties at therapeutic doses. It is initially managed by remov-ing all unnecessary clothing. Sponging with tepid water will promote evaporation; iced water should **not** be used.

Both hypothermia and hyperthermia require urgent hospitalisation for assessment and supportive treat-ment.

Convulsions

Single short-lived convulsions do not require treat-ment. If convulsions are protracted or recur fre-quently, lorazepam 4 mg or diazepam (preferably as emulsion) up to 10 mg should be given by slow intravenous injection into a large vein; the benzo-diazepines should not be given intramuscularly.

Removal and elimination

Removal from the gastro-intestinal tract

The dangers of attempting to empty the stomach have to be balanced against the toxicity of the ingested poison, as assessed by the quantity ingested, the inherent toxicity of the poison, and the time since ingestion. Gastric emptying is clearly unnecessary if the risk of toxicity is small or if the patient presents too late.

Emptying the stomach by *gastric lavage* is of doubtful value if attempted more than 1 hour after ingestion. The chief danger of gastric aspiration and lavage is inhalation of stomach contents, and it should **not** be attempted in drowsy or comatose patients unless there is adequate cough reflex or the airway can be protected by a cuffed endotracheal tube. Stomach tubes should **not** be passed after corrosive poisoning.

Petroleum products are more dangerous in the lungs than in the stomach and therefore removal from the stomach is **not** advised because of the risk of inhalation.

On balance gastric lavage is seldom practicable or desirable before the patient reaches hospital.

Induction of *emesis* (traditionally with an ipecacu-anha mixture) for the treatment of poisoning is **not recommended**. There is no evidence that it prevents significant absorption (even if used within 1–2 hours), its adverse effects may complicate diagnosis and it may increase the likelihood of aspiration.

Salt solutions, copper sulphate, apomorphine, and mustard are dangerous and should **never** be used to induce emesis.

Whole bowel irrigation (by means of a bowel cleansing solution) has been used in poisoning with certain modified-release or enteric-coated formula-tions and in severe poisoning with iron and lithium salts. However, it is not clear that the procedure improves outcome and advice should be sought from a poisons information centre when considering it.

Prevention of absorption

Given by mouth, **activated charcoal** can bind many poisons in the gastro-intestinal system, thereby *reducing their absorption*. The **sooner** it is given the **more effective** it is, but it may still be effective up to 1 hour after ingestion of the poison—longer in the case of modified-release preparations or of drugs with antimuscarinic (anticholinergic) properties. It is relatively safe and is particularly useful for the prevention of absorption of poisons which are toxic in small amounts, e.g. antidepressants.

For the use of charcoal in active elimination techniques, see below.

CHARCOAL, ACTIVATED

Indications: adsorption of poisons in the gastro-intestinal system; see also active elimination techniques, below

Cautions: drowsy or comatose patient (risk of aspiration); reduced gastro-intestinal motility (risk of obstruction); not for poisoning with petroleum distillates, corrosive substances, alcohols, dico-phane (DDT), malathion, and metal salts including iron and lithium salts

Side-effects: black stools

Dose: see under preparations below

Actidose-Aqua® Advance (Cambridge)
Oral suspension, activated charcoal, net price 50-g pack (240 mL) = £12.50
NOTE. The brand name *Actidose-Aqua®* was formerly used

Dose: reduction of absorption, 50–100 g; INFANT under 1 year 1 g/kg (approx. 5 mL/kg), CHILD 1–12 years 25–50 g

Active elimination (see below for ADULT dose); INFANT under 1 year, 1 g/kg (approx. 5 mL/kg) every 4–6 hours; CHILD 1–12 years, 25–50 g every 4–6 hours

Carbomix® (Penn)
Powder, activated charcoal, net price 25-g pack = £8.50, 50-g pack = £11.90

Dose: reduction of absorption, 50 g, repeated if necessary; CHILD under 12 years 25 g (50 g in severe poisoning)

Active elimination, see below

Charcodote® (Dominion)

Oral suspension, activated charcoal, net price 50-g pack = £12.50

Dose: reduction of absorption, 50 g; CHILD under 12 years 25 g (50 g in severe poisoning)

Active elimination, see below

Medicoal® (Concord)

Granules, effervescent, activated charcoal 5 g/sachet. Contains Na⁺ 17.9 mmol/sachet. Net price 5-sachet pack = £6.52, 30-sachet pack = £30.16

Dose: reduction of absorption, initially 2 sachets repeated every 15–20 minutes until dose of charcoal given is 10 times that of poison ingested (if amount known) or until max. 10 sachets/24 hours have been given; each sachet suspended in approx. 100 mL water (may be administered in divided doses for children)

Active elimination techniques

Repeated doses of **activated charcoal** by mouth *enhance the elimination* of some drugs after they have been absorbed; repeated doses are given after overdosage with:

Barbiturates	Quinine
Carbamazepine	Theophylline
Dapsone	

The usual adult dose of activated charcoal is 50 g initially then 50 g every 4 hours. Vomiting should be treated (e.g. with an anti-emetic drug) since it may reduce the efficacy of charcoal treatment. In cases of intolerance, the dose may be reduced and the frequency increased (e.g. 25 g every 2 hours *or* 12.5 g every hour) but this may compromise efficacy.

Other techniques intended to enhance the elimination of poisons after absorption are only practicable in hospital and are only suitable for a small number of severely poisoned patients. Moreover, they only apply to a limited number of poisons. Examples include:

Haemodialysis for salicylates, phenobarbital, methyl alcohol (methanol), ethylene glycol, and lithium

Haemoperfusion for medium- and short-acting barbiturates, chloral hydrate, meprobamate, and theophylline.

Alkalinisation of the urine increases elimination of salicylates, but forced alkaline diuresis is no longer recommended.

Specific drugs

Alcohol

Acute intoxication with alcohol (ethanol) is common in adults but also occurs in children. The features include ataxia, dysarthria, nystagmus, and drowsiness, which may progress to coma, with hypotension and acidosis. Aspiration of vomit is a special hazard and hypoglycaemia may occur in children and some adults. Patients are managed supportively with particular attention to maintaining a clear airway and measures to reduce the risk of aspiration of gastric contents. The blood glucose is measured and glucose given if indicated.

Analgesics (non-opioid)

ASPIRIN. The chief features of salicylate poisoning are hyperventilation, tinnitus, deafness, vasodilatation, and sweating. Coma is uncommon but indicates very severe poisoning. The associated acid-base disturbances are complex.

Treatment must be in hospital where plasma salicylate, pH, and electrolytes can be measured. Fluid losses are replaced and sodium bicarbonate (1.26%) given to enhance urinary salicylate excretion when the plasma-salicylate concentration is greater than:

500 mg/litre (3.6 mmol/litre) in adults *or*

350 mg/litre (2.5 mmol/litre) in children.

Haemodialysis is the treatment of choice for severe salicylate poisoning and should be given serious consideration when the plasma-salicylate concentration is greater than 700 mg/litre (5.1 mmol/litre) or in the presence of severe metabolic acidosis.

NSAIDS. Mefenamic acid has important consequences in overdosage because it can cause convulsions, which if prolonged or recurrent, require treatment with intravenous lorazepam or diazepam. Ibuprofen may cause nausea, vomiting, and tinnitus, but more serious toxicity is very uncommon. Gastric emptying is indicated if more than 400 mg/kg has been ingested within the preceding hour, followed by symptomatic measures.

PARACETAMOL. As little as 10–15 g (20–30 tablets) or 150 mg/kg of paracetamol taken within 24 hours may cause severe hepatocellular necrosis and, less frequently, renal tubular necrosis. Nausea and vomiting, the only early features of poisoning, usually settle within 24 hours. Persistence beyond this time, often associated with the onset of right subcostal pain and tenderness, usually indicates development of hepatic necrosis. Liver damage is maximal 3–4 days after ingestion and may lead to encephalopathy, haemorrhage, hypoglycaemia, cerebral oedema, and death.

Therefore, despite a lack of significant early symptoms, patients who have taken an overdose of paracetamol should be transferred to hospital urgently.

Administration of activated charcoal should be considered if paracetamol in excess of 150 mg/kg or 12 g **whichever is the smaller**, is thought to have been ingested within the previous hour.

Antidotes such as **acetylcysteine** and **methionine** protect the liver if given within 10–12 hours of ingestion; acetylcysteine is effective up to and possibly beyond 24 hours.

Patients at risk of liver damage and therefore requiring treatment can be identified from a single measurement of the plasma-paracetamol concentration, related to the time from ingestion, provided this time interval is not less than 4 hours; earlier samples may be misleading. The concentration is plotted on a paracetamol treatment graph of a reference line ('normal treatment line') joining plots of 200 mg/litre (1.32 mmol/litre) at 4 hours and 6.25 mg/litre (0.04 mmol/litre) at 24 hours (see p. 23). Those whose plasma-paracetamol concentrations are above the *normal treatment line* are treated with acetylcysteine by intravenous infusion (or with methionine by mouth, provided the overdose has been taken **within 10–12 hours** *and* the

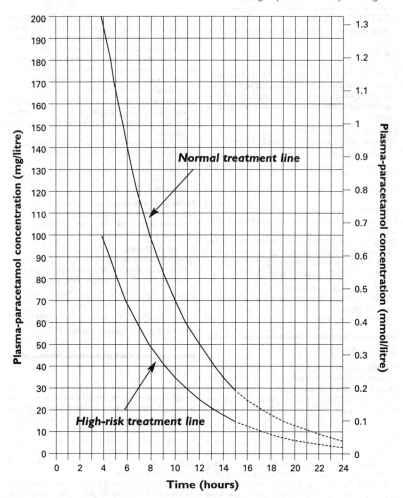

Patients whose plasma-paracetamol concentrations are above the **normal treatment line** should be treated with acetylcysteine by intravenous infusion (or with methionine by mouth, provided the overdose has been taken **within 10–12 hours** and the patient is not vomiting). Patients on enzyme-inducing drugs (e.g. carbamazepine, phenobarbital, phenytoin, rifampicin, and alcohol) or who are malnourished (e.g. in anorexia, in alcoholism, or those who are HIV-positive) should be treated if their plasma-paracetamol concentrations are above the **high-risk treatment line**. The prognostic accuracy after 15 hours is uncertain but a plasma-paracetamol concentration above the relevant treatment line should be regarded as carrying a serious risk of liver damage.
Graph reproduced courtesy of University of Wales College of Medicine Therapeutics and Toxicology Centre

patient is not vomiting). Patients on enzyme-inducing drugs (e.g. carbamazepine, phenobarbital, phenytoin, rifampicin, and alcohol) or who are malnourished (e.g. in anorexia, in alcoholism, or those who are HIV-positive) may develop toxicity at **lower** plasma-paracetamol concentrations and should be treated if concentrations are above the *high-risk treatment line* (which joins plots that are at 50% of the plasma-paracetamol concentrations of the normal treatment line).

The prognostic accuracy after 15 hours is uncertain but a plasma-paracetamol concentration above the relevant treatment line should be regarded as carrying a serious risk of liver damage.

Plasma-paracetamol concentration may be difficult to interpret when paracetamol has been ingested over several hours. If there is doubt about timing or the need for treatment then the patient should be treated with an antidote.

In remote areas methionine (2.5 g) should be given by mouth since it is seldom practicable to give acetylcysteine outside hospital. Once the patient reaches hospital the need to continue treatment with the antidote will be assessed from the plasma-paracetamol concentration (related to the time from ingestion).

See also Co-proxamol, under Analgesics (opioid).

ACETYLCYSTEINE

Indications: paracetamol overdosage, see notes above
Cautions: asthma
Side-effects: rashes, anaphylaxis
Dose: *by intravenous infusion,* in glucose intravenous infusion 5%, initially 150 mg/kg in 200 mL over 15 minutes, followed by 50 mg/kg in 500 mL over 4 hours, then 100 mg/kg in 1000 mL over 16 hours

Parvolex® (Celltech) PoM
Injection, acetylcysteine 200 mg/mL, net price 10-mL amp = £2.65

METHIONINE

Indications: paracetamol overdosage, see notes above
Cautions: hepatic impairment (Appendix 2)
Side-effects: nausea, vomiting, drowsiness, irritability
Dose: ADULT and CHILD over 6 years initially 2.5 g, followed by 3 further doses of 2.5 g every 4 hours, CHILD under 6 years initially 1 g, followed by 3 further doses of 1 g every 4 hours

Methionine (Non-proprietary)
Tablets, DL-methionine 250 mg, net price 200-tab pack = £66.05
Available from Celltech

Analgesics (opioid)

Opioids (narcotic analgesics) cause varying degrees of coma, respiratory depression, and pinpoint pupils. The specific antidote **naloxone** is indicated if there is coma or bradypnoea. Since naloxone has a shorter duration of action than many opioids, close monitoring and repeated injections are necessary according to the respiratory rate and depth of coma. Alternatively, it may be given by continuous intravenous infusion, the rate of administration being adjusted according to response and based on close monitoring of vital signs. The effects of some opioids, such as buprenorphine, are only partially reversed by naloxone. Dextropropoxyphene and methadone have very long durations of action; patients may need to be monitored for long periods following large overdoses.

CO-PROXAMOL. A combination of dextropropoxyphene and paracetamol (co-proxamol) is frequently taken in overdosage. The initial features are those of acute opioid overdosage with coma, respiratory depression, and pinpoint pupils. Patients may die of acute cardiovascular collapse before reaching hospital (particularly if alcohol has also been consumed) unless adequately resuscitated or given **naloxone** as antidote to the dextropropoxyphene (see also above). Paracetamol hepatotoxicity may develop later and should be anticipated and treated as indicated above.

NALOXONE HYDROCHLORIDE

Indications: overdosage with opioids; postoperative respiratory depression (section 15.1.7)
Cautions: physical dependence on opioids; cardiac irritability; naloxone is short-acting, see notes above

Dose: *by intravenous injection,* 0.8–2 mg repeated at intervals of 2–3 minutes to a max. of 10 mg if respiratory function does not improve (then question diagnosis); CHILD 10 micrograms/kg; subsequent dose of 100 micrograms/kg if no response
By subcutaneous or intramuscular injection, as intravenous injection but only if intravenous route not feasible (onset of action slower)
By continuous intravenous infusion using an infusion pump, 10 mg diluted in 50 mL intravenous infusion solution at a rate adjusted according to the response
IMPORTANT. Doses used in acute opioid overdosage may not be appropriate for the management of opioid-induced respiratory depression and sedation in those receiving palliative care and in chronic opioid use, see also section 15.1.7 for management of postoperative respiratory depression

Naloxone (Non-proprietary) PoM
Injection, naloxone hydrochloride 400 micrograms/mL, net price 1-mL amp = £6.92
Available from Antigen, Mayne

Minijet® **Naloxone** (Celltech) PoM
Injection, naloxone hydrochloride 400 micrograms/mL, net price 1-mL disposable syringe = £5.57; 2-mL disposable syringe = £10.71

Narcan® (Bristol-Myers Squibb) PoM
Injection, naloxone hydrochloride 400 micrograms/mL, net price 1-mL amp = £4.54

Neonatal preparations —section 15.1.7

Antidepressants

Tricyclic and related antidepressants cause dry mouth, coma of varying degree, hypotension, hypothermia, hyperreflexia, extensor plantar responses, convulsions, respiratory failure, cardiac conduction defects, and arrhythmias. Dilated pupils and urinary retention also occur. Metabolic acidosis may complicate severe poisoning; delirium with confusion, agitation, and visual and auditory hallucinations, is common during recovery.

Symptomatic treatment and activated charcoal by mouth may reasonably be given in the home before transfer but hospital admission is strongly advised, and supportive measures to ensure a patent airway and adequate ventilation during transfer are mandatory. Intravenous diazepam may be required for control of convulsions (preferably in emulsion form). Although arrhythmias are worrying, some will respond to correction of hypoxia and acidosis; the use of anti-arrhythmic drugs is best avoided. Diazepam given by mouth is usually adequate to sedate delirious patients but large doses may be required.

Antimalarials

Overdosage with chloroquine and hydroxychloroquine is extremely hazardous and difficult to treat. Urgent advice from a poisons information centre is essential. Life-threatening features include arrhythmias (which can have a very rapid onset) and convulsions (which can be intractable). Quinine overdosage is also a severe hazard and calls for urgent advice from a poisons information centre.

Beta-blockers

Therapeutic overdosages with beta-blockers may cause lightheadedness, dizziness, and possibly syncope as a result of bradycardia and hypotension; heart failure may be precipitated or exacerbated. These complications are most likely in patients with conduction system disorders or impaired myocardial function. Bradycardia is the most common arrhythmia caused by beta-blockers, but sotalol may induce ventricular tachyarrhythmias (sometimes of the torsades de pointes type). The effects of massive overdosage may vary from one beta-blocker to another; propranolol overdosage in particular may cause coma and convulsions.

Acute massive overdosage must be managed in hospital and expert advice should be obtained. Maintenance of a clear airway and adequate ventilation is mandatory. An intravenous injection of atropine is required to treat bradycardia and hypotension (3 mg for an adult, 40 micrograms/kg for a child). Cardiogenic shock unresponsive to atropine is probably best treated with an intravenous injection of glucagon 2–10 mg (CHILD 50–150 micrograms/kg) [unlicensed indication and dose] in glucose 5% (with precautions to protect the airway in case of vomiting) followed by an intravenous infusion of 50 micrograms/kg/hour. If glucagon is not available, intravenous isoprenaline or intravenous prenalterol [not on UK market] are alternatives. A cardiac pacemaker may be used to increase the heart rate.

Hypnotics and anxiolytics

BARBITURATES. These cause drowsiness, coma, respiratory depression, hypotension, and hypothermia. The duration and depth of cerebral depression vary greatly with the drug, the dose, and the tolerance of the patient. The severity of poisoning is often greater with a large dose of barbiturate hypnotics than with the longer-acting phenobarbital. The majority of patients survive with supportive measures alone. Repeated doses of activated charcoal (see Active Elimination Techniques, above) may be used for barbiturate poisoning. Charcoal haemoperfusion is the treatment of choice for the small minority of patients with very severe barbiturate poisoning who fail to improve, or who deteriorate despite good supportive care.

BENZODIAZEPINES. Benzodiazepines taken alone cause drowsiness, ataxia, dysarthria, and occasionally minor and short-lived depression of consciousness. They potentiate the effects of other central nervous system depressants taken concomitantly. Flumazenil, a benzodiazepine antagonist, may be used in the *differential diagnosis* of unclear cases of multiple drug overdose but expert advice is **essential** since adverse effects may occur (e.g. convulsions in patients dependent on benzodiazepines).

Iron salts

Iron poisoning is commonest in childhood and is usually accidental. The symptoms are nausea, vomiting, abdominal pain, diarrhoea, haematemesis, and rectal bleeding. Hypotension, coma, and hepatocel-

lular necrosis occur later. Mortality is reduced with intensive and specific therapy with **desferrioxamine**, which chelates iron. The stomach should be emptied by gastric lavage (with a wide-bore tube) within 1 hour of ingesting a significant quantity of iron or if radiography reveals tablets in the stomach; whole bowel irrigation may be considered in severe poisoning but advice should be sought from a poisons information centre. The serum-iron concentration is measured as an emergency and intravenous desferrioxamine given to chelate absorbed iron in excess of the expected iron binding capacity. In **severe toxicity** intravenous desferrioxamine should be given *immediately* without waiting for the result of the serum-iron measurement (contact a poisons information centre for advice).

DESFERRIOXAMINE MESILATE
(Deferoxamine Mesilate)

Indications: iron poisoning; chronic iron overload (section 9.1.3)

Cautions: section 9.1.3

Side-effects: section 9.1.3

Dose: *by continuous intravenous infusion*, up to 15 mg/kg/hour; max. 80 mg/kg in 24 hours

■ Preparations
Section 9.1.3

Lithium

Most cases of lithium intoxication occur as a complication of long-term therapy and are caused by reduced excretion of the drug due to a variety of factors including dehydration, deterioration of renal function, infections, and co-administration of diuretics or NSAIDs (or other drugs that interact). Acute deliberate overdoses may also occur with delayed onset of symptoms (12 hours or more) due to slow entry of lithium into the tissues and continuing absorption from modified-release formulations.

The early clinical features are non-specific and may include apathy and restlessness which could be confused with mental changes due to the patient's depressive illness. Vomiting, diarrhoea, ataxia, weakness, dysarthria, muscle twitching, and tremor may follow. Severe poisoning is associated with convulsions, coma, renal failure, electrolyte imbalance, dehydration, and hypotension.

Therapeutic lithium concentrations are within the range of 0.4–1.0 mmol/litre; concentrations in excess of 2.0 mmol/litre are usually associated with serious toxicity and such cases may need treatment with haemodialysis (if there is renal failure). In acute overdosage much higher serum concentrations may be present without features of toxicity and all that is usually necessary is to take measures to increase urine production (e.g. by ensuring adequate fluid intake; but avoid diuretics). Otherwise treatment is supportive with special regard to electrolyte balance, renal function, and control of convulsions. Whole bowel irrigation should be considered for significant ingestion, but advice should be sought from a poisons information centre.

Phenothiazines and related drugs

Phenothiazines cause less depression of consciousness and respiration than other sedatives. Hypotension, hypothermia, sinus tachycardia, and arrhythmias (particularly with thioridazine) may complicate poisoning. Dystonic reactions can occur with therapeutic doses, (particularly with prochlorperazine and trifluoperazine) and convulsions may occur in severe cases. Arrhythmias may respond to correction of hypoxia, acidosis and other biochemical abnormalities but specialist advice should be sought if arrhythmias result from a prolonged QT interval; the use of some anti-arrhythmic drugs may worsen such arrhythmias. Dystonic reactions are rapidly abolished by injection of drugs such as benzatropine or procyclidine (section 4.9.2).

Stimulants

AMPHETAMINES. These cause wakefulness, excessive activity, paranoia, hallucinations, and hypertension followed by exhaustion, convulsions, hyperthermia, and coma. The early stages can be controlled by diazepam or lorazepam; advice should be sought from a poisons information centre on the management of hypertension. Later, tepid sponging, anticonvulsants, and artificial respiration may be needed.

COCAINE. Cocaine stimulates the central nervous system, causing agitation, dilated pupils, tachycardia, hypertension, hallucinations, hypertonia, and hyperreflexia.

ECSTASY. Ecstasy (methylenedioxymethamfetamine, MDMA) may cause severe reactions, even at doses that were previously tolerated. The most serious effects are delirium, coma, convulsions, ventricular arrhythmias, hyperpyrexia, rhabdomyolysis, acute renal failure, acute hepatitis, disseminated intravascular coagulation, adult respiratory distress syndrome, hyperreflexia, hypotension and intracerebral haemorrhage; hyponatraemia has also been associated with ecstasy use.
    Treatment is supportive, with diazepam to control severe agitation or persistent convulsions and close monitoring including ECG. Self-induced water intoxication should be considered in patients with ecstasy poisoning.

Theophylline

Theophylline and related drugs are often prescribed as modified-release formulations and toxicity may therefore be delayed. They cause vomiting (which may be severe and intractable), agitation, restlessness, dilated pupils, sinus tachycardia, and hyperglycaemia. More serious effects are haematemesis, convulsions, and supraventricular and ventricular arrhythmias. Profound **hypokalaemia** may develop rapidly.
    The stomach should be emptied if the patient presents within 2 hours. Elimination of theophylline is enhanced by repeated doses of activated charcoal by mouth (see also under Active Elimination Techniques). Hypokalaemia is corrected by intravenous infusion of potassium chloride and may be so severe as to require 60 mmol/hour (high doses under ECG monitoring). Convulsions should be controlled by intravenous administration of diazepam (emulsion preferred). Sedation with diazepam may be necessary in agitated patients.
    Provided the patient does **not** suffer from asthma, **propranolol** (section 2.4) may be administered intravenously to reverse extreme tachycardia, hypokalaemia, and hyperglycaemia.

Other poisons

Consult a poisons information centre day and night—p. 20.

Cyanides

Cyanide antidotes include dicobalt edetate, given alone, and sodium nitrite followed by sodium thiosulphate. These antidotes are held for emergency use in hospitals as well as in centres where cyanide poisoning is a risk such as factories and laboratories. Hydroxocobalamin is an alternative antidote but its use should ideally be discussed with a poisons information centre; the usual dose is hydroxocobalamin 70 mg/kg by intravenous infusion (repeated once or twice according to severity). *Cyanokit*®, which provides hydroxocobalamin 2.5 g/bottle, is available but it is not licensed for use in the UK.

DICOBALT EDETATE

Indications: acute poisoning with cyanides
Cautions: owing to toxicity to be used only when patient tending to lose, or has lost, consciousness; not to be used as a precautionary measure
Side-effects: hypotension, tachycardia, and vomiting
Dose: *by intravenous injection*, 300 mg over 1 minute (5 minutes if condition less serious) followed immediately by 50 mL of glucose intravenous infusion 50%; if response inadequate a second dose of both may be given; if no response after further 5 minutes a third dose of both may be given

Dicobalt Edetate (Cambridge) [PoM]
Injection, dicobalt edetate 15 mg/mL, net price 20-mL (300-mg) amp = £9.80

SODIUM NITRITE

Indications: poisoning with cyanides (used in conjunction with sodium thiosulphate)
Side-effects: flushing and headache due to vasodilatation
Dose: see under preparation below

Sodium Nitrite Injection [PoM]
Injection, sodium nitrite 3% (30 mg/mL) in water for injections
Dose: 10 mL by intravenous injection over 3 minutes, followed by 25 mL of sodium thiosulphate injection 50%, by intravenous injection over 10 minutes
'Special-order' [unlicensed] product: contact Martindale, or regional hospital manufacturing unit

SODIUM THIOSULPHATE

Indications: poisoning with cyanides (used in conjunction with sodium nitrite)

Sodium Thiosulphate Injection PoM
Injection, sodium thiosulphate 50% (500 mg/mL) in
water for injections
Dose: see above under Sodium Nitrite Injection
'Special-order' [unlicensed] product: contact Martindale,
or regional hospital manufacturing unit

Ethylene glycol

Ethanol (by mouth or by intravenous infusion) is
used for the treatment of ethylene glycol poisoning.
Fomepizole (*Antizol*®, available on named-patient
basis from poisons information centres or from IDIS)
has also been used for the treatment of ethylene
glycol poisoning. Advice on the treatment of ethylene glycol poisoning should be obtained from a
poisons information centre.

Heavy metals

Heavy metal antidotes include dimercaprol, penicill-
amine, and sodium calcium edetate.Other antidotes
for heavy metal poisoning include succimer
(DMSA) and unithiol (DMPS) [both unlicensed];
their use may be valuable in certain cases and the
advice of a poisons information centre should be
sought.

DIMERCAPROL
(BAL)

Indications: poisoning by antimony, arsenic, bismuth, gold, mercury, possibly thallium; adjunct
(with sodium calcium edetate) in lead poisoning

Cautions: hypertension, renal impairment (discontinue or use with extreme caution if impairment
develops during treatment), elderly, pregnancy and
breast-feeding

Contra-indications: not indicated for iron, cad-
mium, or selenium poisoning; severe hepatic
impairment (unless due to arsenic poisoning)

Side-effects: hypertension, tachycardia, malaise,
nausea, vomiting, salivation, lacrimation, sweating, burning sensation (mouth, throat, and eyes),
feeling of constriction of throat and chest, headache, muscle spasm, abdominal pain, tingling of
extremities; pyrexia in children; local pain and
abscess at injection site

Dose: *by intramuscular injection*, 2.5–3 mg/kg
every 4 hours for 2 days, 2–4 times on the third
day, then 1–2 times daily for 10 days or until
recovery

Dimercaprol (Sovereign) PoM
Injection, dimercaprol 50 mg/mL. Net price 2-mL
amp = £42.73
NOTE. Contains arachis (peanut) oil as solvent

PENICILLAMINE

Indications: lead poisoning
Cautions: see section 10.1.3
Contra-indications: see section 10.1.3
Side-effects: see section 10.1.3
Dose: 1–2 g daily in divided doses before food until
urinary lead is stabilised at less than 500 micr-
ograms/day; CHILD 20 mg/kg daily

▪ Preparations
Section 10.1.3

SODIUM CALCIUM EDETATE
(Sodium Calciumedetate)

Indications: poisoning by heavy metals, especially
lead
Cautions: renal impairment
Side-effects: nausea, diarrhoea, abdominal pain,
pain at site of injection, thrombophlebitis if given
too rapidly, renal damage particularly in overdosage; hypotension, lacrimation, myalgia, nasal
congestion, sneezing, malaise, thirst, fever, chills,
headache also reported
Dose: *by intravenous infusion*, ADULT and CHILD up
to 40 mg/kg twice daily for up to 5 days, repeated if
necessary after 48 hours

Ledclair® (Durbin) PoM
Injection, sodium calcium edetate 200 mg/mL, net
price 5-mL amp = £7.29

Noxious gases

CARBON MONOXIDE. Carbon monoxide
poisoning is usually due to inhalation of smoke,
car exhaust, or fumes caused by blocked flues or
incomplete combustion of fuel gases in confined
spaces. Its toxic effects are entirely due to hypoxia.

Immediate treatment of carbon monoxide
poisoning is essential. The person should be
removed into the fresh air, the airway cleared, and
oxygen 100% administered as soon as available.
Artificial respiration should be given as necessary
and continued until adequate spontaneous breathing
starts, or stopped only after persistent and efficient
treatment of cardiac arrest has failed. Admission to
hospital is desirable because complications may arise
after a delay of hours or days. Cerebral oedema
should be anticipated in severe poisoning and is
treated with an intravenous infusion of mannitol
(section 2.2.5). Referral for hyperbaric oxygen
treatment should be discussed with the poisons
information services if the victim is or has been
unconscious, or has a blood carboxyhaemoglobin
concentration of more than 20%, or is pregnant.

CS SPRAY. CS spray, which is used for riot control,
irritates the eyes (hence 'tear gas') and the respiratory tract; symptoms normally settle spontaneously
within 15 minutes. If symptoms persist, the patient
should be removed to a well-ventilated area, and the
exposed skin washed with soap and water after
removal of contaminated clothing. Contact lenses
should be removed and hard ones washed (soft ones
should be discarded). Eye symptoms should be
treated by irrigating the eyes with physiological
saline (or water if saline not available) and advice
sought from an ophthalmologist. Patients with
features of severe poisoning, particularly respiratory
complications, should be admitted to hospital for
symptomatic treatment.

SULPHUR DIOXIDE, CHLORINE, PHOSGENE,
AMMONIA. All of these gases can cause upper
respiratory tract and conjunctival irritation. Pulmonary oedema, with severe breathlessness and cyanosis may develop suddenly up to 36 hours after
exposure. Death may occur. Patients are kept under
observation and those who develop pulmonary
oedema are given corticosteroids and oxygen.
Assisted ventilation may be necessary in the most
serious cases.

NERVE AGENTS. Treatment of nerve agent poisoning is similar to organophosphorus insecticide poisoning (see below), but advice should be sought from a poisons information centre. In emergencies involving the release of nerve agents, kits ('NAAS pods') which contain **pralidoxime mesilate** may be obtained through the Ambulance Service from the National Blood Service (or the Welsh Blood Service in South Wales or designated hospital pharmacies in Northern Ireland). If the patient does not respond to atropine and pralidoxime it may be appropriate to use **obidoxime**, but advice should be sought from a poisons information centre. In the very rare circumstances where the nerve agent is tabun (GA), obidoxime will also be supplied as part of the pod.

Pesticides

PARAQUAT. Concentrated liquid paraquat preparations (e.g. *Gramoxone*®), available to farmers and horticulturists, contain 10–20% paraquat and are extremely toxic. Granular preparations, for garden use, contain only 2.5% paraquat and have caused few deaths.

Paraquat has local and systemic effects. Splashes in the eyes irritate and ulcerate the cornea and conjunctiva. Copious washing of the eye and instillation of antibacterial eye-drops, should aid healing but it may be a long process. Skin irritation, blistering, and ulceration can occur from prolonged contact both with the concentrated and dilute forms. Inhalation of spray, mist, or dust containing paraquat may cause nose bleeding and sore throat but not systemic toxicity.

Ingestion of concentrated paraquat solutions is followed by nausea, vomiting, and diarrhoea. Painful ulceration of the tongue, lips, and fauces may appear after 36 to 48 hours together with renal failure. Some days later there may be dyspnoea with pulmonary fibrosis due to proliferative alveolitis and bronchiolitis.

Treatment should be started immediately. The single most useful measure is oral administration of repeat-dose **activated charcoal**[1]; the first dose of 100 g is given with a laxative (e.g. magnesium sulphate), followed by activated charcoal 50 g every 4 hours (or more frequently if tolerated) until charcoal is seen in the stool. Vomiting may preclude the use of activated charcoal and an anti-emetic may be required. Gastric lavage is of doubtful value. Intravenous fluids and analgesics are given as necessary. Oxygen therapy should be avoided in the early stages of management since this may exacerbate damage to the lungs, but oxygen may be required in the late stages to palliate symptoms. Measures to enhance elimination of absorbed paraquat are probably valueless but should be discussed with the poisons information centres who will also give guidance on predicting the likely outcome from plasma concentrations. Paraquat absorption can be confirmed by a simple qualitative urine test.

ORGANOPHOSPHORUS INSECTICIDES. Organophosphorus insecticides are usually supplied as powders or dissolved in organic solvents. All are absorbed through the bronchi and intact skin as well as through the gut and inhibit cholinesterase activity thereby prolonging and intensifying the effects of acetylcholine. Toxicity between different compounds varies considerably, and onset may be delayed after skin exposure.

Anxiety, restlessness, dizziness, headache, miosis, nausea, hypersalivation, vomiting, abdominal colic, diarrhoea, bradycardia, and sweating are common. Muscle weakness and fasciculation may develop and progress to generalised flaccid paralysis including the ocular and respiratory muscles. Convulsions, coma, pulmonary oedema with copious bronchial secretions, hypoxia, and arrhythmias occur in severe cases. Hyperglycaemia and glycosuria without ketonuria may also be present.

Further absorption should be prevented by emptying the stomach, removing the patient to fresh air, or removing soiled clothing and washing contaminated skin. In severe poisoning it is vital to ensure a clear airway, frequent removal of bronchial secretions, and adequate ventilation and oxygenation. **Atropine** will reverse the muscarinic effects of acetylcholine and is given in a dose of 2 mg (20 micrograms/kg in a child) as atropine sulphate (intramuscularly or intravenously according to the severity of poisoning) every 5 to 10 minutes until the skin becomes flushed and dry, the pupils dilate, and tachycardia develops.

Pralidoxime mesilate (P2S), a cholinesterase reactivator, is used, as an adjunct to atropine, in moderate or severe poisoning but it is effective only if given within 24 hours. It produces muscle improvement within 30 minutes but further doses may be required; an intravenous infusion may be required in severe cases. Pralidoxime mesilate may be obtained from designated centres, the names of which are held by the poisons information centres (see p. 20).

PRALIDOXIME MESILATE

(P2S)

Indications: adjunct to atropine in the treatment of poisoning by organophosphorus insecticide or nerve agent

Cautions: renal impairment, myasthenia gravis

Contra-indications: poisoning due to carbamates and to organophosphorus compounds without anticholinesterase activity

Side-effects: drowsiness, dizziness, disturbances of vision, nausea, tachycardia, headache, hyperventilation, and muscular weakness

Dose: *by slow intravenous injection* (diluted to 10–15 mL with water for injections) over 5–10 minutes, initially 30 mg/kg followed by 1–2 further doses if necessary *or by intravenous infusion*, 8 mg/kg/hour; usual max. 12 g in 24 hours

CHILD 20–60 mg/kg as required depending on severity of poisoning and response

NOTE. Pralidoxime mesilate doses in BNF may differ from those in product literature

Pralidoxime Mesilate ▣PoM▣

Injection, pralidoxime mesilate 200 mg/mL
Available as 5-mL amps (from designated centres for organophosphorus insecticide poisoning or from the National Blood Service and the Welsh Blood Service for nerve agent poisoning)

---

1. **Fuller's earth** and **bentonite** given by mouth have also been used as adsorbents. A suspension of Fuller's earth 30% was used in 3 doses of 200–500 mL given at 2-hour intervals; magnesium sulphate or mannitol were given with Fuller's earth to promote diarrhoea and empty the gut.

Snake bites and animal stings

SNAKE BITES.   Envenoming from snake bite is uncommon in the UK. Many exotic snakes are kept, some illegally, but the only indigenous venomous snake is the adder (*Vipera berus*). The bite may cause local and systemic effects. Local effects include pain, swelling, bruising, and tender enlargement of regional lymph nodes. Systemic effects include early anaphylactoid symptoms (transient hypotension with syncope, angioedema, urticaria, abdominal colic, diarrhoea, and vomiting), with later persistent or recurrent hypotension, ECG abnormalities, spontaneous systemic bleeding, coagulopathy, adult respiratory distress syndrome, and acute renal failure. Fatal envenoming is rare but the potential for severe envenoming must not be underestimated.

Early anaphylactoid symptoms should be treated with **adrenaline (epinephrine)** (section 3.4.3). Indications for antivenom treatment include systemic envenoming, especially hypotension (see above), ECG abnormalities, vomiting, haemostatic abnormalities, and marked local envenoming such that after bites on the hand or foot, swelling extends beyond the wrist or ankle within 4 hours of the bite. For both **adults** and **children**, the contents of one vial (10 mL) of **European viper venom antiserum** (available from Farillon) is given *by intravenous injection* over 10–15 minutes or *by intravenous infusion* over 30 minutes after diluting in sodium chloride intravenous infusion 0.9% (use 5 mL diluent/kg body-weight). The **same dose** should be used for **adults** and **children**. The dose can be repeated in 1–2 hours if symptoms of **systemic envenoming** persist. Adrenaline (epinephrine) injection must be immediately to hand for treatment of anaphylactic reactions to the antivenom (for the management of anaphylaxis see section 3.4.3).

Antivenom is available for certain foreign snakes, spiders and scorpions. For information on identification, management, and supply, telephone:

Oxford	(01865) 220 968
or	(01865) 221 332
or	(01865) 741 166
Liverpool	(0151) 708 9393
Liverpool (University Hospital Aintree)	
(emergency supply only)	(0151) 525 5980
London (emergency supply only)	(020) 7771 5394

INSECT STINGS. Stings from ants, wasps, hornets, and bees cause local pain and swelling but seldom cause severe direct toxicity unless many stings are inflicted at the same time. If the sting is in the mouth or on the tongue local swelling may threaten the upper airway. The stings from these insects are usually treated by cleaning the area. Bee stings should be removed as quickly as possible. Anaphylactic reactions require immediate treatment with intramuscular **adrenaline (epinephrine)**; self-administered intramuscular adrenaline (e.g. *EpiPen*®) is the best first-aid treatment for patients with severe hypersensitivity. An inhaled bronchodilator should be used for asthmatic reactions. For the management of anaphylaxis, see section 3.4.3. A short course of an **oral antihistamine** or a **topical corticosteroid** may help to reduce inflammation and relieve itching.

MARINE STINGS. The severe pain of weeverfish stings can be relieved by immersing the stung area in uncomfortably hot, but not scalding, water (not more than 45° C). People stung by jellyfish and Portugese man-o'-war around the UK coast should be removed from the sea as soon as possible. Adherent tentacles should be scraped or washed off with seawater. Alcoholic solutions including suntan lotions should **not** be applied because they may cause further discharge of stinging hairs. Ice packs will reduce pain and a slurry of baking soda (sodium bicarbonate), but not vinegar, may be useful for treating stings from UK species.

1: Gastro-intestinal system

1.1 Dyspepsia and gastro-oesophageal reflux disease

Dyspepsia

Dyspepsia covers pain, fullness, early satiety, bloating, or nausea. It can occur with gastric and duodenal ulceration (section 1.3) and gastric cancer but most commonly it is of uncertain origin.

Helicobacter pylori infection may be present but most individuals with non-ulcer dyspepsia do not benefit symptomatically from *H. pylori* eradication. However, eradication therapy (section 1.3) may be considered for dyspepsia if it is ulcer-like and if it is not accompanied by 'alarm symptoms' (e.g. bleeding or weight loss).

Gastro-oesophageal reflux disease

Gastro-oesophageal reflux disease (including non-erosive gastro-oesophageal reflux and erosive oesophagitis) is characterised by symptoms which include heartburn, acid regurgitation, and sometimes, difficulty in swallowing (dysphagia); oesophageal inflammation (oesophagitis), ulceration, and stricture formation may occur and there is an association with asthma.

The management of gastro-oesophageal reflux disease includes drug treatment, lifestyle changes and, in some cases, surgery. Initial treatment is guided by the severity of symptoms and treatment is then adjusted according to response. The extent of healing depends on the severity of the disease, the treatment chosen, and the duration of therapy.

For *mild symptoms* of gastro-oesophageal reflux disease, initial management may include the use of **antacids** and **alginates**. Alginate-containing antacids form a 'raft' that floats on the surface of the stomach contents to reduce reflux and protect the oesophageal mucosa. **Histamine H₂-receptor antagonists** (section 1.3.1) suppress acid secretion and they may relieve symptoms and permit reduction in antacid consumption. For refractory cases, a course of a **proton pump inhibitor** (section 1.3.5) may be considered (as described for severe symptoms, below).

For *severe symptoms* of gastro-oesophageal reflux disease or for patients with a proven or severe pathology (e.g. *oesophagitis, oesophageal ulceration, Barrett's oesophagus*), initial management involves the use of a **proton pump inhibitor** (section 1.3.5); patients need to be reassessed if symptoms persist despite 4–6 weeks of treatment with a proton pump inhibitor. When symptoms abate, treatment is titrated down to a level which maintains remission (e.g. by reducing the dose of the proton pump inhibitor or by giving it intermittently, or by substituting treatment with a histamine H_2-receptor antagonist). However, for endoscopically confirmed *erosive, ulcerative*, or *stricturing* disease, treatment with a proton pump inhibitor usually needs to be maintained at the minimum effective dose.

A prokinetic drug such as **metoclopramide** (section 4.6) may improve gastro-oesophageal sphincter function and accelerate gastric emptying.

Patients with gastro-oesophageal reflux disease need to be advised about lifestyle changes (avoidance of excess alcohol and of aggravating foods such as fats); other measures include weight reduction, smoking cessation, and raising the head of the bed.

CHILDREN. Gastro-oesophageal reflux disease is common in infancy but most symptoms resolve between 12 and 18 months of age. Mild or moderate reflux without complications can be managed initially by changes in posture and thickening of liquid feeds (see Appendix 7 for suitable products) followed if necessary by treatment with an alginate-containing product (low sodium and low aluminium content for infants). For older children, life-style changes similar to those for adults (see above) may be helpful followed if necessary by treatment with an alginate-containing product.

Children who do not respond to these measures or who have problems such as respiratory disorders or suspected oesophagitis need to be referred to hospital; an H_2-receptor antagonist such as cimetidine (section 1.3.1) may be needed to reduce acid secretion. If the oesophagitis is resistant to H_2-receptor blockade, the proton pump inhibitor omeprazole (section 1.3.5) can be tried.

1.1.1 Antacids and dimeticone

Antacids (usually containing aluminium or magnesium compounds) can often relieve symptoms in *ulcer dyspepsia* and in *non-erosive gastro-oesophageal reflux* (see also section 1.1); they are also sometimes used in non-ulcer dyspepsia but the evidence of benefit is uncertain. Antacids are best given when symptoms occur or are expected, usually between meals and at bedtime, 4 or more times daily; additional doses may be required up to once an hour. Conventional doses e.g. 10 mL 3 or 4 times daily of liquid magnesium–aluminium antacids promote ulcer healing, but less well than antisecretory drugs (section 1.3); proof of a relationship between healing and neutralising capacity is lacking. Liquid preparations are more effective than solids.

Aluminium- and magnesium-containing antacids (e.g. aluminium hydroxide, and magnesium carbonate, hydroxide and trisilicate), being relatively insoluble in water, are long-acting if retained in the stomach. They are suitable for most antacid purposes. Magnesium-containing antacids tend to be laxative whereas aluminium-containing antacids may be constipating; antacids containing both magnesium and aluminium may reduce these colonic side-effects. Aluminium accumulation does not appear to be a risk if renal function is normal (see also Appendix 3).

The acid-neutralising capacity of preparations that contain more than one antacid may be the same as simpler preparations. Complexes such as **hydrotalcite** confer no special advantage.

Sodium bicarbonate has been used in the relief of dyspepsia. Some individuals may still use sodium bicarbonate, but it has largely fallen from use as an antacid. However, it retains a place in the management of urinary-tract disorders (section 7.4.3) and acidosis (section 9.2.1.3 and section 9.2.2). Sodium bicarbonate should be avoided in patients on salt-restricted diets.

Bismuth-containing antacids (unless chelates) are not recommended because absorbed bismuth can be neurotoxic, causing encephalopathy; they tend to be constipating. **Calcium-containing** antacids can induce rebound acid secretion: with modest doses the clinical significance is doubtful, but prolonged high doses also cause hypercalcaemia and alkalosis, and can precipitate the milk-alkali syndrome.

Activated **dimeticone** (simethicone) is added to an antacid as an antifoaming agent to relieve flatulence. These preparations may be useful for the relief of hiccup in palliative care. **Alginates** added as protectants against gastro-oesophageal reflux disease (section 1.1) may be useful. The amount of additional ingredient or antacid in individual preparations varies widely, as does their sodium content, so that preparations may not be freely interchangeable

For **preparations** on sale to the public (not prescribable on the NHS), see p. 34.

See also section 1.3 for drugs used in the treatment of peptic ulceration.

INTERACTIONS. Antacids should preferably not be taken at the same time as other drugs since they may impair absorption. Antacids may also damage enteric coatings designed to prevent dissolution in the stomach. See also **Appendix 1** (antacids).

> **Low Na⁺.** The words low Na^+ added after some preparations indicate a sodium content of less than 1 mmol per tablet or 10-mL dose.

Aluminium- and magnesium-containing antacids

ALUMINIUM HYDROXIDE

Indications: dyspepsia; hyperphosphataemia (section 9.5.2.2)

Cautions: see notes above; **interactions:** Appendix 1 (antacids)

Contra-indications: hypophosphataemia; porphyria (section 9.8.2)

Side-effects: see notes above

■ Aluminium-only preparations

Aluminium Hydroxide (Non-proprietary)

Tablets, dried aluminium hydroxide 500 mg. Net price 20 = 28p

Dose: 1–2 tablets chewed 4 times daily and at bedtime or as required

Oral suspension, about 4% w/w Al_2O_3 in water, with a peppermint flavour. Net price 200 mL = 41p

Dose: antacid, 5–10 mL 4 times daily between meals and at bedtime or as required; CHILD 6–12 years, up to 5 mL 3 times daily

NOTE. The brand name *Aludrox®* [NHS] (Pfizer Consumer) is used for aluminium hydroxide mixture; net price 200 mL = £1.42. *Aludrox®* [NHS] tablets also contain magnesium.

Alu-Capⁿ (3M)
Capsules, green/red, dried aluminium hydroxide
475 mg (low Na⁺). Net price 120-cap pack = £4.03
Dose: antacid, 1 capsule 4 times daily and at bedtime;
CHILD not recommended for antacid therapy

■ **Co-magaldrox**
Co-magaldrox is a mixture of aluminium hydroxide and
magnesium hydroxide; the proportions are expressed in the
form x/y where x and y are the strengths in milligrams per
unit dose of magnesium hydroxide and aluminium hydroxide respectively

Maaloxⁿ (Rhône-Poulenc Rorer)
Suspension, sugar-free, co-magaldrox 195/220
(magnesium hydroxide 195 mg, dried aluminium
hydroxide 220 mg/5 mL (low Na⁺)). Net price
500 mL = £2.38
Dose: 10–20 mL 20–60 minutes after meals and at
bedtime or when required; CHILD under 14 years not
recommended

Mucogelⁿ (Forest)
Suspension, sugar-free, co-magaldrox 195/220
(magnesium hydroxide 195 mg, dried aluminium
hydroxide 220 mg/5 mL (low Na⁺)). Net price
500 mL = £1.82
Dose: 10–20 mL 3 times daily, 20–60 minutes after
meals, and at bedtime or when required; CHILD under 12
years not recommended

MAGNESIUM CARBONATE

Indications: dyspepsia
Cautions: renal impairment; see also notes above;
interactions: Appendix 1 (antacids)
Contra-indications: hypophosphataemia
Side-effects: diarrhoea; belching due to liberated
carbon dioxide

Aromatic Magnesium Carbonate Mixture, BP
(Aromatic Magnesium Carbonate Oral
Suspension)
Oral suspension, light magnesium carbonate 3%,
sodium bicarbonate 5%, in a suitable vehicle
containing aromatic cardamom tincture. Contains
about 6 mmol Na⁺/10 mL. Net price 200 mL = 60p
Dose: 10 mL 3 times daily in water
For **preparations** also containing aluminium, see
above and section 1.1.2.

MAGNESIUM TRISILICATE

Indications: dyspepsia
Cautions: see under Magnesium Carbonate
Contra-indications: see under Magnesium Carb-
onate
Side-effects: diarrhoea; silica-based renal stones
reported on long-term treatment

Magnesium Trisilicate Tablets, Compound, BP
Tablets, magnesium trisilicate 250 mg, dried alu-
minium hydroxide 120 mg
Dose: 1–2 tablets chewed when required

Magnesium Trisilicate Mixture, BP
(Magnesium Trisilicate Oral Suspension)
Oral suspension, 5% each of magnesium trisilicate,
light magnesium carbonate, and sodium bicarbonate in a suitable vehicle with a peppermint
flavour. Contains about 6 mmol Na⁺/10 mL
Dose: 10 mL 3 times daily in water
For **preparations** also containing aluminium, see
above and section 1.1.2.

Aluminium-magnesium complexes

HYDROTALCITE
Aluminium magnesium carbonate hydroxide hydrate

Indications: dyspepsia

Cautions: see notes above; **interactions:** Appendix 1 (antacids)

Side-effects: see notes above

Hydrotalcite (Peckforton)
Suspension, hydrotalcite 500 mg/5 mL (low Na⁺).
Net price 500-mL pack = £1.96
Dose: 10 mL between meals and at bedtime; CHILD under
6 years not recommended, 6–12 years 5 mL
NOTE. The brand name *Altacite*ⁿ [NHS] is used for hydro-
talcite suspension; for *Altacite Plus*ⁿ suspension, see
below

Antacid preparations containing dimeticone

Altacite Plusⁿ (Peckforton)
Suspension, sugar-free, co-simalcite 125/500
(activated dimeticone 125 mg, hydrotalcite
500 mg)/5 mL (low Na⁺). Net price 500 mL = £1.96
Dose: 10 mL between meals and at bedtime when
required; CHILD 8–12 years 5 mL
Tablets [NHS], see p. 34

Asiloneⁿ (SSL)
Suspension, sugar-free, dried aluminium hydroxide
420 mg, activated dimeticone 135 mg, light
magnesium oxide 70 mg/5 mL (low Na⁺). Net price
500 mL = £1.95
Dose: 5–10 mL after meals and at bedtime or when
required up to 4 times daily; CHILD under 12 years not
recommended
Tablets [NHS], see p. 34
Liquid [NHS], see p. 34

Maalox Plusⁿ (Rhône-Poulenc Rorer)
Suspension, sugar-free, dried aluminium hydroxide
220 mg, activated dimeticone 25 mg, magnesium
hydroxide 195 mg/5 mL (low Na⁺). Net price
500 mL = £2.38
Dose: 5–10 mL 4 times daily (after meals and at bedtime
or when required); CHILD under 5 years 5 mL 3 times
daily, over 5 years appropriate proportion of adult dose
Tablets [NHS], see p. 34

Dimeticone alone

Activated **dimeticone** (also known as simethicone)
is an antifoaming agent. It is licensed for infantile
colic but evidence of benefit is uncertain.

Dentinoxⁿ (DDD)
Colic drops (= emulsion), activated dimeticone
21 mg/2.5 mL dose. Net price 100 mL = £1.40
Dose: gripes, colic or wind pains, INFANT 2.5 mL with or
after each feed (max. 6 doses in 24 hours); may be added
to bottle feed
NOTE. The brand name *Dentinox*ⁿ is also used for other
preparations including teething gel

Infacol® (Forest) ▰▰
Liquid, sugar-free, activated dimeticone 40 mg/mL (low Na⁺). Net price 50 mL = £1.97. Counselling, use of dropper

Dose: gripes, colic or wind pains, INFANT 0.5–1 mL before feeds

Woodward's Colic Drops® (SSL) ▰▰
Oral drops, activated dimeticone 20 mg/0.3-mL dose, net price 30 mL = £1.78

Dose: gripes, colic or wind pains, CHILD under 2 years 0.3–0.6 mL 4 times daily before feeds

---

1.1.2 Compound alginates and proprietary indigestion preparations

Alginate-containing antacids form a 'raft' that floats on the surface of the stomach contents to reduce reflux and protect the oesophageal mucosa; they are used in the management of mild symptoms of gastro-oesophageal reflux disease.

Indigestion preparations on sale to the public include antacids with other ingredients such as alginates, dimeticone, and peppermint oil.

Compound alginate preparations

Algicon® (Rhône-Poulenc Rorer)
Tablets, aluminium hydroxide-magnesium carbonate co-gel 360 mg, magnesium alginate 500 mg, heavy magnesium carbonate 320 mg, potassium bicarbonate 100 mg, sucrose 1.5 g (low Na⁺). Net price 60-tab pack = £2.64

Cautions: diabetes mellitus (high sugar content)

Dose: 1–2 tablets 4 times daily (chewed after meals and at bedtime); CHILD under 12 years not recommended
Suspension, yellow, aluminium hydroxide-magnesium carbonate co-gel 140 mg, magnesium alginate 250 mg, magnesium carbonate 175 mg, potassium bicarbonate 50 mg/5 mL (low Na⁺). Net price 500 mL (lemon-flavoured) = £3.07

Dose: 10–20 mL 4 times daily (after meals and at bedtime); CHILD under 12 years not recommended

Gastrocote® (SSL)
Tablets, alginic acid 200 mg, dried aluminium hydroxide 80 mg, magnesium trisilicate 40 mg, sodium bicarbonate 70 mg. Contains about 1 mmol Na⁺/tablet. Net price 100-tab pack = £3.51

Cautions: diabetes mellitus (high sugar content)

Dose: 1–2 tablets chewed 4 times daily (after meals and at bedtime); CHILD under 6 years not recommended
Liquid, sugar-free, peach-coloured, dried aluminium hydroxide 80 mg, magnesium trisilicate 40 mg, sodium alginate 220 mg, sodium bicarbonate 70 mg/5 mL. Contains 1.8 mmol Na⁺/5 mL. Net price 500 mL = £2.67

Dose: 5–15 mL 4 times daily (after meals and at bedtime)

Gaviscon® (R&C)
Tablets, sugar-free, alginic acid 500 mg, dried aluminium hydroxide 100 mg, magnesium trisilicate 25 mg, sodium bicarbonate 170 mg. Contains 2 mmol Na⁺/tablet. Net price 60-tab pack (peppermint- or lemon-flavoured) = £2.25

Dose: 1–2 tablets chewed after meals and at bedtime, followed by water; CHILD 2–6 years 1 tablet (on doctor's advice only) and 6–12 years 1 tablet
Liquid, sugar-free, sodium alginate 250 mg, sodium bicarbonate 133.5 mg, calcium carbonate 80 mg/5 mL. Contains about 3 mmol Na⁺/5 mL. Net price 500 mL (aniseed- or peppermint-flavour) = £2.70

Dose: 10–20 mL after meals and at bedtime; CHILD 2–6 years (on doctor's advice only) and 6–12 years 5–10 mL
Gaviscon 250® ▣▣▣, *Gaviscon 500*® *Tablets*, and *Gaviscon*® *Liquid Sachets*, see p. 34

Gaviscon® **Advance** (R&C)
Suspension, sugar-free, sodium alginate 500 mg, potassium bicarbonate 100 mg/5 mL. Contains 2.3 mmol Na⁺, 1 mmol K⁺/5 mL. Net price 500 mL (aniseed- or peppermint-flavour) = £5.40

Dose: ADULT and CHILD over 12 years, 5–10 mL after meals and at bedtime

Gaviscon® **Infant** (R&C)
Oral powder, sugar-free, sodium alginate 225 mg, magnesium alginate 87.5 mg, with colloidal silica and mannitol/dose (half dual-sachet). Contains 0.92 mmol Na⁺/dose. Net price 15 dual-sachets (30 doses) = £2.46

Dose: INFANT under 4.5 kg 1 dose (half dual-sachet) mixed with feeds (or water in breast-fed infants) when required; over 4.5 kg 2 doses (1 dual-sachet); CHILD 2 doses (1 dual-sachet) in water after each meal
NOTE. Not to be used in premature infants, or where excessive water loss likely (e.g. fever, diarrhoea, vomiting, high room temperature), or if intestinal obstruction. Not to be used with other preparations containing thickening agents
IMPORTANT. Each half of the dual-sachet is identified as 'one dose'. To avoid errors prescribe as 'dual-sachet' with directions in terms of 'dose'

Peptac® (IVAX)
Suspension, sugar-free, sodium bicarbonate 133.5 mg, sodium alginate 250 mg, calcium carbonate 80 mg/5 mL. Contains 3.1 mmol Na⁺/5mL. Net price 500 mL (aniseed-flavoured) = £2.16

Dose: 10–20 mL after meals and at bedtime; CHILD 6–12 years 5–10 mL

Rennie® **Duo** (Roche Consumer Health)
Suspension, sugar-free, calcium carbonate 600 mg, magnesium carbonate 70 mg, sodium alginate 150 mg/5 mL. Contains 2.6 mmol Na+/5 mL. Net price 500 mL (mint flavour) = £2.67

Dose: ADULT and CHILD over 12 years, 10 mL after meals and at bedtime; an additional 10 mL may be taken between doses for heartburn if necessary, max. 80 mL daily
Excipients: include propylene glycol
Rennie® ▣▣▣ and *Rennie Deflatine*®, see p. 34

Topal® (Ceuta)
Tablets, alginic acid 200 mg, dried aluminium hydroxide 30 mg, light magnesium carbonate 40 mg with lactose 220 mg, sucrose 880 mg, sodium bicarbonate 40 mg (low Na⁺). Net price 42-tab pack = £1.67

Cautions: diabetes mellitus (high sugar content)

Dose: 1–3 tablets chewed 4 times daily (after meals and at bedtime); CHILD half adult dose

Indigestion preparations

Indigestion **preparations** on sale to the public (not prescribable on the NHS) include:

Actal® (alexitol = aluminium), **Actonorm Gel**® (aluminium, magnesium, activated dimeticone, peppermint oil), **Actonorm Powder**® (section 1.2), **Altacite**® (hydrotalcite = aluminium, magnesium), **Aludrox Liquid**® (aluminium), **Aludrox Tablets**® (aluminium, magnesium), **Andrews Antacid**® (calcium, magnesium), **APP**® (section 1.2), **Asilone Antacid Liquid**® (aluminium, activated dimeticone, magnesium; suspension is prescribable), **Asilone Antacid Tablets**® (aluminium, activated dimeticone), **Asilone Heartburn Liquid**® (sodium alginate, aluminium, magnesium, sodium bicarbonate), **Asilone Heartburn Tablets**® (alginic acid, aluminium, magnesium, sodium bicarbonate), **Asilone Windcheaters**® **Capsules** (activated dimeticone)

Barum Antacid® (calcium), **Birley**® (aluminium, magnesium), **Bismag**® (magnesium, sodium bicarbonate), **Bisma-Rex**® (bismuth, calcium, magnesium, peppermint oil), **Bisodol Heartburn Relief Tablets**® (alginic acid, magaldrate, sodium bicarbonate), **Bisodol Indigestion Relief Powder**® (magnesium, sodium bicarbonate), **Bisodol Indigestion Relief Tablets**® and **Bisodol Extra Strong Mint Tablets**® (calcium, magnesium, sodium bicarbonate), **Bisodol Wind Relief Tablets**® (calcium, magnesium, sodium bicarbonate, activated dimeticone), **Boots Heartburn Relief**® (sodium alginate, calcium, sodium bicarbonate), **Boots Indigestion Tablets**® (calcium, magnesium, sodium bicarbonate), **Boots Gripe Mixture 1 Month Plus**® (sodium bicarbonate)

Carbellon® (magnesium, charcoal, peppermint oil)

De Witt's Antacid Powder® (calcium, magnesium, sodium bicarbonate, light kaolin, peppermint oil), **De Witt's Antacid Tablets**® (calcium, magnesium, peppermint oil), **Dijex**® (aluminium, magnesium), **Dynese**® (magaldrate = aluminium, magnesium)

Eno®, **Eno Lemon**® (sodium bicarbonate, sodium carbonate), **Entrotabs**® (aluminium, attapulgite, pectin)

Gaviscon 250® **Tablets** (alginic acid, aluminium, magnesium, sodium bicarbonate; **Gaviscon**® and **Gaviscon 500**® **Tablets** are prescribable), **Gaviscon**® **Liquid Sachets** (sodium alginate, calcium, sodium bicarbonate), **Gelusil**® (aluminium, magnesium)

Maalox Plus Tablets® (aluminium, magnesium, activated dimeticone; suspension is prescribable), **Maclean**® (aluminium, calcium, magnesium), **Magnatol**® (alexitol, magnesium, potassium bicarbonate, xanthan gum), **Moorland**® (aluminium, bismuth, calcium, magnesium, light kaolin)

Nulacin® (calcium, magnesium, peppermint oil; *contains* gluten)

Opas® (calcium, magnesium, sodium bicarbonate)

Pepto-Bismol® (bismuth), **Phillips' Milk of Magnesia**® (magnesium), **Premiums**® (aluminium, calcium, magnesium, peppermint oil)

Rap-eze® (calcium), **Remegel**®, **Remegel Alpine Mint with Lemon**® and **Remegel Freshmint**® (calcium), **Remegel Wind Relief**® (calcium, activated dimeticone), **Rennie**® (calcium, magnesium), **Rennie Deflatine**® (calcium, magnesium, activated dimeticone), **Roter**® (bismuth, magnesium, sodium bicarbonate, frangula)

Setlers Antacid® (calcium), **Setlers Heartburn and Indigestion Liquid**® (calcium, sodium alginate, sodium bicarbonate), **Simeco**® (aluminium, magnesium, activated dimeticone), **Sovol**® (aluminium, magnesium, activated dimeticone)

Tums® (calcium)

Wind-eze® (activated dimeticone)

1.2 Antispasmodics and other drugs altering gut motility

The smooth muscle relaxant properties of antimuscarinic and other antispasmodic drugs may be useful in *irritable bowel syndrome* and in *diverticular disease*. The gastric antisecretory effects of conventional antimuscarinic drugs are of little practical significance since dosage is limited by atropine-like side-effects. Moreover, they have been superseded by more powerful and specific antisecretory drugs, including the histamine H_2-receptor antagonists and proton pump inhibitors.

The dopamine-receptor antagonists metoclopramide and domperidone stimulate transit in the gut.

Antimuscarinics

Antimuscarinics (formerly termed 'anticholinergics') reduce intestinal motility and may be useful in irritable bowel syndrome and in diverticular disease. Other indications of antimuscarinic drugs include arrhythmias (section 2.3.1), asthma and airways disease (section 3.1.2), motion sickness (section 4.6), parkinsonism (section 4.9.2), urinary incontinence (section 7.4.2), mydriasis and cycloplegia (section 11.5), premedication (section 15.1.3) and as an antidote to organophosphorus poisoning (p. 28).

Antimuscarinics that are used for gastro-intestinal smooth muscle spasm include the tertiary amines **atropine sulphate** and **dicycloverine hydrochloride (dicyclomine hydrochloride)** and the quaternary ammonium compounds **propantheline bromide** and **hyoscine butylbromide**. The quaternary ammonium compounds are less lipid soluble than atropine and so may be less likely to cross the blood-brain barrier; they are also less well absorbed. Although central atropine-like side-effects, such as confusion, are thereby reduced, peripheral side-effects are common with quaternary ammonium compounds.

Propantheline bromide is indicated as an adjunct in the treatment of gastro-intestinal disorders characterised by smooth muscle spasm (including non-ulcer dyspepsia and irritable bowel syndrome); atropine sulphate is also licensed for these indications. Dicycloverine hydrochloride (dicyclomine hydrochloride) has a much less marked antimuscarinic action than atropine and may also have some direct action on smooth muscle. Hyoscine butylbromide is advocated as a gastro-intestinal antispasmodic, but it is poorly absorbed; the injection is useful in endoscopy and radiology. Atropine and the belladonna alkaloids are outmoded treatments, any clinical virtues being outweighed by atropinic side-effects.

CAUTIONS. Antimuscarinics should be used with caution (due to increased risk of side-effects) in Down's syndrome, in children and in the elderly; they should also be used with caution in gastro-oesophageal reflux disease, diarrhoea, ulcerative colitis, acute myocardial infarction, hypertension, conditions characterised by tachycardia (including hyperthyroidism, cardiac insufficiency, cardiac surgery), pyrexia, pregnancy and breast-feeding. **Interactions:** Appendix 1 (antimuscarinics).

CONTRA-INDICATIONS. Antimuscarinics are contra-indicated in angle-closure glaucoma, myasthenia gravis (but may be used to decrease muscarinic side-effects of anticholinesterases—section 10.2.1), paralytic ileus, pyloric stenosis and prostatic enlargement.

SIDE-EFFECTS. Side-effects of antimuscarinics include constipation, transient bradycardia (followed by tachycardia, palpitations and arrhythmias), reduced bronchial secretions, urinary urgency and retention, dilatation of the pupils with loss of accommodation, photophobia, dry mouth, flushing and dryness of the skin. Side-effects that occur occasionally include confusion (particularly in the elderly), nausea, vomiting and giddiness.

ATROPINE SULPHATE ▆

Indications: symptomatic relief of gastro-intestinal disorders characterised by smooth muscle spasm; mydriasis and cycloplegia (section 11.5); pre-medication (section 15.1.3); see also notes above

Cautions: see notes above

Contra-indications: see notes above

Side-effects: see notes above

Atropine (Non-proprietary) PoM
Tablets, atropine sulphate 600 micrograms. Net price 28-tab pack = £6.60
Available from CP
Dose: 0.6–1.2 mg at night

■ Preparations on sale to the public
Preparations on sale to the public (not prescribable on the NHS) containing atropine or related compounds include:
Actonorm Powder® (atropine, aluminium, calcium, magnesium, sodium bicarbonate, peppermint oil), **APP**® (homatropine, aluminium, bismuth, calcium, magnesium)

DICYCLOVERINE HYDROCHLORIDE/ DICYCLOMINE HYDROCHLORIDE

Indications: symptomatic relief of gastro-intestinal disorders characterised by smooth muscle spasm

Cautions: see notes above

Contra-indications: see notes above; infants under 6 months

Side-effects: see notes above

Dose: 10–20 mg 3 times daily; CHILD 6–24 months 5–10 mg up to 3–4 times daily, 15 minutes before feeds, 2–12 years 10 mg 3 times daily

[1]**Merbentyl**® (Florizel) PoM
Tablets, dicycloverine hydrochloride 10 mg, net price 20 = £1.08; 20 mg (*Merbentyl 20*®), 84-tab pack = £9.11
Syrup, dicycloverine hydrochloride 10 mg/5 mL, net price 120 mL = £1.98

1. Dicycloverine hydrochloride can be sold to the public provided that max. single dose is 10 mg and max. daily dose is 60 mg

■ Compound preparations
Kolanticon® (Peckforton)
Gel, sugar-free, dicycloverine hydrochloride 2.5 mg, dried aluminium hydroxide 200 mg, light magnesium oxide 100 mg, activated dimeticone (simethicone USP) 20 mg/5 mL, net price 200 mL = £1.69, 500 mL = £1.85
Dose: 10–20 mL every 4 hours when required

HYOSCINE BUTYLBROMIDE

Indications: symptomatic relief of gastro-intestinal or genito-urinary disorders characterised by smooth muscle spasm

Cautions: see notes above

Contra-indications: see notes above; avoid in porphyria (section 9.8.2)

Side-effects: see notes above

Dose: *by mouth*, 20 mg 4 times daily; CHILD 6–12 years, 10 mg 3 times daily
Irritable bowel syndrome, 10 mg 3 times daily, increased if required up to 20 mg 4 times daily
By intramuscular or intravenous injection, acute spasm and spasm in diagnostic procedures, 20 mg repeated after 30 minutes if necessary (may be repeated more frequently in endoscopy); CHILD not recommended

Buscopan® (Boehringer Ingelheim) PoM
[1]*Tablets* ▆, coated, hyoscine butylbromide 10 mg. Net price 56-tab pack = £2.59
Injection, hyoscine butylbromide 20 mg/mL. Net price 1-mL amp = 20p

1. Hyoscine butylbromide can be sold to the public provided single dose does not exceed 20 mg, daily dose does not exceed 80 mg, and pack does not contain a total of more than 240 mg.

PROPANTHELINE BROMIDE

Indications: symptomatic relief of gastro-intestinal disorders characterised by smooth muscle spasm; urinary frequency (section 7.4.2); gustatory sweating (section 6.1.5)

Cautions: see notes above

Contra-indications: see notes above

Side-effects: see notes above

Dose: 15 mg 3 times daily at least 1 hour before meals and 30 mg at night, max. 120 mg daily; CHILD not recommended

Pro-Banthine® (Hansam) PoM
Tablets, pink, s/c, propantheline bromide 15 mg, net price 112-tab pack = £15.32. Label: 23

Other antispasmodics

Alverine, mebeverine, and **peppermint oil** are believed to be direct relaxants of intestinal smooth muscle and may relieve pain in *irritable bowel syndrome* and *diverticular disease*. They have no serious adverse effects but, like all antispasmodics, should be avoided in paralytic ileus. Peppermint oil occasionally causes heartburn.

ALVERINE CITRATE

Indications: adjunct in gastro-intestinal disorders characterised by smooth muscle spasm; dysmenorrhoea

Cautions: pregnancy and breast-feeding

Contra-indications: paralytic ileus; when combined with sterculia, intestinal obstruction, faecal impaction, colonic atony

Side-effects: nausea, headache, pruritus, rash and dizziness reported

Dose: 60–120 mg 1–3 times daily; CHILD under 12 years not recommended

Spasmonal[᠁] (Norgine)
Capsules, alverine citrate 60 mg (blue/grey), net
price 100-cap pack = £11.69; 120 mg (*Spasmonal*[᠁]
Forte, blue/grey), 60-cap pack = £13.50
NOTE. A proprietary brand of alverine citrate 60 mg
(*Relaxyl*[᠁]) is on sale to the public for irritable bowel
syndrome

■ Compound preparations
Spasmonal Fibre[᠁] (Norgine)
Granules, beige, coated, sterculia 62%, alverine
citrate 0.5%. Net price 500 g = £13.70. Label: 25,
27, counselling, see below

Dose: irritable bowel syndrome, 1–2 heaped 5-mL
spoonfuls swallowed without chewing with water once or
twice daily after meals; CHILD not recommended
COUNSELLING. Preparations that swell in contact with
liquid should always be carefully swallowed with water
and should not be taken immediately before going to bed

MEBEVERINE HYDROCHLORIDE

Indications: adjunct in gastro-intestinal disorders
characterised by smooth muscle spasm

Cautions: pregnancy and breast-feeding; avoid in
porphyria (section 9.8.2.)

Contra-indications: paralytic ileus

Side-effects: rarely allergic reactions (including
rash, urticaria, angioedema)

Dose: ADULT and CHILD over 10 years 135–150 mg
3 times daily preferably 20 minutes before meals

¹**Mebeverine Hydrochloride** (Non-proprietary)
[PoM]
Tablets, mebeverine hydrochloride 135 mg, net
price 20 = £1.55
Available from Alpharma, APS, Arrow, Generics, Hill-
cross, IVAX

1. Mebeverine hydrochloride can be sold to the public for
symptomatic relief of irritable bowel syndrome provided
that max. single dose is 135 mg and max. daily dose is
405 mg; for uses other than symptomatic relief of irritable
bowel syndrome provided that max. single dose is 100 mg
and max. daily dose is 300 mg; proprietary brands on sale
to the public include *Colofac 100*[᠁], *Colofac IBS*[᠁] (135 mg),
Equilon[᠁] (135 mg), *IBS Relief*[᠁]

Colofac[᠁] (Solvay) [PoM]
Tablets, s/c, mebeverine hydrochloride 135 mg. Net
price 20 = £1.67
Liquid, yellow, sugar-free, mebeverine hydrochloride 50 mg (as embonate)/5 mL. Net price
300 mL = £3.50

■ Modified release
Colofac[᠁] **MR** (Solvay) [PoM]
Capsules, m/r, mebeverine hydrochloride 200 mg,
net price 60-cap pack = £7.41. Label: 25
Dose: irritable bowel syndrome, 1 capsule twice daily
preferably 20 minutes before meals; CHILD not
recommended

■ Compound preparations
¹**Fybogel**[᠁] **Mebeverine** (R&C) [PoM]
Granules, buff, effervescent, ispaghula husk 3.5 g,
mebeverine hydrochloride 135 mg/sachet.
Contains 7 mmol K^+/sachet (caution in renal
impairment). Net price 60 sachets = £15.00.
Label: 13, 22, counselling, see below
Dose: irritable bowel syndrome, ADULT, 1 sachet in water,
morning and evening 30 minutes before food; an

additional sachet may also be taken before the midday
meal if necessary; CHILD not recommended
COUNSELLING. Preparations that swell in contact with
liquid should always be carefully swallowed with water
and should not be taken immediately before going to bed

1. 10-sachet pack can be sold to the public

PEPPERMINT OIL

Indications: relief of abdominal colic and distension, particularly in irritable bowel syndrome
Cautions: rarely sensitivity to menthol
Side-effects: heartburn, perianal irritation; rarely,
allergic reactions (including rash, headache, bradycardia, muscle tremor, ataxia)
LOCAL IRRITATION. Capsules should not be broken or
chewed because peppermint oil may irritate mouth or
oesophagus

Colpermin[᠁] (Pharmacia)
Capsules, m/r, e/c, light blue/dark blue, blue band,
peppermint oil 0.2 mL. Net price 100-cap pack =
£10.96. Label: 5, 25
Excipients: include arachis (peanut) oil
Dose: 1–2 capsules, swallowed whole with water, 3 times
daily for up to 2–3 months if necessary; CHILD under 15
years not recommended

Mintec[᠁] (Shire)
Capsules, e/c, green/ivory, peppermint oil 0.2 mL.
Net price 84-cap pack = £7.04. Label: 5, 22, 25
Dose: 1–2 capsules swallowed whole with water, 3 times
daily before meals for up to 2–3 months if necessary;
CHILD not recommended

Motility stimulants

Metoclopramide and **domperidone** (section 4.6)
are dopamine antagonists which stimulate gastric
emptying and small intestinal transit, and enhance
the strength of oesophageal sphincter contraction.
They are used in some patients with *non-ulcer
dyspepsia*. Metoclopramide is also used to speed
the transit of barium during intestinal follow-through
examination, and as accessory treatment for *gastro-
oesophageal reflux disease*. Metoclopramide and
domperidone are useful in non-specific and in cyto-
toxic-induced nausea and vomiting. Metoclopramide
and occasionally domperidone may induce an acute
dystonic reaction, particularly in young women and
children—for further details of this and other side-
effects, see section 4.6.

1.3   Ulcer-healing drugs

1.3.1	H_2-receptor antagonists
1.3.2	Selective antimuscarinics
1.3.3	Chelates and complexes
1.3.4	Prostaglandin analogues
1.3.5	Proton pump inhibitors
1.3.6	Other ulcer-healing drugs

Peptic ulceration commonly involves the stomach,
duodenum, and lower oesophagus; after gastric
surgery it involves the gastro-enterostomy stoma.
Healing can be promoted by general measures,
stopping smoking and taking antacids and by antisecretory drug treatment, but relapse is common
when treatment ceases. Nearly all duodenal ulcers
and most gastric ulcers not associated with NSAIDs
are caused by *Helicobacter pylori*.

The management of *H. pylori* infection and of NSAID-associated ulcers is discussed below.

Helicobacter pylori infection

Long-term healing of gastric and duodenal ulcers can be achieved rapidly by eradicating *Helicobacter pylori*; it is recommended that the presence of *H. pylori* is confirmed before starting eradication treatment. Acid inhibition combined with antibacterial treatment is highly effective in the eradication of *H. pylori*; reinfection is rare. Antibiotic-induced colitis is an uncommon risk.

One-week triple-therapy regimens that comprise a proton pump inhibitor, amoxicillin, and either clarithromycin or metronidazole, eradicate *H. pylori* in over 90% of cases. There is normally no need to continue antisecretory treatment (with a proton pump inhibitor or H$_2$-receptor antagonist) unless the ulcer is complicated by haemorrhage or perforation. Resistance to clarithromycin or to metronidazole is much more common than to amoxicillin and can develop during treatment. A regimen containing amoxicillin and clarithromycin is therefore recommended for initial therapy and one containing amoxicillin and metronidazole for eradication failure. Ranitidine bismuth citrate may be substituted for a proton pump inhibitor. Other regimens, including those combining clarithromycin and metronidazole are best used in specialist settings. Treatment failure usually indicates antibacterial resistance or poor compliance.

Two-week triple-therapy regimens offer the possibility of higher eradication rates compared to one-week regimens, but adverse effects are common and poor compliance is likely to offset any possible gain.

Two-week dual-therapy regimens using a proton pump inhibitor and a single antibacterial are licensed, but produce low rates of *H. pylori* eradication and are **not** recommended.

A two-week regimen using tripotassium dicitratobismuthate *plus* a proton pump inhibitor *plus* two antibacterials may have a role in the treatment of resistant cases after confirmation of the presence of *H. pylori*.

Tinidazole or tetracycline are also used occasionally for *H. pylori* eradication; they should be used in combination with antisecretory drugs and other antibacterials.

There is insufficient evidence to support eradication therapy in patients infected with *H. pylori* who continue to take NSAIDs.

Test for *Helicobacter pylori*

^{13}C-Urea breath test kits are available for the diagnosis of gastro-duodenal infection with *Helicobacter pylori*. The test involves collection of breath samples before and after ingestion of an oral solution of ^{13}C-urea; the samples are sent for analysis by an appropriate laboratory. The test should not be performed within 4 weeks of treatment with an antibacterial or within 2 weeks of treatment with an antisecretory drug.

diabact UBT® (MDE) [PoM]
Tablets, ^{13}C-urea 50 mg, net price 1 kit (including 2 tablets, 4 breath-sample containers, straws) = £19.55 (analysis included), 10-kit pack (hosp. only) = £175 (analysis included)

Recommended regimens for *Helicobacter pylori* eradication

Acid suppressant	Antibacterial			Price for 7–day course
	Amoxicillin	Clarithromycin	Metronidazole	
Esomeprazole	1 g twice daily	500 mg twice daily	—	£34.24
20 mg twice daily	—	500 mg twice daily	400 mg twice daily	£33.36
Lansoprazole	1 g twice daily	500 mg twice daily	—	£36.87
30 mg twice daily	1 g twice daily	—	400 mg twice daily	£13.88
	—	500 mg twice daily	400 mg twice daily	£35.99
Omeprazole	1 g twice daily	500 mg twice daily	—	£36.59
20 mg twice daily	500 mg 3 times daily	—	400 mg 3 times daily	£14.29
	—	500 mg twice daily	400 mg twice daily	£35.71
Pantoprazole	1 g twice daily	500 mg twice daily	—	£36.82
40 mg twice daily	—	500 mg twice daily	400 mg twice daily	£35.94
Rabeprazole	1 g twice daily	500 mg twice daily	—	£36.37
20 mg twice daily	—	500 mg twice daily	400 mg twice daily	£35.49
Ranitidine bismuth	1 g twice daily	500 mg twice daily	—	£37.99
citrate	1 g twice daily	—	400 mg twice daily	£15.00
400 mg twice daily	—	500 mg twice daily	400 mg twice daily	£37.11

Regimens that include amoxicillin with either clarithromycin or metronidazole are suitable for use in the community. Regimens that combine clarithromycin with metronidazole are best used in specialist settings (see also notes above)

Helicobacter Test Hp-Plus® (Espire) [PoM]
Soluble tablets, ^{13}C-urea 100 mg, net price 1 kit (including 4 breath-sample containers, straws, citric acid test meal) = £19.75 (analysis included)

Helicobacter Test INFAI® (Infai) [PoM]
Oral powder, ^{13}C-urea 75 mg for dissolving in water, net price 1 kit (including 4 breath-sample containers, straws) = £21.01 (analysis included)

Pylobactell® (Torbet) [PoM]
Soluble tablets, ^{13}C-urea 100 mg, net price 1 kit (including 6 breath-sample containers, 30-mL mixing and administration straws) = £20.75 (analysis included)

NSAID-associated ulcers

Gastro-intestinal bleeding and ulceration can occur with NSAID use (section 10.1.1). Wherever possible, NSAIDs should be **withdrawn** if an ulcer occurs.

A proton pump inhibitor or misoprostol may be considered for protection against NSAID-associated gastric and duodenal ulcers; colic and diarrhoea may limit the dose of misoprostol. An H$_2$-receptor antagonist may be effective for protection against NSAID-associated duodenal ulcers only.

NSAID use and *H. pylori* infection are independent risk factors for gastro-intestinal bleeding and ulceration. In patients already on an NSAID, eradication of *H. pylori* is not recommended because it is unlikely to reduce the risk of NSAID-induced bleeding or ulceration. However, in patients about to start long-term NSAID treatment who are *H. pylori* positive and have dyspepsia or a history of gastric or duodenal ulcer, eradication of *H. pylori* may reduce the risk of NSAID-induced ulceration.

If the *NSAID can be discontinued* in a patient who has developed an ulcer, a proton pump inhibitor usually produces the most rapid healing, but the ulcer can be treated with an H$_2$-receptor antagonist or misoprostol.

If *NSAID treatment needs to continue*, NSAID-associated ulceration is most effectively treated with a proton pump inhibitor (see also guidance issued by NICE, section 1.3.5 and section 10.1.1); on healing, the dose of proton pump inhibitor should **not** normally be reduced because asymptomatic ulcer deterioration may occur. Misoprostol is an alternative for maintenance treatment.

1.3.1 H$_2$-receptor antagonists

All H$_2$-receptor antagonists heal *gastric and duodenal ulcers* by reducing gastric acid output as a result of histamine H$_2$-receptor blockade; they can also be expected to relieve *gastro-oesophageal reflux disease* (section 1.1). High doses of H$_2$-receptor antagonists have been used in the *Zollinger–Ellison syndrome*, but a proton pump inhibitor may now be preferred.

Maintenance treatment with low doses has largely been replaced in *Helicobacter pylori* positive patients by eradication regimens (section 1.3). Maintenance treatment may occasionally be used for those with frequent severe recurrences and for the elderly who suffer ulcer complications.

Treatment of *undiagnosed dyspepsia* with H$_2$-receptor antagonists may be acceptable in younger patients but care is required in older people because of the possibility of gastric cancer in these patients.

H$_2$-receptor antagonist therapy can promote healing of *NSAID-associated ulcers* (particularly duodenal) (section 1.3).

Treatment has not been shown to be beneficial in haematemesis and melaena, but prophylactic use reduces the frequency of bleeding from *gastroduodenal erosions in hepatic coma*, and possibly in other conditions requiring intensive care. Treatment also reduces the risk of *acid aspiration* in obstetric patients at delivery (Mendelson's syndrome).

CAUTIONS. H$_2$-receptor antagonists should be used with caution in hepatic impairment (Appendix 2), in renal impairment (Appendix 3), pregnancy (Appendix 4), and in breast-feeding (Appendix 5). H$_2$-receptor antagonists might mask symptoms of gastric cancer; particular care is required in those whose symptoms change and in those who are middle-aged or over.

SIDE-EFFECTS. Side-effects of the H$_2$-receptor antagonists include diarrhoea and other gastro-intestinal disturbances, altered liver function tests (rarely liver damage), headache, dizziness, rash, and tiredness. Rare side-effects include acute pancreatitis, bradycardia, AV block, confusion, depression, and hallucinations particularly in the elderly or the very ill, hypersensitivity reactions (including fever, arthralgia, myalgia, anaphylaxis), and blood disorders (including agranulocytosis, leucopenia, pancytopenia, thrombocytopenia). There have been occasional reports of gynaecomastia and impotence.

INTERACTIONS. Cimetidine retards oxidative hepatic drug metabolism by binding to microsomal cytochrome P450. It should be avoided in patients stabilised on warfarin, phenytoin, and theophylline (or aminophylline), but other interactions (see **Appendix 1**) may be of less clinical relevance. Famotidine, nizatidine, and ranitidine do not share the drug metabolism inhibitory properties of cimetidine.

CIMETIDINE

Indications: benign gastric and duodenal ulceration, stomal ulcer, reflux oesophagitis, Zollinger–Ellison syndrome, other conditions where gastric acid reduction is beneficial (see notes above and section 1.9.4)

Cautions: see notes above; also preferably avoid intravenous injection (use intravenous infusion) particularly in high dosage and in cardiovascular impairment (risk of arrhythmias); **interactions:** Appendix 1 (histamine H$_2$-antagonists) and notes above

Side-effects: see notes above; also alopecia; rarely tachycardia, interstitial nephritis

Dose: *by mouth*, 400 mg twice daily (with breakfast and at night) *or* 800 mg at night (benign gastric and duodenal ulceration) for at least 4 weeks (6 weeks in gastric ulceration, 8 weeks in NSAID-associated ulceration); when necessary the dose may be increased to 400 mg 4 times daily or rarely (as in stress ulceration) to max. 2.4 g daily in divided doses; INFANT under 1 year 20 mg/kg daily in divided doses has been used; CHILD over 1 year 25–30 mg/kg daily in divided doses

Maintenance, 400 mg at night *or* 400 mg morning and night

Reflux oesophagitis, 400 mg 4 times daily for 4–8 weeks

Zollinger–Ellison syndrome (but see notes above), 400 mg 4 times daily or occasionally more

Gastric acid reduction (prophylaxis of acid aspiration; do not use syrup), obstetrics 400 mg at start of labour, then up to 400 mg every 4 hours if required (max. of 2.4 g daily); surgical procedures 400 mg 90–120 minutes before induction of general anaesthesia

Short-bowel syndrome, 400 mg twice daily (with breakfast and at bedtime) adjusted according to response

To reduce degradation of pancreatic enzyme supplements, 0.8–1.6 g daily in 4 divided doses according to response 1–1½ hours before meals

By intramuscular injection, 200 mg every 4–6 hours; max. 2.4 g daily

By slow intravenous injection (but see Cautions above) over at least 5 minutes, 200 mg; may be repeated every 4–6 hours; if larger dose needed or if cardiovascular impairment, dilute and give injection over at least 10 minutes (infusion preferable); max. 2.4 g daily

By intravenous infusion, 400 mg (may be repeated every 4–6 hours) *or by continuous intravenous infusion* usually at a rate of 50–100 mg/hour over 24 hours, max. 2.4 g daily; INFANT under 1 year, *by slow intravenous injection or by intravenous infusion*, 20 mg/kg daily in divided doses has been used; CHILD over 1 year, 25–30 mg/kg daily in divided doses

[1]**Cimetidine** (Non-proprietary) PoM
Tablets, cimetidine 200 mg, net price 120-tab pack = £2.78; 400 mg, 60-tab pack = £5.59; 800 mg, 30-tab pack = £5.72

Available from Alpharma, APS, Ashbourne (*Peptimax*®), Berk (*Ultec*®), BHR (*Phimetin*®), CP, Dexcel Pharma, Eastern (*Zita*®), Hillcross, IVAX, Kent, Opus (*Acitak*®), Sovereign

Oral solution, cimetidine 200 mg/5 mL, net price 300 mL = £14.24

Available from Rosemont (sugar-free)

1. Cimetidine can be sold to the public for adults and children over 16 years (provided packs do not contain more than 2 weeks' supply) for the short-term symptomatic relief of heartburn, dyspepsia, and hyperacidity (max. single dose 200 mg, max. daily dose 800 mg), and for the prophylactic management of nocturnal heartburn (single night-time dose 100 mg); a proprietary brand (*Tagamet 100*® containing cimetidine 100 mg) is on sale to the public

Dyspamet® (Goldshield) PoM
Suspension, sugar-free, cimetidine 200 mg/5 mL. Contains sorbitol 2.79 g/5 mL. Net price 600 mL = £24.08

Tagamet® (GSK) PoM
Tablets, all green, f/c, cimetidine 200 mg, net price 120-tab pack = £19.58; 400 mg, 60-tab pack = £22.62; 800 mg, 30-tab pack = £22.62
Syrup, orange, cimetidine 200 mg/5 mL. Net price 600 mL = £28.49
Injection, cimetidine 100 mg/mL. Net price 2-mL amp = 36p

FAMOTIDINE

Indications: see under Dose

Cautions: see notes above; **interactions:** Appendix 1 (histamine H$_2$-antagonists) and notes above

Side-effects: see notes above; also rarely anxiety, toxic epidermal necrolysis, urticaria, anorexia, dry mouth, cholestatic jaundice

Dose: benign gastric and duodenal ulceration, treatment, 40 mg at night for 4–8 weeks; maintenance (duodenal ulceration), 20 mg at night; CHILD not recommended
Reflux oesophagitis, 20–40 mg twice daily for 6–12 weeks; maintenance, 20 mg twice daily
Zollinger–Ellison syndrome (but see notes above), 20 mg every 6 hours (higher dose in those who have previously been receiving another H$_2$-antagonist); up to 800 mg daily in divided doses has been used

[1]**Famotidine** (Non-proprietary) PoM
Tablets, famotidine 20 mg, net price 28-tab pack = £12.40; 40 mg, 28-tab pack = £23.12

Available from APS, Arrow, Generics, Lagap, Niche

1. Famotidine can be sold to the public for adults and children over 16 years (provided packs do not contain more than 2 weeks' supply) for the short-term symptomatic relief of heartburn, dyspepsia, and hyperacidity, and for the prevention of these symptoms when associated with consumption of food or drink including when they cause sleep disturbance (max. single dose 10 mg, max. daily dose 20 mg); proprietary brands (*Boots Excess Acid Control*®, *Pepcid*® AC, *Pepcid*® AC Chewable all containing famotidine 10 mg) are on sale to the public; a combination of famotidine and antacids (*Pepcidtwo*®) is also available for sale to the public

Pepcid® (MSD) PoM
Tablets, f/c, famotidine 20 mg (beige), net price 28-tab pack = £13.37; 40 mg (brown), 28-tab pack = £25.40

NIZATIDINE

Indications: see under Dose

Cautions: see notes above; also avoid rapid intravenous injection (risk of arrhythmias and postural hypotension); **interactions:** Appendix 1 (histamine H$_2$-antagonists) and notes above

Side-effects: see notes above; also sweating; rarely vasculitis, hyperuricaemia, exfoliative dermatitis

Dose: *by mouth*, benign gastric, duodenal or NSAID-associated ulceration, treatment, 300 mg in the evening *or* 150 mg twice daily for 4–8 weeks; maintenance, 150 mg at night; CHILD not recommended
Gastro-oesophageal reflux disease, 150–300 mg twice daily for up to 12 weeks

By intravenous infusion, for short-term use in peptic ulcer hospital inpatients as alternative to oral route, *by intermittent intravenous infusion* over 15 minutes, 100 mg 3 times daily, *or by continuous intravenous infusion*, 10 mg/hour; max. 480 mg daily; CHILD not recommended

¹**Nizatidine** (Non-proprietary) PoM
Capsules, nizatidine 150 mg, net price 30-cap pack = £6.63; 300 mg, 30-cap pack = £13.24
Available from APS, Ashbourne (*Zinga*®), Generics, Niche

1. Nizatidine can be sold to the public for the prevention and treatment of symptoms of food-related heartburn and meal-induced indigestion in adults and children over 16 years; max. single dose 75 mg, max. daily dose 150 mg for max. 14 days

Axid® (Lilly) PoM
Capsules, nizatidine 150 mg (pale yellow/dark yellow), net price 28-cap pack (hosp. only) = £6.87, 30-cap pack = £8.27; 300 mg (pale yellow/brown), 30-cap pack = £16.40
Injection, nizatidine 25 mg/mL. For dilution and use as an intravenous infusion. Net price 4-mL amp = £1.14

RANITIDINE

Indications: see under Dose, other conditions where reduction of gastric acidity is beneficial (see notes above and section 1.9.4)

Cautions: see notes above; also avoid in porphyria (section 9.8.2); **interactions:** Appendix 1 (histamine H$_2$-antagonists) and notes above

Side-effects: see notes above; also rarely tachycardia, agitation, visual disturbances, erythema multiforme, alopecia

Dose: *by mouth*, 150 mg twice daily *or* 300 mg at night (benign gastric and duodenal ulceration) for 4 to 8 weeks, up to 6 weeks in chronic episodic dyspepsia, and up to 8 weeks in NSAID-associated ulceration (in duodenal ulcer 300 mg can be given twice daily for 4 weeks to achieve a higher healing rate); maintenance, 150 mg at night; CHILD (peptic ulcer) 2–4 mg/kg twice daily, max. 300 mg daily
Duodenal ulceration associated with *H. pylori* (but see p. 37 for recommended regimens), ranitidine 300 mg daily in 1–2 divided doses (plus amoxicillin 750 mg 3 times daily and metronidazole 500 mg 3 times daily) for 2 weeks; ranitidine treatment continued for a further 2 weeks
Prophylaxis of NSAID-induced duodenal ulcer, 150 mg twice daily
Reflux oesophagitis, 150 mg twice daily *or* 300 mg at night for up to 8 weeks, or if necessary 12 weeks (moderate to severe, 150 mg 4 times daily for up to 12 weeks); long-term treatment of healed oesophagitis, 150 mg twice daily
Zollinger–Ellison syndrome (but see notes above), 150 mg 3 times daily; doses up to 6 g daily in divided doses have been used
Gastric acid reduction (prophylaxis of acid aspiration) in obstetrics, *by mouth*, 150 mg at onset of labour, then every 6 hours; surgical procedures, *by intramuscular or slow intravenous injection*, 50 mg 45–60 minutes before induction of anaesthesia (intravenous injection diluted to 20 mL and given over at least 2 minutes), or *by mouth*, 150 mg 2 hours before induction of anaesthesia, and also, when possible on the preceding evening

By intramuscular injection, 50 mg every 6–8 hours

By slow intravenous injection, 50 mg diluted to 20 mL and given over at least 2 minutes; may be repeated every 6–8 hours

By intravenous infusion, 25 mg/hour for 2 hours; may be repeated every 6–8 hours

Prophylaxis of stress ulceration, initial slow intravenous injection of 50 mg (as above) then *continuous infusion*, 125–250 micrograms/kg per hour (may be followed by 150 mg twice daily *by mouth* when oral feeding commences)

¹**Ranitidine** (Non-proprietary) PoM
Tablets, ranitidine (as hydrochloride) 150 mg, net price 60-tab pack = £8.16; 300 mg, 30-tab pack = £8.16
Available from Alpharma, APS, Ashbourne (*Zaedoc*®), Berk (*Rantec*®), CP, Dominion, Galen, Generics, Genus, Goldshield, Hillcross, IVAX, Ranbaxy, Sovereign, Sterwin, Tillomed (*Ranitic*®)
Effervescent tablets, ranitidine (as hydrochloride) 150 mg, net price 60-tab pack = £26.46; 300 mg, 30-tab pack = £25.84. Label: 13
Excipients: may include sodium (check with supplier)
Available from Alpharma, Lagap
Oral solution, ranitidine (as hydrochloride) 75 mg/5 mL, net price 300 mL = £22.32
Available from Rosemont (sugar-free, contains alcohol 8%)

1. Ranitidine can be sold to the public for adults and children over 16 years (provided packs do not contain more than 2 weeks' supply) for the short-term symptomatic relief of heartburn, dyspepsia, and hyperacidity, and for the prevention of these symptoms when associated with consumption of food or drink (max. single dose 75 mg, max. daily dose 300 mg); proprietary brands (*Zantac*® 75, *Ranzac*® containing ranitidine (as hydrochloride) 75 mg) are on sale to the public

Zantac® (GSK) PoM
Tablets, f/c, ranitidine (as hydrochloride) 150 mg, net price 60-tab pack = £19.52; 300 mg, 30-tab pack = £19.20
Effervescent tablets, pale yellow, ranitidine (as hydrochloride) 150 mg (contains 14.3 mmol Na⁺/tablet), net price 60-tab pack = £27.89; 300 mg (contains 20.8 mmol Na⁺/tablet), 30-tab pack = £27.43. Label: 13
NOTE. The effervescent tablets contain aspartame (section 9.4.1)
Syrup, sugar-free, ranitidine (as hydrochloride) 75 mg/5 mL. Net price 300 mL = £22.32
NOTE. Contains alcohol 8%
Injection, ranitidine (as hydrochloride) 25 mg/mL. Net price 2-mL amp = 64p

RANITIDINE BISMUTH CITRATE
(Ranitidine Bismutrex)

Indications: see under Dose

Cautions: see notes above; see also under Tripotassium Dicitratobismuthate; **interactions:** Appendix 1 (histamine H$_2$-antagonists) and notes above

Contra-indications: moderate to severe renal impairment; pregnancy (Appendix 4); breast-feeding (Appendix 5); porphyria (section 9.8.2)

Side-effects: see notes above; may darken tongue or blacken faeces; rarely tachycardia, agitation, visual disturbances, erythema multiforme, alopecia

Dose: 400 mg twice daily, preferably with food, for 8 weeks in benign gastric ulceration or 4–8 weeks in duodenal ulceration; CHILD not recommended
Eradication of *Helicobacter pylori*, see eradication regimens on p. 37; ranitidine bismuth citrate treatment may be continued for a total of 4 weeks; long-term (maintenance) treatment not recommended (max. total of 16 weeks treatment in any 1 year); CHILD not recommended
COUNSELLING. May darken tongue and blacken faeces

Pylorid® (GSK) PoM
Tablets, blue, f/c, ranitidine bismuth citrate 400 mg.
Net price 14-tab pack = £13.00; Counselling
(discoloration of tongue and faeces)

1.3.2 Selective antimuscarinics

Pirenzepine is a selective antimuscarinic drug which
was used for the treatment of gastric and duodenal
ulcers. It has been discontinued.

1.3.3 Chelates and complexes

Tripotassium dicitratobismuthate is a bismuth
chelate effective in healing gastric and duodenal
ulcers, but not on its own in maintaining remission.
For the role of tripotassium dicitratobismuthate in a
Helicobacter pylori eradication regimen for those
who have not responded to first-line regimens, see
section 1.3.

The bismuth content of tripotassium dicitratobismuthate is low but absorption has been reported;
encephalopathy (described with older high-dose
bismuth preparations) has not been reported.

Ranitidine bismuth citrate (section 1.3.1) is used in
the management of gastric and duodenal ulcers, and
in combination with two antibacterials for the
eradication of *H. pylori* (section 1.3).

Sucralfate may act by protecting the mucosa from
acid-pepsin attack in gastric and duodenal ulcers. It is
a complex of aluminium hydroxide and sulphated
sucrose but has minimal antacid properties. It should
be used with caution in patients under intensive care
(**important:** reports of bezoar formation, see CSM
advice below)

TRIPOTASSIUM DICITRATOBISMUTHATE

Indications: benign gastric and duodenal ulceration; see also *Helicobacter pylori* infection,
section 1.3
Cautions: see notes above; **interactions:** Appendix
1 (tripotassium dicitratobismuthate)
Contra-indications: renal impairment, pregnancy
Side-effects: may darken tongue and blacken
faeces; nausea and vomiting reported

De-Noltab® (Yamanouchi)
Tablets, f/c, tripotassium dicitratobismuthate
120 mg. Net price 112-tab pack = £7.11.
Counselling, see below
Dose: 2 tablets twice daily *or* 1 tablet 4 times daily; taken
for 28 days followed by further 28 days if necessary;
maintenance not indicated but course may be repeated
after interval of 1 month; CHILD not recommended
COUNSELLING. Each dose to be swallowed with half a
tumblerful of water; twice daily dosage to be taken 30
minutes before breakfast and main evening meal; four
times daily dosage to be taken as follows: one dose 30
minutes before breakfast, midday meal and main evening
meal, and one dose 2 hours after main evening meal; milk
should not be drunk by itself during treatment but small
quantities may be taken in tea or coffee or on cereal;
antacids should not be taken half an hour before or after a
dose; may darken tongue and blacken faeces

SUCRALFATE

Indications: see under Dose
Cautions: renal impairment (avoid if severe, see
Appendix 3); pregnancy and breast-feeding;
administration of sucralfate and enteral feeds
should be separated by 1 hour; **interactions:**
Appendix 1 (sucralfate)
BEZOAR FORMATION. Following reports of bezoar formation associated with sucralfate, the **CSM** has advised
caution in seriously ill patients, especially those receiving
concomitant enteral feeds or those with predisposing
conditions such as delayed gastric emptying
Side-effects: constipation, diarrhoea, nausea, indigestion, gastric discomfort, dry mouth, rash,
hypersensitivity reactions, back pain, dizziness,
headache, vertigo and drowsiness, bezoar formation (see above)
Dose: benign gastric and duodenal ulceration and
chronic gastritis, 2 g twice daily (on rising and at
bedtime) *or* 1 g 4 times daily 1 hour before meals
and at bedtime, taken for 4–6 weeks or in resistant
cases up to 12 weeks; max. 8 g daily
Prophylaxis of stress ulceration, 1 g 6 times daily
(max. 8 g daily)
CHILD not recommended

Sucralfate (Non-proprietary) PoM
Tablets, sucralfate 1 g. Net price 112-tab pack =
£9.80. Label: 5
Available from Hillcross

Antepsin® (Chugai) PoM
Tablets, scored, sucralfate 1 g. Net price 112-tab
pack = £9.80. Label: 5
COUNSELLING. Tablets may be dispersed in water
Suspension, sucralfate, 1 g/5 mL. Net price 250 mL
(aniseed- and caramel-flavoured) = £4.37. Label: 5

1.3.4 Prostaglandin analogues

Misoprostol, a synthetic prostaglandin analogue has
antisecretory and protective properties, promoting
healing of *gastric and duodenal ulcers*. It can
prevent NSAID-associated ulcers, its use being most
appropriate for the frail or very elderly from whom
NSAIDs cannot be withdrawn.

For comment on the use of misoprostol to induce
abortion or labour [unlicensed indications], see
section 7.1.1.

MISOPROSTOL

Indications: see notes above and under Dose
Cautions: conditions where hypotension might
precipitate severe complications (e.g. cerebrovascular disease, cardiovascular disease)
Contra-indications: pregnancy or planning
pregnancy (increases uterine tone)—**important:**
women of childbearing age, see also below, and
breast-feeding
WOMEN OF CHILDBEARING AGE. Manufacturer advises
that misoprostol should not be used in women of childbearing age unless the patient requires non-steroidal anti-
inflammatory (NSAID) therapy and is at high risk of
complications from NSAID-induced ulceration. In such
patients it is advised that misoprostol should only be used
if the patient takes *effective contraceptive measures* and
has been advised of the *risks of taking misoprostol if
pregnant.*

Side-effects: diarrhoea (may occasionally be severe and require withdrawal, reduced by giving single doses not exceeding 200 micrograms and by avoiding magnesium-containing antacids); also reported: abdominal pain, dyspepsia, flatulence, nausea and vomiting, abnormal vaginal bleeding (including intermenstrual bleeding, menorrhagia, and postmenopausal bleeding), rashes, dizziness

Dose: benign gastric and duodenal ulceration and NSAID-associated ulceration, 800 micrograms daily (in 2–4 divided doses) with breakfast (or main meals) and at bedtime; treatment should be continued for at least 4 weeks and may be continued for up to 8 weeks if required
Prophylaxis of NSAID-induced gastric and duodenal ulcer, 200 micrograms 2–4 times daily taken with the NSAID

CHILD not recommended

Cytotec® (Pharmacia) [PoM]
Tablets, scored, misoprostol 200 micrograms, net price 60-tab pack = £10.03, 140-tab pack = £23.40. Label: 21

■ With diclofenac or naproxen
Section 10.1.1

1.3.5 Proton pump inhibitors

The proton pump inhibitors **omeprazole**, **esomeprazole**, **lansoprazole**, **pantoprazole** and **rabeprazole** inhibit gastric acid by blocking the hydrogen-potassium adenosine triphosphatase enzyme system (the 'proton pump') of the gastric parietal cell. Proton pump inhibitors are effective short-term treatments for *gastric and duodenal ulcers*; they are also used in combination with antibacterials for the eradication of *Helicobacter pylori* (see p. 37 for specific regimens). An initial short course of a proton pump inhibitor is the treatment of choice in *gastro-oesophageal reflux disease* with severe symptoms; patients with endoscopically confirmed *erosive*, *ulcerative*, or *stricturing oesophagitis* usually need to be maintained on a proton pump inhibitor (section 1.1).

Proton pump inhibitors are also used in the prevention and treatment of NSAID-associated ulcers (see p. 38 and guidance issued by NICE, below). In patients who need to continue NSAID treatment after an ulcer has healed, the dose of proton pump inhibitor should normally not be reduced because asymptomatic ulcer deterioration may occur.

Omeprazole is effective in the treatment of the *Zollinger-Ellison syndrome* (including cases resistant to other treatment); lansoprazole is also indicated for this condition.

CAUTIONS. Proton pump inhibitors should be used with caution in patients with liver disease (Appendix 2), in pregnancy (Appendix 4) and in breast-feeding. Proton pump inhibitors may mask symptoms of gastric cancer; particular care is required in those whose symptoms change and in those over 45 years of age; the presence of gastric malignancy should be excluded before treatment.

SIDE-EFFECTS. Side-effects of the proton pump inhibitors include gastro-intestinal disturbances (including diarrhoea, nausea and vomiting, constipation, flatulence, abdominal pain), headache, hypersensitivity reactions (including rash, urticaria, angioedema, bronchospasm, anaphylaxis), pruritus, dizziness, peripheral oedema, muscle and joint pain, malaise, blurred vision, depression and dry mouth. Proton pump inhibitors decrease gastric acidity and may increase the risk of gastro-intestinal infections.

> **NICE advice (proton pump inhibitors).** NICE has provided guidance (July 2000) on the use of proton pump inhibitors for the following indications:
>
> - Gastro-oesophageal reflux disease—use only for severe symptoms (reduce dose when symptoms abate) and in disease complicated by stricture, ulceration, or haemorrhage (full dose should be maintained);
>
> - NSAID-associated ulceration in patients who need to continue NSAID treatment—on healing of the ulcer a lower dose of proton pump inhibitor may be used [but see notes above].

OMEPRAZOLE

Indications: see under Dose

Cautions: see notes above; **interactions:** Appendix 1 (proton pump inhibitors)

Side-effects: see notes above; also reported, bullous eruption, Stevens-Johnson syndrome, toxic epidermal necrolysis, fever, photosensitivity, paraesthesia, vertigo, interstitial nephritis, alopecia, somnolence, insomnia, sweating, gynaecomastia, rarely impotence, taste disturbance, stomatitis, liver enzyme changes and liver dysfunction, encephalopathy in severe liver disease; haematological changes (including agranulocytosis, leucopenia, pancytopenia, thrombocytopenia), hyponatraemia; reversible confusion, agitation, and hallucinations in the severely ill; visual impairment reported with high-dose injection

Dose: *by mouth*, benign gastric and duodenal ulcers, 20 mg once daily for 4 weeks in duodenal ulceration or 8 weeks in gastric ulceration; in severe or recurrent cases increase to 40 mg daily; maintenance for recurrent duodenal ulcer, 20 mg once daily; prevention of relapse in duodenal ulcer, 10 mg daily increasing to 20 mg once daily if symptoms return

NSAID-associated duodenal or gastric ulcer and gastroduodenal erosions, 20 mg once daily for 4 weeks, followed by a further 4 weeks if not fully healed; prophylaxis in patients with a history of NSAID-associated duodenal or gastric ulcers, gastroduodenal lesions, or dyspeptic symptoms who require continued NSAID treatment, 20 mg once daily

Duodenal ulcer associated with *Helicobacter pylori*, see eradication regimens on p. 37

Benign gastric ulcer associated with *H. pylori*, omeprazole 40 mg daily in 1–2 divided doses (plus amoxicillin 0.75–1 g twice daily) for 2 weeks

Zollinger–Ellison syndrome, initially 60 mg once daily; usual range 20–120 mg daily (above 80 mg in 2 divided doses)

Gastric acid reduction during general anaesthesia (prophylaxis of acid aspiration), 40 mg on the preceding evening then 40 mg 2–6 hours before surgery

Gastro-oesophageal reflux disease, 20 mg once daily for 4 weeks, followed by a further 4–8 weeks if not fully healed; 40 mg once daily has been given for 8 weeks in gastro-oesophageal reflux disease refractory to other treatment; may be continued at 20 mg once daily

Acid reflux disease (long-term management), 10 mg daily increasing to 20 mg once daily if symptoms return

Acid-related dyspepsia, 10–20 mg once daily for 2–4 weeks according to response

CHILD over 2 years, severe ulcerating reflux oesophagitis, 0.7–1.4 mg/kg daily for 4–12 weeks; max. 40 mg daily (to be initiated by hospital paediatrician)

By intravenous injection over 5 minutes or by intravenous infusion, gastric acid reduction during anaesthesia (prophylaxis of acid aspiration), 40 mg completed 1 hour before surgery

Benign gastric ulcer, duodenal ulcer and gastro-oesophageal reflux, 40 mg once daily until oral administration possible

CHILD not recommended

COUNSELLING. Swallow whole, *or* disperse *MUPS*® tablets in water, *or* mix capsule contents or *MUPS*® tablets with fruit juice or yoghurt

Omeprazole (Non-proprietary) PoM
Capsules, enclosing e/c granules, omeprazole 10 mg, net price 28-cap pack = £16.73; 20 mg, 28-cap pack = £24.18; 40 mg, 7-cap pack = £13.06. Label: 5, counselling, administration
Available from Alpharma, APS, Generics, Kent, Ratiopharm
Tablets, e/c, omeprazole 10 mg, net price 28-tab pack = £17.28; 20 mg, 28-tab pack = £26.17; 40 mg, 7-tab pack = £13.11. Label: 25
Available from Alpharma, Dexcel

Losec® (AstraZeneca) PoM
MUPS®(multiple-unit pellet system = dispersible tablets), f/c, omeprazole 10 mg (light pink), net price 28-tab pack = £18.91; 20 mg (pink), 28-tab pack = £28.56; 40 mg (red-brown), 7-tab pack = £14.28. Counselling, administration
Capsules, enclosing e/c granules, omeprazole 10 mg (pink), net price 28-cap pack = £18.91; 20 mg (pink/brown), 28-cap pack = £28.56; 40 mg (brown), 7-cap pack = £14.28. Counselling, administration
Intravenous infusion ▼, powder for reconstitution, omeprazole (as sodium salt), net price 40-mg vial = £5.21
Injection ▼, powder for reconstitution, omeprazole (as sodium salt), net price 40-mg vial (with solvent) = £5.21

ESOMEPRAZOLE

Indications: see under Dose
Cautions: see notes above; renal impairment (Appendix 3); **interactions:** Appendix 1 (proton pump inhibitors)
Side-effects: see notes above; also reported, dermatitis
Dose: duodenal ulcer associated with *Helicobacter pylori,* see eradication regimens on p. 37

Gastro-oesophageal reflux disease, 40 mg once daily for 4 weeks, followed by a further 4 weeks if not fully healed or symptoms persist; maintenance 20 mg daily; symptomatic treatment in the absence of oesophagitis, 20 mg daily for up to 4 weeks, followed by 20 mg daily when required

CHILD not recommended
COUNSELLING. Swallow whole *or* disperse in water

Nexium® (AstraZeneca) PoM
Tablets, f/c, esomeprazole (as magnesium trihydrate) 20 mg (light pink), net price 28-tab pack = £18.50 (also 7–tab pack, hosp. only); 40 mg (pink), 28-tab pack = £28.56 (also 7–tab pack, hosp. only). Counselling, administration

LANSOPRAZOLE

Indications: see under Dose
Cautions: see notes above; **interactions:** Appendix 1 (proton pump inhibitors)
Side-effects: see notes above; also reported, Stevens-Johnson syndrome, toxic epidermal necrolysis, bullous eruption, alopecia, photosensitivity, paraesthesia, interstitial nephritis, liver dysfunction, haematological changes (including agranulocytosis, eosinophilia, leucopenia, pancytopenia, thrombocytopenia), bruising, purpura, petechiae, fatigue, taste disturbance, vertigo, hallucinations, confusion, rarely gynaecomastia, impotence
Dose: benign gastric ulcer, 30 mg daily in the morning for 8 weeks

Duodenal ulcer, 30 mg daily in the morning for 4 weeks; maintenance 15 mg daily

NSAID-associated duodenal or gastric ulcer, 15–30 mg once daily for 4 weeks, followed by a further 4 weeks if not fully healed; prophylaxis, 15–30 mg once daily

Duodenal ulcer associated with *Helicobacter pylori,* see eradication regimens on p. 37

Zollinger-Ellison syndrome (and other hypersecretory conditions), initially 60 mg once daily adjusted according to response; daily doses of 120 mg or more given in two divided doses

Gastro-oesophageal reflux disease, 30 mg daily in the morning for 4 weeks, followed by a further 4 weeks if not fully healed; maintenance 15–30 mg daily

Acid-related dyspepsia, 15–30 mg daily in the morning for 2–4 weeks

CHILD not recommended

Zoton® (Wyeth) PoM
Capsules, enclosing e/c granules, lansoprazole 15 mg (yellow), net price 28-cap pack = £12.98, 56-cap pack = £25.96; 30 mg (lilac/purple), 14-cap pack = £11.88, 28-cap pack = £23.75, 56-cap pack = £47.50 (also 7-cap pack, hosp. only). Label: 5, 25
FasTab® (= orodispersible tablet), lansoprazole 15 mg, net price 28-tab pack = £12.98; 30 mg, 7-tab pack = £5.94, 14-tab pack = £11.88, 28-tab pack = £23.75. Label: 5, counselling, administration
Excipients: include aspartame (section 9.4.1)
COUNSELLING. Tablets should be placed on the tongue, allowed to disperse and swallowed or may be swallowed whole with a glass of water; tablets should not be crushed or chewed.
Suspension, pink, powder for reconstitution, lansoprazole 30 mg/sachet (strawberry flavour), net price 28-sachet pack = £34.14. Label: 5, 13

■ **With antibacterials**
For additional cautions, contra-indications and side-effects see Amoxicillin (section 5.1.1), Clarithromycin (section 5.1.5), and Metronidazole (section 5.1.11)

HeliClear® (Wyeth) PoM
Triple pack, lansoprazole capsules 30 mg (*Zoton*®), amoxicillin (as trihydrate) capsules 500 mg, clarithromycin tablets 500 mg (*Klaricid*®). Net price 7-day pack (14 × lansoprazole caps, 28 × amoxicillin caps, 14 × clarithromycin tabs) = £36.82. Label: 5, 9, 25
Dose: eradication of *Helicobacter pylori* in patients with duodenal ulcer, lansoprazole 30 mg twice daily, clarithromycin 500 mg twice daily, and amoxicillin 1 g twice daily for 7–14 days; CHILD not recommended

HeliMet® (Wyeth) PoM
Triple pack, lansoprazole capsules 30 mg (*Zoton*®), clarithromycin tablets 500 mg (*Klaricid*®), metronidazole tablets 400 mg, net price 7-day pack (14 × lansoprazole caps, 14 × clarithromycin tabs, 14 × metronidazole tabs) = £35.42. Label: 4, 5, 9, 25, 27
Dose: eradication of *Helicobacter pylori* in patients with duodenal ulcer, lansoprazole 30 mg twice daily, clarithromycin 500 mg twice daily, and metronidazole 400 mg twice daily for 7 days; CHILD not recommended

PANTOPRAZOLE

Indications: see under Dose

Cautions: see notes above; also renal impairment (Appendix 3); **interactions:** Appendix 1 (proton pump inhibitors)

Side-effects: see notes above; also reported fever, liver dysfunction, raised triglycerides

Dose: *By mouth,* benign gastric ulcer, 40 mg daily in the morning for 4 weeks, continued for further 4 weeks if not fully healed
Gastro-oesophageal reflux disease, 20–40 mg daily in the morning for 4 weeks, continued for further 4 weeks if not fully healed; may be continued at 20 mg daily (long-term management), increased to 40 mg daily if symptoms return
Duodenal ulcer, 40 mg daily in the morning for 2 weeks, continued for further 2 weeks if not fully healed
Duodenal ulcer associated with *Helicobacter pylori,* see eradication regimens on p. 37
Prophylaxis of NSAID-associated gastric or duodenal ulcer in patients with an increased risk of gastroduodenal complications who require continued NSAID treatment, 20 mg daily

CHILD not recommended

By intravenous injection over at least 2 minutes *or by intravenous infusion,* duodenal ulcer, gastric ulcer, and gastro-oesophageal reflux, 40 mg daily until oral administration can be resumed

CHILD not recommended

Protium® (Abbott) PoM
Tablets, e/c, pantoprazole (as sodium sesquihydrate) 20 mg, net price 28-tab pack = £12.88; 40 mg 28-tab pack = £23.65. Label: 25
Injection, powder for reconstitution, pantoprazole (as sodium sesquihydrate), net price 40-mg vial = £5.71

RABEPRAZOLE SODIUM

Indications: see under Dose

Cautions: see notes above; **interactions:** Appendix 1 (proton pump inhibitors)

Side-effects: see notes above; also reported, stomatitis, chest pain, cough, rhinitis, sinusitis, leucocytosis, insomnia, nervousness, drowsiness, asthenia, taste disturbance, pharyngitis, anorexia, influenza-like syndrome, sweating, weight gain

Dose: benign gastric ulcer, 20 mg daily in the morning for 6 weeks, followed by a further 6 weeks if not fully healed
Duodenal ulcer, 20 mg daily in the morning for 4 weeks, followed by a further 4 weeks if not fully healed
Gastro-oesophageal reflux disease, 10–20 mg daily in the morning for 4–8 weeks; may be continued at 10–20 mg daily
Duodenal and benign gastric ulcer associated with *Helicobacter pylori,* see eradication regimens on p. 37

CHILD not recommended

Pariet® (Eisai, Janssen-Cilag) PoM
Tablets, e/c, rabeprazole sodium 10 mg (pink), net price 28-tab pack = £12.43; 20 mg (yellow), 28-tab pack = £22.75. Label: 25

1.3.6 Other ulcer-healing drugs

Carbenoxolone is a synthetic derivative of glycyrrhizinic acid (a constituent of liquorice).

The only oral preparation of carbenoxolone remaining on the UK market is in the form of a combination with antacids for *oesophageal ulceration and inflammation.*

Side-effects of carbenoxolone (commonly sodium and water retention and occasionally hypokalaemia) may cause or exacerbate hypertension, oedema, cardiac failure, and muscle weakness. For these reasons other drugs are preferred; if used, regular monitoring of weight, blood pressure, and electrolytes is advisable during treatment. Carbenoxolone may act by protecting the mucosal barrier from acid–pepsin attack and increasing mucosal mucin production.

CARBENOXOLONE SODIUM ▱

Indications: oesophageal inflammation and ulceration

Cautions: cardiac disease, hypertension, hepatic and renal disease (see contra-indications); elderly (see under preparation); not recommended in children; see also notes above; **interactions:** Appendix 1 (carbenoxolone)

Contra-indications: hypokalaemia, cardiac failure and in those receiving cardiac glycosides (unless electrolyte levels monitored weekly and measures taken to avoid hypokalaemia); hepatic and renal impairment (see Appendixes 2 and 3); pregnancy

Side-effects: sodium and water retention (provoking hypertension and cardiac failure), hypokalaemia (leading to impaired neuromuscular function and muscle damage and to renal damage if prolonged)

Dose: see under preparations

TREATMENT OF ACUTE ULCERATIVE COLITIS AND CROHN'S DISEASE. Acute mild to moderate disease affecting the rectum (proctitis) or the recto-sigmoid (distal colitis) is treated initially with local application of a corticosteroid or an aminosalicylate; foam preparations are especially useful where patients have difficulty retaining liquid enemas.

Diffuse inflammatory bowel disease or disease that does not respond to local therapy requires oral treatment; mild disease affecting the colon may be treated with an aminosalicylate alone but refractory or moderate disease usually requires adjunctive use of an oral corticosteroid such as **prednisolone** for 4–8 weeks. Modified-release **budesonide** is licensed for Crohn's disease affecting the ileum and the ascending colon; it causes fewer systemic side-effects than oral prednisolone.

Severe inflammatory bowel disease calls for hospital admission and treatment with intravenous corticosteroid; other therapy may include intravenous fluid and electrolyte replacement, blood transfusion, and possibly parenteral nutrition and antibiotics. Specialist supervision is required for patients who fail to respond adequately to these measures. Patients with ulcerative colitis may benefit from a short course of ciclosporin (section 8.2.2) [unlicensed indication]. Patients with unresponsive or chronically active Crohn's disease may benefit from azathioprine, mercaptopurine (see below), or once-weekly methotrexate (section 8.1.3) [all unlicensed indications].

Infliximab (*Remicade*®, Schering-Plough) has been introduced for the treatment of severe active Crohn's disease refractory to treatment with a corticosteroid and an immunosuppressant, and for the treatment of refractory fistulas of Crohn's disease. Infliximab is a monoclonal antibody which inhibits the pro-inflammatory cytokine, tumour necrosis factor α. Infliximab has been associated with the development of tuberculosis (often in extrapulmonary sites) and with worsening of heart failure. It should be used by specialists where adequate resuscitation facilities are available.

Metronidazole (section 5.1.11) may be beneficial for the treatment of active Crohn's disease with perianal involvement, possibly through its antibacterial activity. Metronidazole in doses of 0.6–1.5 g daily in divided doses has been used; it is usually given for a month but no longer than 3 months because of concerns about developing peripheral neuropathy. Other antibacterials should be given if specifically indicated (e.g. sepsis associated with fistulas and perianal disease) and for managing bacterial overgrowth in the small bowel.

MAINTENANCE OF REMISSION OF ACUTE ULCERATIVE COLITIS AND CROHN'S DISEASE. **Aminosalicylates** are of great value in the maintenance of remission of ulcerative colitis. They are of less value in the maintenance of remission of Crohn's disease; an oral formulation of mesalazine is licensed for the long-term management of ileal disease. Corticosteroids are **not** suitable for maintenance treatment because of side-effects. In resistant or frequently relapsing cases either **azathioprine** (section 8.2.1), 2–2.5 mg/kg daily [unlicensed indication] or **mercaptopurine** (section 8.1.3), 1–1.5 mg/kg daily [unlicensed indication], given under close supervision may be helpful.

ADJUNCTIVE TREATMENT OF INFLAMMATORY BOWEL DISEASE. Due attention should be paid to diet; high-fibre or low-residue diets should be used as appropriate. Irritable bowel syndrome during remission of ulcerative colitis calls for avoidance of a high-fibre diet and possible treatment with an antispasmodic (section 1.2).

Antimotility drugs such as codeine and loperamide, and antispasmodic drugs should **not** be used in active ulcerative colitis because they can precipitate paralytic ileus and megacolon; treatment of the inflammation is more logical. Laxatives may be required in proctitis. Diarrhoea resulting from the loss of bile-salt absorption (e.g. in terminal ileal disease or bowel resection) may improve with **colestyramine** (section 1.9.2), which binds bile salts.

Antibiotic-associated colitis

Antibiotic-associated colitis (pseudomembranous colitis) is caused by colonisation of the colon with *Clostridium difficile* which may follow antibiotic therapy. It is usually of acute onset, but may run a chronic course; it is a particular hazard of clindamycin but few antibiotics are free of this side-effect. Oral **vancomycin** (see section 5.1.7) or **metronidazole** (see section 5.1.11) are used as specific treatment; vancomycin may be preferred for very sick patients.

Diverticular disease

Diverticular disease is treated with a high-fibre diet, **bran supplements**, and **bulk-forming drugs**. **Antispasmodics** may provide symptomatic relief when colic is a problem (section 1.2). **Antibacterials** are used only when the diverticula in the intestinal wall become infected (specialist referral). **Antimotility** drugs which slow intestinal motility, e.g. codeine, diphenoxylate, and loperamide could possibly exacerbate the symptoms of diverticular disease and are **contra-indicated**.

Aminosalicylates

Sulfasalazine is a combination of 5-aminosalicylic acid ('5-ASA') and sulfapyridine; sulfapyridine acts only as a carrier to the colonic site of action but still causes side-effects. In the newer aminosalicylates, **mesalazine** (5-aminosalicylic acid), **balsalazide** (a prodrug of 5-aminosalicylic acid) and **olsalazine** (a dimer of 5-aminosalicylic acid which cleaves in the lower bowel), the sulphonamide-related side-effects of sulfasalazine are avoided, but 5-aminosalicylic acid alone can still cause side-effects including blood disorders (see recommendation below) and lupoid phenomenon also seen with sulfasalazine. Olsalazine may also be particularly prone to cause watery diarrhoea. Some manufacturers of sulfasalazine and mesalazine recommend renal function tests, but evidence of practical value is unsatisfactory.

CAUTIONS. Aminosalicylates should be used with caution during pregnancy (Appendix 4) and breast-feeding (Appendix 5); blood disorders can occur (see recommendation below).

> **Blood disorders**
> It is recommended that patients receiving aminosali-
> cylates should be advised to report any unexplained
> bleeding, bruising, purpura, sore throat, fever or
> malaise that occurs during treatment. A blood count
> should be performed and the drug stopped immedi-
> ately if there is suspicion of a blood dyscrasia.

CONTRA-INDICATIONS. Aminosalicylates should
be avoided in salicylate hypersensitivity and in
moderate or severe renal impairment.

SIDE-EFFECTS. Side-effects of the aminosalicylates
include diarrhoea, nausea, headache, exacerbation of
symptoms of colitis, hypersensitivity reactions
(including rash, urticaria, interstitial nephritis and
lupus erythematosus-like syndrome); side-effects
that occur rarely include acute pancreatitis, hepatitis,
nephrotic syndrome, blood disorders (including
agranulocytosis, aplastic anaemia, leucopenia, neutropenia, thrombocytopenia—see also recommendation above).

BALSALAZIDE SODIUM

Indications: treatment of mild to moderate ulcerative colitis and maintenance of remission

Cautions: see notes above; also history of asthma;
interactions: Appendix 1 (aminosalicylates)

Contra-indications: see notes above; also severe
hepatic impairment
BLOOD DISORDERS. See recommendation above

Side-effects: see notes above; also abdominal pain,
vomiting, cholelithiasis

Dose: acute attack, 2.25 g 3 times daily until
remission occurs or for up to max. 12 weeks
Maintenance, 1.5 g twice daily, adjusted according
to response (max. 6 g daily)
CHILD not recommended

Colazide (Shire) PoM
Capsules, beige, balsalazide sodium 750 mg. Net
price 130-cap pack = £39.00. Label: 21, 25,
counselling, blood disorder symptoms (see
recommendation above)

MESALAZINE

Indications: treatment of mild to moderate ulcerative colitis and maintenance of remission; see also
under preparations

Cautions: see notes above; elderly; **interactions:**
Appendix 1 (aminosalicylates)

Contra-indications: see notes above; also severe
hepatic impairment; blood clotting abnormalities
BLOOD DISORDERS. See recommendation above

Side-effects: see notes above; also abdominal pain;
rarely allergic lung reactions, allergic myocarditis,
methaemoglobinaemia

Dose: see under preparations, below
NOTE. The delivery characteristics of enteric-coated
mesalazine preparations may vary; these preparations
should not be considered interchangeable

Asacol MR (Procter & Gamble Pharm.) PoM
Tablets, red, e/c, mesalazine 400 mg, net price 90-
tab pack = £31.22, 120-tab pack = £41.62. Label: 5,
25, counselling, blood disorder symptoms (see
recommendation above)
Dose: ulcerative colitis, acute attack, 6 tablets daily in
divided doses; maintenance of remission of ulcerative

colitis and Crohn's ileo-colitis, 3–6 tablets daily in
divided doses; CHILD not recommended
NOTE. Preparations that lower stool pH (e.g. lactulose)
may prevent release of mesalazine

Foam enema, mesalazine 1 g/metered application.
Net price 14 g (14 applications) with disposable
applicators and plastic bags = £37.82. Counselling,
blood disorder symptoms (see recommendation
above)
Dose: acute attack affecting the rectosigmoid region, 1
metered application (mesalazine 1 g) into the rectum daily
for 4–6 weeks; acute attack affecting the descending
colon, 2 metered applications (mesalazine 2 g) once daily
for 4–6 weeks; CHILD not recommended

Suppositories, mesalazine 250 mg, net price 20-
suppos pack = £6.83; 500 mg, 10 = £6.83.
Counselling, blood disorder symptoms (see
recommendation above)
Dose: 3–6 suppositories of 250 mg (max. 3 suppositories
of 500 mg) daily in divided doses, with last dose at
bedtime; CHILD not recommended

Ipocol (Lagap) PoM
Tablets, e/c, mesalazine 400 mg, net price 120-tab
pack = £41.62. Label: 5, 25, counselling, blood
disorder symptoms (see recommendation above)
Dose: acute attack, 6 tablets daily in divided doses;
maintenance of remission, 3–6 tablets daily in divided
doses; CHILD not recommended
NOTE. Preparations that lower stool pH (e.g. lactulose)
may prevent release of mesalazine

Pentasa (Ferring) PoM
Slow Release tablets, m/r, scored, mesalazine
500 mg (grey), net price 100-tab pack = £25.82.
Counselling, administration, see dose, blood
disorder symptoms (see recommendation above)
Dose: acute attack, up to 4 g daily in 2–3 divided doses;
maintenance, 1.5 g daily in 2–3 divided doses; tablets
may be dispersed in water, but should not be chewed;
CHILD under 15 years not recommended

Granules, m/r, pale brown, mesalazine 1 g/sachet,
net price 50-sachet pack = £31.60. Counselling,
administration, see dose, blood disorder symptoms
(see recommendation above)
Dose: acute attack, up to 4 g daily in 2–4 divided doses;
maintenance, 2 g daily in 2 divided doses; granules should
be placed on tongue and washed down with water or
orange juice without chewing; CHILD under 12 years not
recommended

Retention enema, mesalazine 1 g in 100-mL pack.
Net price 7 enemas = £19.45. Counselling, blood
disorder symptoms (see recommendation above)
Dose: 1 enema at bedtime; CHILD not recommended

Suppositories, mesalazine 1 g. Net price 28-suppos
pack = £44.68. Counselling, blood disorder
symptoms (see recommendation above)
Dose: ulcerative proctitis, acute attack, 1 suppository
daily for 2–4 weeks; maintenance, 1 suppository daily;
CHILD under 15 years not recommended

Salofalk (Provalis) PoM
Tablets, e/c, yellow, mesalazine 250 mg. Net price
100-tab pack = £18.41. Label: 5, 25, counselling,
blood disorder symptoms (see recommendation
above)
Dose: acute attack, 6 tablets daily in 3 divided doses;
maintenance 3–6 tablets daily in divided doses; CHILD not
recommended

Suppositories, mesalazine 500 mg. Net price 30-
suppos pack = £16.75. Counselling, blood disorder
symptoms (see recommendations above)
Dose: acute attack, 1–2 suppositories 2–3 times daily
adjusted according to response; CHILD not recommended

It is also important for those who complain of constipation to understand that bowel habit can vary considerably in frequency without doing harm. Some people tend to consider themselves constipated if they do not have a bowel movement each day. A useful definition of constipation is the passage of hard stools less frequently than the patient's own normal pattern and this can be explained to the patient.

Misconceptions about bowel habits have led to excessive laxative use. Abuse may lead to hypokalaemia and an atonic non-functioning colon.

Thus, laxatives should generally be avoided except where straining will exacerbate a condition (such as angina) or increase the risk of rectal bleeding as in haemorrhoids. Laxatives are also of value in *drug-induced constipation*, for the expulsion of *parasites* after anthelmintic treatment, and to clear the alimentary tract before *surgery and radiological procedures*. Prolonged treatment of constipation is seldom necessary except occasionally in the elderly.

CHILDREN. The use of laxatives in children should be discouraged unless prescribed by a doctor. Infrequent defaecation may be normal in breast-fed babies or in response to poor intake of fluid or fibre. Delays of greater than 3 days between stools may increase the likelihood of pain on passing hard stools leading to anal fissure, anal spasm and eventually to a learned response to avoid defaecation.

If increased fluid and fibre intake is insufficient, an osmotic laxative such as lactulose or a bulk-forming laxative such as methylcellulose may be effective; methylcellulose is given in a dose of 0.5–1 g twice daily for a child over 7 years [unlicensed use]—an appropriate formulation for a younger child is not readily available. If there is evidence of minor faecal retention, the addition of a stimulant laxative such as senna may overcome withholding but may lead to colic or, in the presence of faecal impaction in the rectum, an increase of faecal overflow. Referral to hospital may be needed unless the child evacuates the impacted mass spontaneously. In hospital, enemas or suppositories may clear the mass but their use is frequently distressing for the child and may lead to a persistence of withholding. Enemas may be administered under heavy sedation in hospital or alternatively a bowel cleansing solution (section 1.6.5) may be tried. In severe cases or where the child is afraid, a manual evacuation under anaesthetic may be appropriate.

Long-term use of stimulant laxatives such as senna or sodium picosulfate (sodium picosulphate, section 1.6.2) is essential to prevent recurrence of the faecal impaction. Parents should be encouraged to use them regularly for many months; intermittent use may provoke a series of relapses.

The laxatives that follow have been divided into 5 main groups (sections 1.6.1–1.6.5). This simple classification disguises the fact that some laxatives have a complex action.

1.6.1 # Bulk-forming laxatives

Bulk-forming laxatives relieve constipation by increasing faecal mass which stimulates peristalsis;

the full effect may take some days to develop and patients should be told this.

Bulk-forming laxatives are of particular value in those with small hard stools, but should not be required unless fibre cannot be increased in the diet. A balanced diet, including adequate fluid intake and fibre is of value in preventing constipation.

Bulk-forming laxatives are useful in the management of patients with *colostomy, ileostomy, haemorrhoids, anal fissure, chronic diarrhoea associated with diverticular disease, irritable bowel syndrome*, and as adjuncts in *ulcerative colitis* (section 1.5). Adequate fluid intake must be maintained to avoid intestinal obstruction. Unprocessed wheat **bran**, taken with food or fruit juice, is a most effective bulk-forming preparation. Finely ground bran, though more palatable, has poorer water-retaining properties, but can be taken as bran bread or biscuits in appropriately increased quantities. Oat bran is also used.

Methylcellulose, ispaghula, and **sterculia** are useful in patients who cannot tolerate bran. Methylcellulose also acts as a faecal softener.

ISPAGHULA HUSK

Indications: see notes above; hypercholesterolaemia (section 2.12)

Cautions: adequate fluid intake should be maintained to avoid intestinal obstruction—it may be necessary to supervise elderly or debilitated patients or those with intestinal narrowing or decreased motility

Contra-indications: difficulty in swallowing, intestinal obstruction, colonic atony, faecal impaction

Side-effects: flatulence, abdominal distension, gastro-intestinal obstruction or impaction; hypersensitivity reported

Dose: see preparations below

COUNSELLING. Preparations that swell in contact with liquid should always be carefully swallowed with water and should not be taken immediately before going to bed

Fybogel® (R&C)
Granules, buff, effervescent, sugar- and gluten-free, ispaghula husk 3.5 g/sachet (low Na$^+$), net price 60 sachets (plain, lemon, or orange flavour) = £4.24, 150 g (orange flavour) = £3.44. Label: 13, counselling, see above
Excipients: include aspartame 16 mg/sachet (see section 9.4.1)
Dose: 1 sachet or 2 level 5-mL spoonfuls in water twice daily preferably after meals; CHILD (but see section 1.6) 6–12 years ½–1 level 5-mL spoonful (children under 6 years on doctor's advice only)

Isogel® (Pfizer Consumer)
Granules, brown, sugar- and gluten-free, ispaghula husk 90%. Net price 200 g = £2.35. Label: 13, counselling, see above
Dose: constipation, 2 teaspoonfuls in water once or twice daily, preferably at mealtimes; CHILD (but see section 1.6) 1 teaspoonful
Diarrhoea (section 1.4.1), 1 teaspoonful 3 times daily

Ispagel® (Richmond)
Powder, beige, sugar- and gluten-free, ispaghula husk 3.5 g/sachet, net price 30 sachets (orange flavour) = £2.10. Label: 13, counselling, see above
Excipients: include aspartame (section 9.4.1)
Dose: 1 sachet in water 1–3 times daily; CHILD (but see section 1.6) 6–12 years ½ adult dose (children under 6 years on doctor's advice only)

Cautions: elderly and debilitated; see also notes above

Contra-indications: acute gastro-intestinal conditions

Side-effects: local irritation

Dose: see under preparations

Carbalax® (Forest)
Suppositories, sodium acid phosphate (anhydrous) 1.3 g, sodium bicarbonate 1.08 g, net price 12 = £2.14
Dose: constipation, 1 suppository, inserted 30 minutes before evacuation required; moisten with water before use; CHILD under 12 years not recommended

Fleet® **Ready-to-use Enema** (De Witt)
Enema, sodium acid phosphate 21.4 g, sodium phosphate 9.4 g/118 mL. Net price single-dose pack (standard tube) = 46p
Dose: ADULT and CHILD (but see section 1.6) over 12 years, 118 mL; CHILD 3–12 years, on doctor's advice only (under 3 years not recommended)

Fletchers' Phosphate Enema® (Forest)
Enema, sodium acid phosphate 12.8 g, sodium phosphate 10.24 g, purified water, freshly boiled and cooled, to 128 mL (corresponds to Phosphates Enema Formula B). Net price 128 mL with standard tube = 44p, with long rectal tube = 61p
Dose: 128 mL; CHILD (but see section 1.6) over 3 years, reduced according to body weight (under 3 years not recommended)

SODIUM CITRATE (RECTAL)

Indications: rectal use in constipation

Cautions: elderly and debilitated; see also notes above

Contra-indications: acute gastro-intestinal conditions

Dose: see under preparations

Micolette Micro-enema® (Dexcel)
Enema, sodium citrate 450 mg, sodium lauryl sulphoacetate 45 mg, glycerol 625 mg, together with citric acid, potassium sorbate, and sorbitol in a viscous solution, in 5-mL single-dose disposable packs with nozzle. Net price 5 mL = 31p
Dose: ADULT and CHILD over 3 years, 5–10 mL (but see section 1.6)

Micralax Micro-enema® (Celltech)
Enema, sodium citrate 450 mg, sodium alkylsulphoacetate 45 mg, sorbic acid 5 mg, together with glycerol and sorbitol in a viscous solution in 5-mL single-dose disposable packs with nozzle. Net price 5 mL = 33p
Dose: ADULT and CHILD over 3 years, 5 mL (but see section 1.6)

Relaxit Micro-enema® (Crawford)
Enema, sodium citrate 450 mg, sodium lauryl sulphate 75 mg, sorbic acid 5 mg, together with glycerol and sorbitol in a viscous solution in 5-mL single-dose disposable packs with nozzle. Net price 5 mL = 32p
Dose: ADULT and CHILD (but see section 1.6) 5 mL (insert only half nozzle length in child under 3 years)

1.6.5   Bowel cleansing solutions

Bowel cleansing solutions are used before colonic surgery, colonoscopy, or radiological examination to ensure the bowel is free of solid contents. They are **not** treatments for constipation.

BOWEL CLEANSING SOLUTIONS

Indications: see above

Cautions: pregnancy; renal impairment; heart disease; ulcerative colitis; diabetes mellitus; reflux oesophagitis; impaired gag reflex; unconscious or semiconscious or possibility of regurgitation or aspiration

Contra-indications: gastro-intestinal obstruction, gastric retention, gastro-intestinal ulceration, perforated bowel, congestive cardiac failure; toxic colitis, toxic megacolon or ileus

Side-effects: nausea and bloating; less frequently abdominal cramps (usually transient—reduced by taking more slowly); vomiting

Dose: see under preparations

Citramag® (Sanochemia)
Powder, effervescent, magnesium carbonate 11.57 g, anhydrous citric acid 17.79 g/sachet, net price 10-sachet pack (lemon and lime flavour) = £11.92. Label: 10, patient information leaflet, 13, counselling, see below
Dose: bowel evacuation for surgery, colonoscopy or radiological examination, on day before procedure, 1 sachet at 8 a.m. and 1 sachet between 2 and 4 p.m.; CHILD 5–9 years one-third adult dose; over 10 years and frail ELDERLY one-half adult dose
COUNSELLING. The patient information leaflet advises that hot water (200 mL) is needed to make the solution and provides guidance on the timing and procedure for reconstitution; it also mentions need for high fluid, low residue diet beforehand (according to hospital advice), and explains that only clear fluids can be taken after *Citramag*® until procedure completed

Fleet Phospho-soda® (De Witt)
Oral solution, sugar-free, sodium dihydrogen phosphate dihydrate 24.4 g, disodium phosphate dodecahydrate 10.8 g/45 mL. Net price 2 × 45-mL bottles = £4.79. Label: 10, patient information leaflet, counselling
Dose: 45 mL diluted with half a glass (120 mL) of cold water, followed by one full glass (240 mL) of cold water
Timing of doses is dependent on the time of the procedure
For morning procedure, first dose should be taken at 7 a.m. and second at 7 p.m. on day before the procedure
For afternoon procedure, first dose should be taken at 7 p.m. on day before and second dose at 7 a.m. on day of the procedure
Solid food must not be taken during dosing period; clear liquids or water should be substituted for meals
CHILD and ADOLESCENT under 15 years not recommended

Klean-Prep® (Norgine)
Oral powder, macrogol '3350' (polyethylene glycol '3350') 59 g, anhydrous sodium sulphate 5.685 g, sodium bicarbonate 1.685 g, sodium chloride 1.465 g, potassium chloride 743 mg/sachet. Contains aspartame (see section 9.4.1). Net price 4 sachets = £8.39. Label: 10, patient information leaflet, counselling
Four sachets when reconstituted with water to 4 litres

provides an iso-osmotic solution for bowel cleansing before surgery, colonoscopy or radiological procedures
Dose: 250 mL (1 tumblerful) of reconstituted solution every 10–15 minutes, or by nasogastric tube 20–30 mL/minute, until 4 litres has been consumed or watery stools are free of solid matter; CHILD not recommended

The solution from all 4 sachets should be drunk within 4–6 hours (250 mL drunk rapidly every 10–15 minutes); flavouring such as clear fruit cordials may be added if required; to facilitate gastric emptying domperidone or metoclopramide may be given 30 minutes before starting. Alternatively the administration may be divided into two, e.g. taking the solutions from 2 sachets on the evening before examination and the remaining 2 on the morning of the examination

After reconstitution the solution should be kept in a refrigerator and discarded if unused after 24 hours

NOTE. Allergic reactions reported

Picolax® (Nordic)
Oral powder, sugar-free, sodium picosulfate 10 mg/sachet, with magnesium citrate (for bowel evacuation before radiological procedure, endoscopy, and surgery), net price 2-sachet pack = £3.95. Label: 10, patient information leaflet, 13, counselling, see below
Dose: ADULT and CHILD over 9 years, 1 sachet in water in morning (before 8 a.m.) and a second in afternoon (between 2 and 4 p.m.) of day preceding procedure; CHILD 1–2 years quarter sachet morning and afternoon, 2–4 years half sachet morning and afternoon, 4–9 years 1 sachet morning and half sachet afternoon

Acts within 3 hours of first dose

NOTE. Low residue diet recommended for 2 days before procedure and copious intake of water or other clear fluids recommended during treatment

COUNSELLING. Patients should be warned that heat is generated on addition to water; for this reason the powder should be added initially to 30 mL (2 tablespoonfuls) of water; after 5 minutes (when reaction complete) the solution should be further diluted to 150 mL (about a tumblerful)

1.7 Local preparations for anal and rectal disorders

1.7.1	Soothing haemorrhoidal preparations
1.7.2	Compound haemorrhoidal preparations with corticosteroids
1.7.3	Rectal sclerosants

Anal and perianal pruritus, soreness, and excoriation are best treated by application of bland ointments and suppositories (section 1.7.1). These conditions occur commonly in patients suffering from haemorrhoids, fistulas, and proctitis. Careful local toilet with attention to any minor faecal soiling, adjustment of the diet to avoid hard stools, the use of bulk-forming materials such as bran (section 1.6.1) and a high residue diet are helpful. In proctitis these measures may supplement treatment with corticosteroids or sulfasalazine (see section 1.5).

When necessary topical preparations containing **local anaesthetics** (section 1.7.1) or **corticosteroids** (section 1.7.2) are used provided perianal thrush has been excluded. Perianal thrush is best treated with **nystatin** by mouth and by local application (see section 5.2, section 7.2.2, and section 13.10.2).

The management of *anal fissures* requires stool softening by increasing dietary fibre in the form of bran or by using a bulk-forming laxative. Short-term use of local anaesthetic preparations may help (section 1.7.1). If these measures are inadequate, the patient should be referred for specialist treatment in hospital; surgery or the use of a topical nitrate (e.g. glyceryl trinitrate 0.2–0.3% ointment) may be considered [unlicensed indication].

1.7.1 Soothing haemorrhoidal preparations

Soothing preparations containing mild astringents such as bismuth subgallate, zinc oxide, and hamamelis may give symptomatic relief in haemorrhoids. Many proprietary preparations also contain lubricants, vasoconstrictors, or mild antiseptics.

Local anaesthetics are used to relieve pain associated with *haemorrhoids,* and *pruritus ani* but good evidence is lacking. Lidocaine (lignocaine) ointment (section 15.2) is used before emptying the bowel to relieve pain associated with *anal fissure.* Alternative local anaesthetics include tetracaine (amethocaine), cinchocaine, and pramocaine (pramoxine), but they are more irritant. Local anaesthetic ointments can be absorbed through the rectal mucosa therefore excessive application should be **avoided**, particularly in infants and children. They should be used for short periods only (no longer than a few days) since they may cause sensitisation of the anal skin.

■ Preparations on sale to the public

Soothing haemorrhoidal preparations on sale to the public together with their significant ingredients include:

Anacal® (heparinoid, laureth '9'), **Anodesyn®** (allantoin, lidocaine (lignocaine)), **Anusol® cream** (bismuth oxide, Peru balsam, zinc oxide), **Anusol® ointment** and **suppositories** (bismuth oxide, bismuth subgallate, Peru balsam, zinc oxide)

Boots Haemorrhoid Ointment® (lidocaine (lignocaine), zinc oxide), **Boots Suppositories for Haemorrhoids®** (benzyl alcohol, glycol monosalicylate, methyl salicylate, zinc oxide)

Germoloids® (lidocaine (lignocaine), zinc oxide)

Hemocane® (benzoic acid, bismuth oxide, cinnamic acid, lidocaine (lignocaine), zinc oxide)

Lanacane® cream (benzocaine, chlorothymol)

Nupercainal® (cinchocaine)

Preparation H® gel (hamamelis water), **Preparation H® ointment and suppositories** (shark liver oil, yeast cell extract)

1.7.2 Compound haemorrhoidal preparations with corticosteroids

Corticosteroids are often combined with local anaesthetics and soothing agents in preparations for haemorrhoids. They are suitable for occasional short-term use after exclusion of infections, such as

Ursofalk® (Provalis) [PoM]
Capsules, ursodeoxycholic acid 250 mg. Net price 60 = £32.95. Label: 21
Suspension, sugar-free, ursodeoxycholic acid 250 mg/5 mL, net price 250 mL = £30.20. Label: 21
Dose: primary biliary cirrhosis, 10–15 mg/kg daily in 2–4 divided doses
Dissolution of gallstones, see Dose, above

Ursogal® (Galen) [PoM]
Tablets, scored, ursodeoxycholic acid 150 mg, net price 60-tab pack = £17.05. Label: 21
Capsules, ursodeoxycholic acid 250 mg, net price 60-cap pack = £30.50. Label: 21

Other preparations for biliary disorders

A **terpene** mixture (*Rowachol*®) raises biliary cholesterol solubility. It is not considered to be a useful adjunct.

Rowachol® (Rowa) [PoM] ▭
Capsules, green, e/c, borneol 5 mg, camphene 5 mg, cineole 2 mg, menthol 32 mg, menthone 6 mg, pinene 17 mg in olive oil. Net price 50-cap pack = £7.35. Label: 22
Dose: 1–2 capsules 3 times daily before food (but see notes above)
Interactions: Appendix 1 (*Rowachol*®)

1.9.2 Bile acid sequestrants

Colestyramine (cholestyramine) is an anion-exchange resin that is not absorbed from the gastro-intestinal tract. It relieves diarrhoea and pruritus by forming an insoluble complex with bile acids in the intestine. Colestyramine can interfere with the absorption of a number of drugs. Colestyramine is also used in hypercholesterolaemia (section 2.12).

COLESTYRAMINE
(Cholestyramine)
Indications: pruritus associated with partial biliary obstruction and primary biliary cirrhosis; diarrhoea associated with Crohn's disease, ileal resection, vagotomy, diabetic vagal neuropathy, and radiation; hypercholesterolaemia (section 2.12)
Cautions: see section 2.12
Contra-indications: see section 2.12
Side-effects: see section 2.12
Dose: pruritus, 4–8 g daily in water (or other suitable liquid)
Diarrhoea, after initial introduction over 3–4 week period, 12–24 g daily mixed with water (or other suitable liquid) in 1–4 divided doses, then adjusted as required; max. 36 g daily
CHILD 6–12 years, consult product literature
COUNSELLING. Other drugs should be taken at least 1 hour before or 4–6 hours after colestyramine to reduce possible interference with absorption

■ Preparations
Section 2.12

1.9.3 Aprotinin

Section 2.11.

1.9.4 Pancreatin

Supplements of pancreatin are given by mouth to compensate for reduced or absent exocrine secretion in cystic fibrosis, and following pancreatectomy, total gastrectomy, or chronic pancreatitis. They assist the digestion of starch, fat, and protein.

Pancreatin is inactivated by gastric acid therefore pancreatin preparations are best taken with food (or immediately before or after food). Gastric acid secretion may be reduced by giving cimetidine or ranitidine an hour beforehand (section 1.3). Concurrent use of antacids also reduces gastric acidity. Enteric-coated preparations deliver a higher enzyme concentration in the duodenum (provided the capsule contents are swallowed whole without chewing). Higher-strength versions are now also available (**important:** see CSM advice below).

Since pancreatin is also inactivated by heat, excessive heat should be avoided if preparations are mixed with liquids or food; the resulting mixtures should not be kept for more than one hour.

Dosage is adjusted according to size, number, and consistency of stools, so that the patient thrives; extra allowance may be needed if snacks are taken between meals.

Pancreatin can irritate the perioral skin and buccal mucosa if retained in the mouth, and excessive doses can cause perianal irritation. The most frequent side-effects are gastro-intestinal, including nausea, vomiting, and abdominal discomfort; hyperuricaemia and hyperuricosuria have been associated with very high doses. Hypersensitivity reactions occur occasionally and may affect those handling the powder.

PANCREATIN
NOTE. The pancreatin preparations which follow are all of porcine origin

Indications: see also above

Cautions: see also above and (for higher-strength preparations) see below

Side-effects: see also above and (for higher-strength preparations) see below

Dose: see preparations

Creon® 10 000 (Solvay)
Capsules, brown/clear, enclosing buff-coloured e/c granules of pancreatin, providing: protease 600 units, lipase 10 000 units, amylase 8000 units. Net price 100-cap pack = £16.66. Counselling, see dose
Dose: ADULT and CHILD initially 1–2 capsules with meals either taken whole or contents mixed with fluid or soft food (then swallowed immediately without chewing)

Nutrizym GR® (Merck)
Capsules, green/orange, enclosing e/c pellets of pancreatin, providing minimum of: protease 650 units, lipase 10 000 units, amylase 10 000 units. Net price 100 = £14.47. Counselling, see dose
Dose: ADULT and CHILD 1–2 capsules with meals swallowed whole or contents sprinkled on soft food (then swallowed immediately without chewing); higher doses may be required according to response

digoxin dosage, whereas elimination of digitoxin depends on metabolism by the liver.

Unwanted effects depend both on the concentration of the cardiac glycoside in the plasma and on the sensitivity of the conducting system or of the myocardium, which is often increased in heart disease. Thus plasma concentration alone cannot indicate toxicity reliably but the likelihood of toxicity increases progressively through the range 1.5 to 3 micrograms/litre for digoxin. Cardiac glycosides should be used with special care in the elderly who may be particularly susceptible to digitalis toxicity.

Regular monitoring of plasma-digoxin concentration during maintenance treatment is not necessary unless problems occur. Care should be taken to avoid hypokalaemia if a diuretic is used with a cardiac glycoside because hypokalaemia predisposes the patient to digitalis toxicity. Hypokalaemia is managed by giving a potassium-sparing diuretic or, if necessary, potassium supplements (or foods rich in potassium).

Toxicity can often be managed by discontinuing digoxin and correcting hypokalaemia if appropriate; serious manifestations require urgent specialist management. **Digoxin-specific antibody fragments** are available for reversal of life-threatening overdosage (see below).

CHILDREN. The dose is based on body-weight; they require a relatively larger dose of digoxin than adults.

DIGOXIN

Indications: heart failure, supraventricular arrhythmias (particularly atrial fibrillation)

Cautions: recent infarction; sick sinus syndrome; thyroid disease; reduce dose in the elderly and in renal impairment; avoid hypokalaemia; avoid rapid intravenous administration (nausea and risk of arrhythmias); pregnancy (see also Appendix 4); **interactions:** Appendix 1 (cardiac glycosides)

Contra-indications: intermittent complete heart block, second degree AV block; supraventricular arrhythmias caused by Wolff-Parkinson-White syndrome; hypertrophic obstructive cardiomyopathy (unless concomitant atrial fibrillation and heart failure—but with caution)

Side-effects: usually associated with excessive dosage; include: anorexia, nausea, vomiting, diarrhoea, abdominal pain; visual disturbances, headache, fatigue, drowsiness, confusion, delirium, hallucinations, depression; arrhythmias, heart block; rarely rash, intestinal ischaemia; gynaecomastia on long-term use; thrombocytopenia reported; see also notes above

Dose: *by mouth*, rapid digitalisation, 1–1.5 mg in divided doses over 24 hours; less urgent digitalisation, 250–500 micrograms daily (higher dose may be divided)
Maintenance, 62.5–500 micrograms daily (higher dose may be divided) according to renal function and, in atrial fibrillation, on heart-rate response; usual range, 125–250 micrograms daily (lower dose may be appropriate in elderly)

Emergency loading dose *by intravenous infusion*, 0.75–1 mg over at least 2 hours (see also Cautions) then maintenance dose *by mouth* on the following day

NOTE. The above doses may need to be reduced if digoxin (or another cardiac glycoside) has been given in the preceding 2 weeks. Digoxin doses in the BNF may differ from those in product literature. For plasma concentration monitoring, blood should ideally be taken at least 6 hours after a dose

Digoxin (Non-proprietary) PoM
Tablets, digoxin 62.5 micrograms, net price 20 = 55p; 125 micrograms, 20 = 43p; 250 micrograms, 20 = 43p
Injection, digoxin 250 micrograms/mL, net price 2-mL amp = 70p
Available from Antigen
Paediatric injection, digoxin 100 micrograms/mL (hosp. only, available from BCM Specials)

Lanoxin® (GSK) PoM
Tablets, digoxin 125 micrograms, net price 20 = 32p; 250 micrograms (scored), 20 = 32p
Injection, digoxin 250 micrograms/mL. Net price 2-mL amp = 65p

Lanoxin-PG® (GSK) PoM
Tablets, blue, digoxin 62.5 micrograms. Net price 20 = 32p
Elixir, yellow, digoxin 50 micrograms/mL. Do not dilute, measure with pipette. Net price 60 mL = £5.23. Counselling, use of pipette

---

DIGITOXIN

Indications: heart failure, supraventricular arrhythmias (particularly atrial fibrillation)

Cautions: see under Digoxin but not necessary to reduce dose in mild to moderate renal impairment

Contra-indications: see under Digoxin

Side-effects: see under Digoxin

Dose: maintenance, 100 micrograms daily *or* on alternate days; may be increased to 200 micrograms daily if necessary

Digitoxin (Non-proprietary) PoM
Tablets, digitoxin 100 micrograms, net price 20 = £2.94

Digoxin-specific antibody

Digoxin-specific antibody fragments are indicated for the treatment of known or strongly suspected digoxin or digitoxin overdosage, where measures beyond the withdrawal of the cardiac glycoside and correction of any electrolyte abnormality are felt to be necessary (see also notes above).

Digibind® (GSK) PoM
Injection, powder for preparation of infusion, digoxin-specific antibody fragments (F(ab)) 38 mg. Net price per vial = £91.85 (hosp. and poisons centres only)
Dose: consult product literature

2.1.2 Phosphodiesterase inhibitors

Enoximone and **milrinone** are selective phosphodiesterase inhibitors which exert most of their effect on the myocardium. Sustained haemodynamic benefit has been observed after administration, but there is no evidence of any beneficial effect on survival.

ENOXIMONE

Indications: congestive heart failure where cardiac output reduced and filling pressures increased

Cautions: heart failure associated with hypertrophic cardiomyopathy, stenotic or obstructive valvular disease or other outlet obstruction; monitor blood pressure, heart rate, ECG, central venous pressure, fluid and electrolyte status, renal function, platelet count, hepatic enzymes; renal impairment (Appendix 3); avoid extravasation; pregnancy and breast-feeding

Side-effects: ectopic beats; less frequently ventricular tachycardia or supraventricular arrhythmias (more likely in patients with pre-existing arrhythmias); hypotension; also headache, insomnia, nausea and vomiting, diarrhoea; occasionally, chills, oliguria, fever, urinary retention; upper and lower limb pain

Dose: *by slow intravenous injection* (rate not exceeding 12.5 mg/minute), diluted before use, initially 0.5–1 mg/kg, then 500 micrograms/kg every 30 minutes until satisfactory response or total of 3 mg/kg given; maintenance, initial dose of up to 3 mg/kg may be repeated every 3–6 hours as required

By intravenous infusion, initially 90 micrograms/kg/minute over 10–30 minutes, followed by continuous or intermittent infusion of 5–20 micrograms/kg/minute

Total dose over 24 hours should not usually exceed 24 mg/kg

Perfan® (Myogen) PoM
Injection, enoximone 5 mg/mL. For dilution before use. Net price 20-mL amp = £15.02
Excipients: include alcohol, propylene glycol
NOTE. Plastic apparatus should be used; crystal formation if glass used

MILRINONE

Indications: short-term treatment of severe congestive heart failure unresponsive to conventional maintenance therapy (not immediately after myocardial infarction); acute heart failure, including low output states, following heart surgery

Cautions: see under Enoximone; also correct hypokalaemia, monitor renal function

Side-effects: see under Enoximone; also chest pain, tremor, bronchospasm, anaphylaxis and rash reported

Dose: *by intravenous injection* over 10 minutes, diluted before use, 50 micrograms/kg followed by *intravenous infusion* at a rate of 375–750 nanograms/kg/minute, usually for up to 12 hours following surgery or for 48–72 hours in congestive heart failure; max. daily dose 1.13 mg/kg

Primacor® (Sanofi-Synthelabo) PoM
Injection, milrinone (as lactate) 1 mg/mL. For dilution before use. Net price 10-mL amp = £16.61

2.2　Diuretics

2.2.1	Thiazides and related diuretics
2.2.2	Loop diuretics
2.2.3	Potassium-sparing diuretics
2.2.4	Potassium-sparing diuretics with other diuretics
2.2.5	Osmotic diuretics
2.2.6	Mercurial diuretics
2.2.7	Carbonic anhydrase inhibitors
2.2.8	Diuretics with potassium

Thiazides (section 2.2.1) are used to relieve oedema due to chronic heart failure (section 2.5.5) and, in lower doses, to reduce blood pressure.

Loop diuretics (section 2.2.2) are used in pulmonary oedema due to left ventricular failure and in patients with chronic heart failure (section 2.5.5).

Combination diuretic therapy may be effective in patients with oedema resistant to treatment with one diuretic. Vigorous diuresis, particularly with loop diuretics, may induce acute hypotension; rapid reduction of plasma volume should be avoided.

ELDERLY. Lower initial doses of diuretics should be used in the elderly because they are particularly susceptible to the side-effects. The dose should then be adjusted according to renal function. Diuretics should not be used continuously on a long-term basis to treat simple gravitational oedema (which will usually respond to increased movement, raising the legs, and support stockings).

POTASSIUM LOSS. Hypokalaemia may occur with both thiazide and loop diuretics. The risk of hypokalaemia depends on the duration of action as well as the potency and is thus greater with thiazides than with an equipotent dose of a loop diuretic.

Hypokalaemia is dangerous in severe coronary artery disease and in patients also being treated with cardiac glycosides. Often the use of potassium-sparing diuretics (section 2.2.3) avoids the need to take potassium supplements.

In hepatic failure hypokalaemia caused by diuretics can precipitate encephalopathy, particularly in alcoholic cirrhosis; diuretics may also increase the risk of hypomagnesaemia in alcoholic cirrhosis, leading to arrhythmias.

Potassium supplements are seldom necessary when thiazides are used in the routine treatment of hypertension (see also section 9.2.1.1).

2.2.1　Thiazides and related diuretics

Thiazides and related compounds are moderately potent diuretics; they inhibit sodium reabsorption at the beginning of the distal convoluted tubule. They act within 1 to 2 hours of oral administration and most have a duration of action of 12 to 24 hours; they are usually administered early in the day so that the diuresis does not interfere with sleep.

In the management of *hypertension* a low dose of a thiazide, e.g. bendroflumethiazide (bendrofluazide) 2.5 mg daily, produces a maximal or near-maximal blood pressure lowering effect, with very little biochemical disturbance. Higher doses cause more marked changes in plasma potassium, uric acid, glucose, and lipids, with no advantage in blood pressure control, and should not be used. For reference to the use of thiazides in chronic heart failure see section 2.5.5.

Bendroflumethiazide (bendrofluazide) is widely used for mild or moderate heart failure and for hypertension—alone in the treatment of mild hypertension or with other drugs in more severe hypertension.

Chlortalidone (chlorthalidone), a thiazide-related compound, has a longer duration of action than the thiazides and may be given on alternate days to control oedema. It is also useful if acute retention is liable to be precipitated by a more rapid diuresis or if patients dislike the altered pattern of micturition promoted by other diuretics.

Other thiazide diuretics (including benzthiazide, clopamide, cyclopenthiazide, hydrochlorothiazide and hydroflumethiazide) do not offer any significant advantage over bendroflumethiazide and chlortalidone.

Metolazone is particularly effective when combined with a loop diuretic (even in renal failure); profound diuresis may occur and the patient should therefore be monitored carefully.

Xipamide and **indapamide** are chemically related to chlortalidone. Indapamide is claimed to lower blood pressure with less metabolic disturbance, particularly less aggravation of diabetes mellitus.

BENDROFLUMETHIAZIDE/BENDROFLUAZIDE

Indications: oedema, hypertension (see also notes above)

Cautions: may cause hypokalaemia, aggravates diabetes and gout; may exacerbate systemic lupus erythematosus; elderly; pregnancy (Appendix 4) and breast-feeding; hepatic and renal impairment (avoid if severe, see Appendixes 2 and 3); see also notes above; porphyria (section 9.8.2); **interactions:** Appendix 1 (diuretics)

Contra-indications: refractory hypokalaemia, hyponatraemia, hypercalcaemia; severe renal and hepatic impairment; symptomatic hyperuricaemia; Addison's disease

Side-effects: postural hypotension and mild gastrointestinal effects; impotence (reversible on withdrawal of treatment); hypokalaemia (see also notes above), hypomagnesaemia, hyponatraemia, hypercalcaemia, hypochloraemic alkalosis, hyperuricaemia, gout, hyperglycaemia, and altered plasma lipid concentration; less commonly rashes, photosensitivity; blood disorders (including neutropenia and thrombocytopenia—when given in late pregnancy neonatal thrombocytopenia has been reported); pancreatitis, intrahepatic cholestasis, and hypersensitivity reactions (including pneumonitis, pulmonary oedema, severe skin reactions) also reported

Dose: oedema, initially 5–10 mg in the morning, daily *or* on alternate days; maintenance 5–10 mg 1–3 times weekly

Hypertension, 2.5 mg in the morning; higher doses rarely necessary (see notes above)

Bendroflumethiazide/Bendrofluazide (Non-proprietary) PoM
Tablets, bendroflumethiazide 2.5 mg, net price 20 = 53p; 5 mg, 20 = 52p
Available from Alpharma, APS, Generics, Goldshield (*Neo-NaClex®*, 5 mg only), Hillcross, IVAX, Sovereign (*Aprinox®*)

CHLORTALIDONE
(Chlorthalidone)

Indications: ascites due to cirrhosis in stable patients (under close supervision), oedema due to nephrotic syndrome, hypertension (see also notes above), mild to moderate chronic heart failure; diabetes insipidus (see section 6.5.2)

Cautions: see under Bendroflumethiazide

Contra-indications: see under Bendroflumethiazide

Side-effects: see under Bendroflumethiazide

Dose: oedema, up to 50 mg daily for limited period
Hypertension, 25 mg in the morning, increased to 50 mg if necessary (but see notes above)
Heart failure, 25–50 mg in the morning, increased if necessary to 100–200 mg daily

Hygroton® (Alliance) PoM
Tablets, yellow, scored, chlortalidone 50 mg, net price 28-tab pack = £1.68

CYCLOPENTHIAZIDE

Indications: oedema, hypertension (see also notes above)

Cautions: see under Bendroflumethiazide

Contra-indications: see under Bendroflumethiazide

Side-effects: see under Bendroflumethiazide

Dose: heart failure, 250–500 micrograms daily in the morning increased if necessary to 1 mg daily (reduce to lowest effective dose for maintenance)
Hypertension, initially 250 micrograms daily in the morning, increased if necessary to 500 micrograms daily (but see notes above)
Oedema, up to 500 micrograms daily for a short period

Navidrex® (Goldshield) PoM
Tablets, scored, cyclopenthiazide 500 micrograms. Net price 28-tab pack = £1.27
Excipients: include gluten

INDAPAMIDE

Indications: essential hypertension

Cautions: renal impairment (stop if deterioration); monitor plasma potassium and urate concentrations in elderly, hyperaldosteronism, gout, or with concomitant cardiac glycosides; hyperparathyroidism (discontinue if hypercalcaemia); pregnancy and breast-feeding; **interactions:** Appendix 1 (diuretics)

Contra-indications: recent cerebrovascular accident, severe hepatic impairment

Side-effects: hypokalaemia, headache, dizziness, fatigue, muscular cramps, nausea, anorexia, diarrhoea, constipation, dyspepsia, rashes (erythema multiforme, epidermal necrolysis reported); rarely postural hypotension, palpitations, increase in liver enzymes, blood disorders (including thrombocytopenia), hyponatraemia, metabolic alkalosis, hyperglycaemia, increased plasma urate concen-

Cautions: see under Amiloride Hydrochloride; may cause blue fluorescence of urine

Contra-indications: see under Amiloride Hydrochloride

Side-effects: include gastro-intestinal disturbances, dry mouth, rashes; slight decrease in blood pressure, hyperkalaemia, hyponatraemia; photosensitivity and blood disorders also reported; triamterene found in kidney stones

Dose: initially 150–250 mg daily, reducing to alternate days after 1 week; taken in divided doses after breakfast and lunch; lower initial dose when given with other diuretics

COUNSELLING. Urine may look slightly blue in some lights

Dytac® (Goldshield) PoM
Capsules, maroon, triamterene 50 mg. Net price 30-cap pack = £17.35 Label: 14, (see above), 21

▪ Compound preparations with thiazides or loop diuretics
See section 2.2.4

Aldosterone antagonists

SPIRONOLACTONE

Indications: oedema and ascites in cirrhosis of the liver, malignant ascites, nephrotic syndrome, congestive heart failure (section 2.5.5); primary hyperaldosteronism

Cautions: potential metabolic products carcinogenic in *rodents*; elderly; hepatic impairment; renal impairment (avoid if moderate to severe; Appendix 3); monitor electrolytes (discontinue if hyperkalaemia); porphyria (section 9.8.2); **interactions:** Appendix 1 (diuretics)

Contra-indications: hyperkalaemia, hyponatraemia; pregnancy and breast-feeding; Addison's disease

Side-effects: gastro-intestinal disturbances; impotence, gynaecomastia; menstrual irregularities; lethargy, headache, confusion; rashes; hyperkalaemia (discontinue); hyponatraemia; hepatotoxicity, osteomalacia, and blood disorders reported

Dose: 100–200 mg daily, increased to 400 mg if required; CHILD initially 3 mg/kg daily in divided doses
Heart failure, see section 2.5.5

Spironolactone (Non-proprietary) PoM
Tablets, spironolactone 25 mg, net price 20 = £1.50; 50 mg, 20 = £3.21; 100 mg, 20 = £3.31
Available from Alpharma, APS, Ashbourne (*Spirospare*®), Hillcross, IVAX
Oral suspensions, sugar-free, spironolactone 5 mg/5 mL, 10 mg/5 mL, 25 mg/5 mL, 50 mg/5 mL and 100 mg/5 mL available from Rosemont (special order)

Aldactone® (Searle) PoM
Tablets, all f/c, spironolactone 25 mg (buff), net price 100-tab pack = £8.89; 50 mg (off-white), 100-tab pack = £17.78; 100 mg (buff), 28-tab pack = £9.96

▪ With thiazides or loop diuretics
See section 2.2.4

2.2.4 Potassium-sparing diuretics with other diuretics

Although it is preferable to prescribe thiazides (section 2.2.1) and potassium-sparing diuretics (section 2.2.3) separately, the use of fixed combinations may be justified if compliance is a problem. Potassium-sparing diuretics are not usually necessary in the routine treatment of hypertension, unless hypokalaemia develops. For **interactions**, see Appendix 1 (diuretics).

▪ Amiloride with thiazides

Co-amilozide (Non-proprietary) PoM
Tablets, co-amilozide 2.5/25 (amiloride hydrochloride 2.5 mg, hydrochlorothiazide 25 mg), net price 28-tab pack = £1.85
Available from CP, Bristol-Myers Squibb (*Moduret 25*®)
Dose: hypertension, initially 1 tablet daily, increased if necessary to max. 2 tablets daily
Congestive heart failure, initially 1 tablet daily, increased if necessary to max. 4 tablets daily
Oedema and ascites in cirrhosis of the liver, initially 2 tablets daily, increased if necessary to max. 4 tablets daily; reduce for maintenance if possible
Tablets, co-amilozide 5/50 (amiloride hydrochloride 5 mg, hydrochlorothiazide 50 mg), net price 28 = £1.99
Available from Alpharma, APS, CP, Bristol-Myers Squibb (*Moduretic*®), Hillcross, IVAX (*Amil-Co*®)
Dose: hypertension, initially ½ tablet daily, increased if necessary to max. 1 tablet daily
Congestive heart failure, initially ½ tablet daily, increased if necessary to max. 2 tablets daily
Oedema and ascites in cirrhosis of the liver, initially 1 tablet daily, increased if necessary to max. 2 tablets daily; reduce for maintenance if possible

Navispare® (Novartis) PoM
Tablets, f/c, orange, amiloride hydrochloride 2.5 mg, cyclopenthiazide 250 micrograms. Net price 28-tab pack = £2.25
Excipients: include gluten
Dose: hypertension, 1–2 tablets in the morning

▪ Amiloride with loop diuretics

Co-amilofruse (Non-proprietary) PoM
Tablets, co-amilofruse 2.5/20 (amiloride hydrochloride 2.5 mg, furosemide 20 mg). Net price 28-tab pack = £4.43, 56-tab pack = £3.25
Available from Alpharma, CP, Helios (*Frumil LS*®), Hillcross, Lagap
Dose: oedema, 1 tablet in the morning
Tablets, co-amilofruse 5/40 (amiloride hydrochloride 5 mg, furosemide 40 mg). Net price 28-tab pack = £2.58
Available from Alpharma, APS, Ashbourne (*Froop-Co*®), Borg (*Lasoride*®), CP, Helios (*Frumil*®), Hillcross, IVAX (*Fru-Co*), Lagap, Sovereign
Dose: oedema, 1–2 tablets in the morning
Tablets, co-amilofruse 10/80 (amiloride hydrochloride 10 mg, furosemide 80 mg). Net price 28-tab pack = £7.49, 56-tab pack = £14.98
Available from CP (*Aridil*®), Helios (*Frumil Forte*®)
Dose: oedema, 1 tablet in the morning

Burinex A® (Leo) PoM
Tablets, ivory, scored, amiloride hydrochloride 5 mg, bumetanide 1 mg. Net price 28-tab pack = £3.06
Dose: oedema, 1–2 tablets daily

■ Triamterene with thiazides
COUNSELLING. Urine may look slightly blue in some lights

Co-triamterzide (Non-proprietary) PoM
Tablets, co-triamterzide 50/25 (triamterene 50 mg, hydrochlorothiazide 25 mg), net price 30-tab pack = £1.75. Label: 14, (see above), 21

Dose: hypertension, 1 tablet daily after breakfast, increased if necessary, max. 4 daily

Oedema, 2 tablets daily (1 after breakfast and 1 after midday meal) increased to 3 daily if necessary (2 after breakfast and 1 after midday meal); usual maintenance in oedema, 1 daily or 2 on alternate days; max. 4 daily
Available from Ashbourne (*TriamaxCo*®), IVAX (*Triam-Co*®)

Dyazide® (Goldshield) PoM
Tablets, peach, scored, co-triamterzide 50/25 (triamterene 50 mg, hydrochlorothiazide 25 mg). Net price 30-tab pack = £1.75. Label: 14, (see above), 21

Dose: hypertension, 1 tablet daily after breakfast, increased if necessary, max. 4 daily

Oedema, 2 tablets daily (1 after breakfast and 1 after midday meal) increased to 3 daily if necessary (2 after breakfast and 1 after midday meal); usual maintenance in oedema, 1 daily or 2 on alternate days; max. 4 daily

Dytide® (Goldshield) PoM
Capsules, clear/maroon, triamterene 50 mg, benzthiazide 25 mg. Net price 30-cap pack = £17.35. Label: 14, (see above), 21

Dose: oedema, initially 3 capsules daily (2 after breakfast and 1 after midday meal) for 1 week then 1 or 2 on alternate days

Kalspare® (Dominion) PoM
Tablets, orange, f/c, scored, triamterene 50 mg, chlortalidone 50 mg. Net price 28-tab pack = £3.05. Label: 14, (see above), 21

Dose: hypertension, oedema, 1–2 tablets in the morning

■ Triamterene with loop diuretics
COUNSELLING. Urine may look slightly blue in some lights

Frusene® (Orion) PoM
Tablets, yellow, scored, triamterene 50 mg, furosemide 40 mg. Net price 56-tab pack = £5.67. Label: 14, (see above), 21

Dose: oedema, ½–2 tablets daily in the morning

■ Spironolactone with thiazides

Co-flumactone (Non-proprietary) PoM ▭
Tablets, co-flumactone 25/25 (hydroflumethiazide 25 mg, spironolactone 25 mg). Net price 100-tab pack = £20.23
Available from Searle (*Aldactide 25*®)

Dose: congestive heart failure, initially 4 tablets daily; range 1–8 daily (but not recommended because spironolactone generally given in lower dose)
Tablets, co-flumactone 50/50 (hydroflumethiazide 50 mg, spironolactone 50 mg). Net price 28-tab pack = £10.70
Available from Searle (*Aldactide 50*®)

Dose: congestive heart failure, initially 2 tablets daily; range 1–4 daily (but not recommended because spironolactone generally given in lower dose)

■ Spironolactone with loop diuretics
Lasilactone® (Borg) PoM
Capsules, blue/white, spironolactone 50 mg, furosemide 20 mg. Net price 28-cap pack = £8.91

Dose: resistant oedema, 1–4 capsules daily

2.2.5 Osmotic diuretics

Osmotic diuretics are rarely used in heart failure as they may acutely expand the blood volume. **Mannitol** is used in cerebral oedema—a typical dose is 1 g/kg as a 20% solution given by rapid intravenous infusion.

MANNITOL

Indications: see notes above; glaucoma (section 11.6)
Cautions: extravasation causes inflammation and thrombophlebitis
Contra-indications: congestive cardiac failure, pulmonary oedema
Side-effects: chills, fever
Dose: *by intravenous infusion*, diuresis, 50–200 g over 24 hours, preceded by a test dose of 200 mg/kg by slow intravenous injection
Cerebral oedema, see notes above

Mannitol (Non-proprietary) PoM
Intravenous infusion, mannitol 10% and 20%
Available from Baxter

2.2.6 Mercurial diuretics

Mercurial diuretics are effective but are now almost never used because of their nephrotoxicity.

2.2.7 Carbonic anhydrase inhibitors

The carbonic anhydrase inhibitor **acetazolamide** is a weak diuretic and is little used for its diuretic effect. It is used for prophylaxis against mountain sickness [unlicensed indication] but is not a substitute for acclimatisation.
Acetazolamide and eye drops of dorzolamide and brinzolamide inhibit the formation of aqueous humour and are used in glaucoma (section 11.6).

2.2.8 Diuretics with potassium

Many patients on diuretics do not need potassium supplements (section 9.2.1.1). For many of those who do, the amount of potassium in combined preparations may not be enough, and for this reason their use is to be discouraged.
Diuretics with potassium and potassium-sparing diuretics should **not** usually be given together.
COUNSELLING. Modified-release potassium tablets should be swallowed whole with plenty of fluid during meals while sitting or standing

Burinex K® (Leo) PoM ▭
Tablets, bumetanide 500 micrograms, potassium 7.7 mmol for modified release. Net price 20 = 80p. Label: 25, 27, counselling, see above

Centyl K® (Leo) PoM ▭
Tablets, green, s/c, bendroflumethiazide 2.5 mg, potassium 7.7 mmol for modified release, net price 56-tab pack = £7.50. Label: 25, 27, counselling, see above

may be dazzled by headlights at night. Because of the possibility of phototoxic reactions, patients should be advised to shield the skin from light and to use a wide-spectrum sunscreen (section 13.8.1) to protect against both long ultraviolet and visible light.

Amiodarone contains iodine and can cause disorders of thyroid function; both hypothyroidism and hyperthyroidism may occur. Clinical assessment alone is unreliable, and laboratory tests should be performed before treatment and every 6 months. Thyroxine (T4) may be raised in the absence of hyperthyroidism; therefore tri-iodothyronine (T3), T4, and thyroid-stimulating hormone (thyrotrophin, TSH) should all be measured. A raised T3 and T4 with a very low or undetectable TSH concentration suggests the development of thyrotoxicosis. The thyrotoxicosis may be very refractory, and amiodarone should usually be withdrawn at least temporarily to help achieve control; treatment with carbimazole may be required. Hypothyroidism can be treated with replacement therapy without withdrawing amiodarone if it is essential.

Pneumonitis should always be suspected if new or progressive shortness of breath or cough develops in a patient taking amiodarone. Fresh neurological symptoms should raise the possibility of peripheral neuropathy.

Amiodarone is also associated with hepatotoxicity and treatment should be discontinued if severe liver function abnormalities or clinical signs of liver disease develop.

Beta-blockers act as anti-arrhythmic drugs principally by attenuating the effects of the sympathetic system on automaticity and conductivity within the heart, for details see section 2.4. For special reference to the role of **sotalol** in ventricular arrhythmias, see also p. 77.

Disopyramide may be given by intravenous injection to control arrhythmias after myocardial infarction (including those not responding to lidocaine (lignocaine)), but it impairs cardiac contractility. Oral administration of disopyramide is useful but it has an antimuscarinic effect which limits its use in patients with glaucoma or prostatic hypertrophy.

Flecainide belongs to the same general class as lidocaine. It may be of value in serious symptomatic ventricular arrhythmias. It may also be indicated for junctional re-entry tachycardias and for paroxysmal atrial fibrillation. As with quinidine it may precipitate serious arrhythmias in a small minority of patients (including those with otherwise normal hearts).

Procainamide is given by intravenous injection to control ventricular arrhythmias.

Propafenone is used for the prophylaxis and treatment of ventricular arrhythmias and also for some supraventricular arrhythmias. It has complex mechanisms of action, including weak beta-blocking activity (therefore caution is needed in obstructive airways disease—contra-indicated if severe).

Quinidine may be effective in suppressing supraventricular and ventricular arrhythmias. It may itself precipitate rhythm disorders, and is best used on specialist advice; it can cause hypersensitivity reactions and gastro-intestinal upsets.

Drugs for supraventricular arrhythmias include **adenosine, cardiac glycosides** and **verapamil**, see above under Supraventricular Arrhythmias. Drugs for ventricular arrhythmias include **bretylium**, lido-caine, **mexiletine**, and **phenytoin**, see below under Ventricular Arrhythmias.

AMIODARONE HYDROCHLORIDE

Indications: see notes above (should be initiated in hospital or under specialist supervision)

Cautions: liver-function and thyroid-function tests required before treatment and then every 6 months (see notes above for tests of thyroid function); chest x-ray required before treatment; heart failure; renal impairment; elderly; severe bradycardia and conduction disturbances in excessive dosage; intravenous use may cause moderate and transient fall in blood pressure (circulatory collapse precipitated by rapid administration or overdosage); porphyria (section 9.8.2); **interactions:** Appendix 1 (amiodarone)

Contra-indications: sinus bradycardia, sino-atrial heart block; unless pacemaker fitted avoid in severe conduction disturbances or sinus node disease; history of thyroid dysfunction; pregnancy and breast-feeding (see also Appendixes 4 and 5); iodine sensitivity; avoid *intravenous use* in severe respiratory failure, circulatory collapse, severe arterial hypotension; avoid bolus injection in congestive heart failure or cardiomyopathy; avoid injections containing benzyl alcohol in neonates

Side-effects: reversible corneal microdeposits (sometimes with night glare), rarely impaired vision due to optic neuritis; peripheral neuropathy and myopathy (usually reversible on withdrawal); bradycardia and conduction disturbances (see Cautions); phototoxicity and rarely persistent slate-grey skin discoloration (see also notes); hypothyroidism, hyperthyroidism, diffuse pulmonary alveolitis, pneumonitis, and fibrosis; raised serum transaminases (may require dose reduction or withdrawal if accompanied by acute liver disorders); jaundice, hepatitis and cirrhosis reported; rarely nausea, vomiting, metallic taste, tremor, hot flushes, sweating, nightmares, vertigo, headache, sleeplessness, fatigue, alopecia, paraesthesia, benign raised intracranial pressure, impotence, epididymo-orchitis; ataxia, rashes (including exfoliative dermatitis); hypersensitivity including vasculitis, renal involvement and thrombocytopenia; haemolytic or aplastic anaemia; anaphylaxis on rapid injection, also bronchospasm or apnoea in respiratory failure

Dose: *by mouth,* 200 mg 3 times daily for 1 week reduced to 200 mg twice daily for a further week; maintenance, usually 200 mg daily or the minimum required to control the arrhythmia

By intravenous infusion via caval catheter, initially 5 mg/kg over 20–120 minutes with ECG monitoring; subsequent infusion given if necessary according to response up to max. 1.2 g in 24 hours

Ventricular fibrillation or pulseless ventricular tachycardia, *by intravenous injection* over at least 3 minutes, 300 mg (section 2.7.3)

Amiodarone (Non-proprietary) ▣PoM
Tablets, amiodarone hydrochloride 100 mg, net price 28-tab pack = £4.28; 200 mg, 28-tab pack = £6.45. Label: 11
Available from Alpharma, APS, Generics, Hillcross, IVAX, Lexon (*Amyben*®), Sterwin

Injection, amiodarone hydrochloride 30 mg/mL, net price 10-mL prefilled syringe = £10.00
Excipients: may include benzyl alcohol (avoid in neonates, see Excipients, p. 2)
Available from Aurum

Sterile concentrate, amiodarone hydrochloride 50 mg/mL, net price 3-mL amp= £1.43, 6-mL amp = £2.86. For dilution and use as an infusion
Excipients: may include benzyl alcohol (avoid in neonates, see Excipients, p. 2)
Available from Mayne

Cordarone X® (Sanofi-Synthelabo) PoM
Tablets, both scored, amiodarone hydrochloride 100 mg, net price 28-tab pack = £4.78; 200 mg, 28-tab pack = £7.82. Label: 11
Sterile concentrate, amiodarone hydrochloride 50 mg/mL. Net price 3-mL amp = £1.43. For dilution and use as an infusion
Excipients: include benzyl alcohol (avoid in neonates, see Excipients, p. 2)

DISOPYRAMIDE

Indications: ventricular arrhythmias, especially after myocardial infarction; supraventricular arrhythmias

Cautions: discontinue if hypotension, hypoglyc-aemia, ventricular tachycardia, ventricular fibrilla-tion or torsades de pointes develop; atrial flutter or tachycardia with partial block, bundle branch block, heart failure (avoid if severe); prostatic enlargement; glaucoma; hepatic and renal impair-ment (see Appendixes 2 and 3); pregnancy and breast-feeding (see Appendixes 4 and 5); **interac-tions:** Appendix 1 (disopyramide)

Contra-indications: second-and third-degree heart block and sinus node dysfunction (unless pace-maker fitted); cardiogenic shock; severe uncom-pensated heart failure

Side-effects: ventricular tachycardia, ventricular fibrillation or torsades de pointes (usually asso-ciated with prolongation of QRS complex or QT interval—see Cautions above), myocardial depres-sion, hypotension, AV block; antimuscarinic effects include dry mouth, blurred vision, urinary retention; gastro-intestinal irritation; psychosis, cholestatic jaundice, hypoglycaemia also reported (see Cautions above)

Dose: *by mouth*, 300–800 mg daily in divided doses
By slow intravenous injection, 2 mg/kg over at least 5 minutes to a max. of 150 mg, with ECG monitor-ing, followed immediately *either* by 200 mg *by mouth*, then 200 mg every 8 hours for 24 hours *or* 400 micrograms/kg/hour *by intravenous infusion*; max. 300 mg in first hour and 800 mg daily

Disopyramide (Non-proprietary) PoM
Capsules, disopyramide (as phosphate) 100 mg, net price 20 = £3.76; 150 mg, 20 = £4.99
Available from Hillcross, IVAX (100 mg)

Rythmodan® (Borg) PoM
Capsules, disopyramide 100 mg (green/beige), net price 84-cap pack = £15.82; 150 mg, 84-cap pack = £20.99
Injection, disopyramide (as phosphate) 10 mg/mL, net price 5-mL amp = £2.92

■ Modified release

Isomide® **CR** (Tillomed) PoM
Capsules, m/r, disopyramide (as phosphate) 250 mg, net price 56-cap pack = £31.00. Label: 25
Dose: 250 mg every 12 hours

Rythmodan Retard® (Borg) PoM
Tablets, m/r, scored, f/c, disopyramide (as phosphate) 250 mg. Net price 56-tab pack = £31.02. Label: 25
Dose: 250–375 mg every 12 hours

FLECAINIDE ACETATE

Indications: (should be initiated in hospital)
Tablets and injection: AV nodal reciprocating tachy-cardia, arrhythmias associated with Wolff-Parkin-son-White syndrome and similar conditions with accessory pathways, paroxysmal atrial fibrillation in patients with disabling symptoms (arrhythmias of recent onset will respond more readily)
Tablets only: symptomatic sustained ventricular tachycardia, premature ventricular contractions and/or non-sustained ventricular tachycardia caus-ing disabling symptoms in patients resistant to or intolerant of other therapy
Injection only: ventricular tachyarrhythmias resistant to other treatment

Cautions: patients with pacemakers (especially those who may be pacemaker dependent because stimulation threshold may rise appreciably); avoid in sinus node dysfunction, atrial conduction defects, second-degree or greater AV block, bundle branch block or distal block unless pacing rescue available; atrial fibrillation following heart sur-gery; elderly (accumulation may occur); hepatic impairment (Appendix 2); renal impairment (monitor plasma-flecainide concentration, see also Appendix 3); pregnancy (Appendix 4) and breast-feeding (Appendix 5); **interactions:** Appendix 1 (flecainide)

Contra-indications: heart failure; history of myo-cardial infarction and either asymptomatic ventri-cular ectopics or asymptomatic non-sustained ventricular tachycardia; long-standing atrial fibril-lation where no attempt has been made to convert to sinus rhythm; haemodynamically significant valvular heart disease

Side-effects: nausea, vomiting; pro-arrhythmic effects; dyspnoea; visual disturbances; less com-monly gastro-intestinal disturbances, jaundice, hepatic dysfunction, AV block, heart failure, myo-cardial infarction, hypotension, pneumonitis, hal-lucinations, depression, convulsions, peripheral neuropathy, paraesthesia, ataxia, dyskinesia, hypoaesthesia, tinnitus, vertigo, reduction in red blood cells, in white blood cells and in platelets, corneal deposits, rashes, alopecia, sweating, urti-caria, photosensitivity, increased antinuclear anti-bodies

Dose: *by mouth*, ventricular arrhythmias, initially 100 mg twice daily (max. 400 mg daily usually reserved for rapid control or in heavily built patients), reduced after 3–5 days if possible
Supraventricular arrhythmias, 50 mg twice daily, increased if required to max. 300 mg daily
By slow intravenous injection, 2 mg/kg over 10–30 minutes, max. 150 mg, with ECG monitoring; followed if required by *infusion* at a rate of 1.5 mg/kg/hour for 1 hour, subsequently reduced to 100–250 micrograms/kg/hour for up to 24 hours; max. cumulative dose in first 24 hours, 600 mg; transfer to *oral* treatment, as above
NOTE. Plasma-flecainide concentration for optimum response 0.2–1 mg/litre

Many beta-blockers are now available and in general they are all equally effective. There are, however, differences between them which may affect choice in treating particular diseases or individual patients; esmolol and sotalol are used for the management of arrhythmia only (see below).

Intrinsic sympathomimetic activity (ISA, partial agonist activity) represents the capacity of beta-blockers to stimulate as well as to block adrenergic receptors. **Oxprenolol**, **pindolol**, **acebutolol** and **celiprolol** have intrinsic sympathomimetic activity; they tend to cause less bradycardia than the other beta-blockers and may also cause less coldness of the extremities.

Some beta-blockers are lipid soluble and some are water soluble. **Atenolol**, **celiprolol**, **nadolol**, and **sotalol** are the most water-soluble; they are less likely to enter the brain, and may therefore cause less sleep disturbance and nightmares. Water-soluble beta-blockers are excreted by the kidneys; they accumulate in renal impairment and dosage reduction is therefore often necessary.

Beta-blockers with a relatively short duration of action have to be given two or three times daily. Many of these are, however, available in modified-release formulations so that administration once daily is adequate for hypertension. For angina twice-daily treatment may sometimes be needed even with a modified-release formulation. Some beta-blockers such as atenolol, betaxolol, bisoprolol, carvedilol, celiprolol, and nadolol have an intrinsically longer duration of action and need to be given only once daily.

Beta-blockers slow the heart and can depress the myocardium; they are contra-indicated in patients with second- or third-degree heart block. Beta-blockers should also be avoided in patients with worsening unstable heart failure; care is required when initiating a beta-blocker in those with stable heart failure (see also section 2.5.5). **Sotalol** may prolong the QT interval, and it occasionally causes life-threatening ventricular arrhythmias (**important:** particular care is required to avoid hypokalaemia in patients taking sotalol).

Labetalol, **celiprolol**, **carvedilol** and **nebivolol** are beta-blockers which have, in addition, an arteriolar vasodilating action, by diverse mechanisms, and thus lower peripheral resistance. There is no evidence that these drugs have important advantages over other beta-blockers in the treatment of hypertension.

Beta-blockers may precipitate asthma and this effect can be dangerous. Beta-blockers should be **avoided** in patients with a history of asthma or chronic obstructive airways disease; if there is no alternative, a cardioselective beta-blocker may be used with extreme caution under specialist supervision. **Atenolol**, **betaxolol**, **bisoprolol**, **metoprolol**, **nebivolol** and (to a lesser extent) **acebutolol**, have less effect on the beta$_2$ (bronchial) receptors and are, therefore, relatively *cardioselective*, but they are **not** *cardiospecific*. They have a lesser effect on airways resistance but are **not** free of this side-effect.

Beta-blockers are also associated with fatigue, coldness of the extremities (may be less common with those with ISA, see above), and sleep disturbances with nightmares (may be less common with the water-soluble ones, see above).

Beta-blockers are not contra-indicated in diabetes; however they can lead to a small deterioration in glucose tolerance and interfere with metabolic and autonomic responses to hypoglycaemia. Cardioselective beta-blockers (see above) may be preferable and beta-blockers should be avoided altogether in those with frequent episodes of hypoglycaemia.

HYPERTENSION. Beta-blockers are effective antihypertensives but their mode of action is not understood; they reduce cardiac output, alter baroceptor reflex sensitivity, and block peripheral adrenoceptors. Some beta-blockers depress plasma renin secretion. It is possible that a central effect may also explain their mode of action. Blood pressure can usually be controlled with relatively few side-effects. In general the dose of beta-blocker does not have to be high; for example **atenolol** is given in a dose of 50 mg daily and it is usually not necessary to increase the dose to 100 mg.

Combined thiazide and beta-blocker preparations may help compliance but combined preparations should only be used when blood pressure is not adequately controlled by a thiazide or a beta-blocker alone. Beta-blockers reduce, but do not abolish, the tendency for diuretics to cause hypokalaemia.

Beta-blockers can be used to control the pulse rate in patients with *phaeochromocytoma* (section 2.5.4). However, they should never be used alone as beta-blockade without concurrent alpha-blockade may lead to a hypertensive crisis. For this reason phenoxybenzamine should always be used together with the beta-blocker.

ANGINA. By reducing cardiac work beta-blockers improve exercise tolerance and relieve symptoms in patients with *angina* (for further details on the management of stable and unstable angina see section 2.6). As with hypertension there is no good evidence of the superiority of any one drug, although occasionally a patient will respond better to one beta-blocker than to another. There is some evidence that sudden withdrawal may cause an exacerbation of angina and therefore gradual reduction of dose is preferable when beta-blockers are to be stopped. There is a risk of precipitating heart failure when beta-blockers and verapamil are used together in established ischaemic heart disease (**important**: see p. 106).

MYOCARDIAL INFARCTION. For advice on the management of myocardial infarction see section 2.10.1.

Several studies have shown that some beta-blockers can reduce the recurrence rate of *myocardial infarction*. However, uncontrolled heart failure, hypotension, bradyarrhythmias, and obstructive airways disease render beta-blockers unsuitable in some patients following a myocardial infarction. **Atenolol** and **metoprolol** may reduce early mortality after intravenous and subsequent oral administration in the acute phase, while **acebutolol**, **metoprolol**, **propranolol**, and **timolol** have protective value when started in the early convalescent phase. The evidence relating to other beta-blockers is less convincing; some have not been tested in trials of secondary protection. It is also not known whether the protective effect of beta-blockers continues after 2–3 years; it is possible that sudden cessation may cause a rebound worsening of myocardial ischaemia.

ARRHYTHMIAS. Beta-blockers act as *anti-arrhythmic drugs* principally by attenuating the effects of the sympathetic system on automaticity and conductivity within the heart. They may be used in conjunction with digoxin to control the ventricular response in atrial fibrillation, especially in patients with thyrotoxicosis. Beta-blockers are also useful in the management of supraventricular tachycardias, and are used to control those following myocardial infarction, see above.

Esmolol is a relatively cardioselective beta-blocker with a very short duration of action, used intravenously for the short-term treatment of supraventricular arrhythmias, sinus tachycardia, or hypertension, particularly in the peri-operative period. It may also be used in other situations, such as acute myocardial infarction, where sustained beta blockade might be hazardous.

Sotalol, a non-cardioselective beta-blocker with additional class III anti-arrhythmic activity, is used for prophylaxis in paroxysmal supraventricular arrhythmias. It also suppresses ventricular ectopic beats and non-sustained ventricular tachycardia. It has been shown to be more effective than lidocaine (lignocaine) in the termination of spontaneous sustained ventricular tachycardia due to coronary disease or cardiomyopathy. However, it may induce torsades de pointes in susceptible patients.

HEART FAILURE. Beta-blockers may produce benefit in heart failure by blocking sympathetic activity. **Bisoprolol** and **carvedilol** (as well as modified-release **metoprolol** [unlicensed indication]) reduce mortality in any grade of stable heart failure. Treatment should be initiated by those experienced in the management of heart failure (see section 2.5.5 for details on heart failure).

THYROTOXICOSIS. Beta-blockers are used in pre-operative preparation for thyroidectomy. Administration of propranolol can reverse clinical symptoms of *thyrotoxicosis* within 4 days. Routine tests of increased thyroid function remain unaltered. The thyroid gland is rendered less vascular thus making surgery easier (section 6.2.2).

OTHER USES. Beta-blockers have been used to alleviate some symptoms of *anxiety*; probably patients with palpitations, tremor, and tachycardia respond best (see also section 4.1.2 and section 4.9.3). Beta-blockers are also used in the *prophylaxis of migraine* (section 4.7.4.2). Betaxolol, carteolol, levobunolol, metipranolol and timolol are used topically in *glaucoma* (section 11.6).

PROPRANOLOL HYDROCHLORIDE

Indications: see under Dose

Cautions: pregnancy and breast-feeding (see also Appendixes 4 and 5); avoid abrupt withdrawal especially in angina; first-degree AV block; reduce oral dose of propranolol in liver disease; portal hypertension (risk of deterioration in liver function); renal impairment (Appendix 3); diabetes; history of obstructive airways disease (introduce cautiously and monitor lung function—see also Bronchospasm below); myasthenia gravis; history of hypersensitivity—may increase sensitivity to allergens and result in more serious hypersensitivity response, also may reduce response to adr-

enaline (epinephrine) (see also section 3.4.3); see also notes above; **interactions:** Appendix 1 (beta-blockers), **important:** verapamil interaction, see also p. 106

Contra-indications: asthma (**important:** see Bronchospasm below), uncontrolled heart failure, Prinzmetal's angina, marked bradycardia, hypotension, sick sinus syndrome, second- or third-degree AV block, cardiogenic shock, metabolic acidosis, severe peripheral arterial disease; phaeochromocytoma (apart from specific use with alpha-blockers, see also notes above)

BRONCHOSPASM. The CSM has advised that beta-blockers, including those considered to be cardioselective, should not be given to patients with a history of asthma or bronchospasm. However, in these patients there are very rare situations where there is no alternative to the use of a beta-blocker, when a cardioselective one is given with extreme caution and under specialist supervision

Side-effects: bradycardia, heart failure, hypotension, conduction disorders, bronchospasm, peripheral vasoconstriction (including exacerbation of intermittent claudication and Raynaud's phenomenon), gastro-intestinal disturbances, fatigue, sleep disturbances; rare reports of rashes and dry eyes (reversible on withdrawal), sexual dysfunction, and exacerbation of psoriasis; see also notes above; **overdosage:** see Emergency Treatment of Poisoning, p. 25

Dose: *by mouth*, hypertension, initially 80 mg twice daily, increased at weekly intervals as required; maintenance 160–320 mg daily

Portal hypertension, initially 40 mg twice daily, increased to 80 mg twice daily according to heart-rate; max. 160 mg twice daily

Phaeochromocytoma (only with an alpha-blocker), 60 mg daily for 3 days before surgery *or* 30 mg daily in patients unsuitable for surgery

Angina, initially 40 mg 2–3 times daily; maintenance 120–240 mg daily

Arrhythmias, hypertrophic obstructive cardiomyopathy, anxiety tachycardia, and thyrotoxicosis (adjunct), 10–40 mg 3–4 times daily

Anxiety with symptoms such as palpitations, sweating, tremor, 40 mg once daily, increased to 40 mg 3 times daily if necessary

Prophylaxis after myocardial infarction, 40 mg 4 times daily for 2–3 days, then 80 mg twice daily, beginning 5 to 21 days after infarction

Migraine prophylaxis and essential tremor, initially 40 mg 2–3 times daily; maintenance 80–160 mg daily

By intravenous injection, arrhythmias and thyrotoxic crisis, 1 mg over 1 minute; if necessary repeat at 2-minute intervals; max. 10 mg (5 mg in anaesthesia)

NOTE. Excessive bradycardia can be countered with intravenous injection of atropine sulphate 0.6–2.4 mg in divided doses of 600 micrograms; for **overdosage** see Emergency Treatment of Poisoning, p. 25

Propranolol (Non-proprietary) PoM

Tablets, propranolol hydrochloride 10 mg, net price 20 = 42p; 40 mg, 20 = 46p; 80 mg, 20 = 34p; 160 mg, 20 = 85p. Label: 8

Available from Alpharma, APS, DDSA (*Angilol*®), Hillcross

Oral solution, propranolol hydrochloride 5 mg/5 mL, net price 150 mL = £13.30; 10 mg/5 mL, 150 mL = £17.50; 50 mg/5 mL, 150 mL = £21.25

Available from Rosemont (*Syprol*®)

Eucardic® (Roche) ▼ PoM
Tablets, all scored, carvedilol 3.125 mg (pink), net price 28-tab pack =£8.14; 6.25 mg (yellow), 28-tab pack = £9.04; 12.5 mg (peach), 28-tab pack = £10.05; 25 mg, 28-tab pack = £12.56. Label: 8

CELIPROLOL HYDROCHLORIDE

Indications: mild to moderate hypertension

Cautions: see under Propranolol Hydrochloride

Contra-indications: see under Propranolol Hydrochloride; also avoid in severe renal impairment

Side-effects: headache, dizziness, fatigue, nausea and somnolence; also bradycardia, bronchospasm; depression and pneumonitis reported rarely

Dose: 200 mg once daily in the morning, increased to 400 mg once daily if necessary

Celiprolol (Non-proprietary) PoM
Tablets, celiprolol hydrochloride 200 mg, net price 28-tab pack = £14.61; 400 mg, 28-tab pack = £32.97. Label: 8, 22
Available from APS, Generics, IVAX, Sovereign

Celectol® (Pantheon) PoM
Tablets, both f/c, scored, celiprolol hydrochloride 200 mg (yellow), net price 28-tab pack = £17.19; 400 mg, 28-tab pack = £34.38. Label: 8, 22

ESMOLOL HYDROCHLORIDE

Indications: short-term treatment of supraventricular arrhythmias (including atrial fibrillation, atrial flutter, sinus tachycardia); tachycardia and hypertension in peri-operative period

Cautions: see under Propranolol Hydrochloride; renal impairment

Contra-indications: see under Propranolol Hydrochloride

Side-effects: see under Propranolol Hydrochloride

Dose: *by intravenous infusion*, usually within range 50–200 micrograms/kg/minute (consult product literature for details of dose titration and doses during peri-operative period)

Brevibloc® (Baxter) PoM
Injection, esmolol hydrochloride 10 mg/mL, net price 10-mL vial = £6.49, 250-mL infusion bag = £74.75
Injection concentrate, esmolol hydrochloride 250 mg/mL (for dilution before infusion), 10-mL amp = £72.49

LABETALOL HYDROCHLORIDE

Indications: hypertension (including hypertension in pregnancy, hypertension with angina, and hypertension following acute myocardial infarction); hypertensive crisis (but see section 2.5); controlled hypotension in anaesthesia

Cautions: see under Propranolol Hydrochloride; interferes with laboratory tests for catecholamines; liver damage (see below)
LIVER DAMAGE. Severe hepatocellular damage reported after both short-term and long-term treatment. Appropriate laboratory testing needed at first symptom of liver dysfunction and if laboratory evidence of damage (or if jaundice) labetalol should be stopped and not restarted

Contra-indications: see under Propranolol Hydrochloride

Side-effects: postural hypotension (avoid upright position during and for 3 hours after intravenous administration), tiredness, weakness, headache, rashes, scalp tingling, difficulty in micturition; epigastric pain, nausea, vomiting; liver damage (see above); rarely lichenoid rash

Dose: *by mouth*, initially 100 mg (50 mg in elderly) twice daily with food, increased at intervals of 14 days to usual dose of 200 mg twice daily; up to 800 mg daily in 2 divided doses (3–4 divided doses if higher); max. 2.4 g daily
By intravenous injection, 50 mg over at least 1 minute, repeated after 5 minutes if necessary; max. 200 mg
NOTE. Excessive bradycardia can be countered with intravenous injection of atropine sulphate 0.6–2.4 mg in divided doses of 600 micrograms; for **overdosage** see Emergency Treatment of Poisoning, p. 25
By intravenous infusion, 2 mg/minute until satisfactory response then discontinue; usual total dose 50–200 mg, (**not** recommended for phaeochromocytoma, see under Phaeochromocytoma, section 2.5.4)
Hypertension of pregnancy, 20 mg/hour, doubled every 30 minutes; usual max. 160 mg/hour
Hypertension following myocardial infarction, 15 mg/hour, gradually increased to max. 120 mg/hour

Labetalol Hydrochloride (Non-proprietary) PoM
Tablets, all f/c, labetalol hydrochloride 100 mg, net price 20 = £1.70; 200 mg, 20 = £2.30; 400 mg, 20 = £3.97. Label: 8, 21
Available from Alpharma, Hillcross, Ivax

Trandate® (Celltech) PoM
Tablets, all orange, f/c, labetalol hydrochloride 50 mg, net price 56-tab pack = £5.05; 100 mg, 56-tab pack = £5.56; 200 mg, 56-tab pack = £9.02; 400 mg, 56-tab pack = £12.56. Label: 8, 21
Injection, labetalol hydrochloride 5 mg/mL. Net price 20-mL amp = £2.83

METOPROLOL TARTRATE

Indications: see under Dose

Cautions: see under Propranolol Hydrochloride; reduce dose in hepatic impairment

Contra-indications: see under Propranolol Hydrochloride

Side-effects: see under Propranolol Hydrochloride

Dose: *by mouth*, hypertension, initially 100 mg daily, maintenance 100–200 mg daily in 1–2 doses
Angina, 50–100 mg 2–3 times daily
Arrhythmias, usually 50 mg 2–3 times daily; up to 300 mg daily in divided doses if necessary
Migraine prophylaxis, 100–200 mg daily in divided doses
Hyperthyroidism (adjunct), 50 mg 4 times daily
By intravenous injection, arrhythmias, up to 5 mg at rate 1–2 mg/minute, repeated after 5 minutes if necessary, total dose 10–15 mg
NOTE. Excessive bradycardia can be countered with intravenous injection of atropine sulphate 0.6–2.4 mg in divided doses of 600 micrograms; for **overdosage** see Emergency Treatment of Poisoning, p. 25
In surgery, 2–4 mg *by slow intravenous injection* at induction or to control arrhythmias developing during anaesthesia; 2-mg doses may be repeated to a max. of 10 mg
Early intervention within 12 hours of infarction, 5 mg *by intravenous injection* every 2 minutes to a

max. of 15 mg, followed after 15 minutes by 50 mg *by mouth* every 6 hours for 48 hours; maintenance 200 mg daily in divided doses

Metoprolol Tartrate (Non-proprietary) [PoM]
Tablets, metoprolol tartrate 50 mg, net price 20 = 63p; 100 mg, 20 = £1.15. Label: 8
Available from Alpharma, APS, Hillcross, IVAX

Betaloc® (AstraZeneca) [PoM]
Tablets, both scored, metoprolol tartrate 50 mg, net price 100-tab pack = £3.30; 100 mg, 100-tab pack = £6.13. Label: 8
Injection, metoprolol tartrate 1 mg/mL. Net price 5-mL amp = 42p

Lopresor® (Novartis) [PoM]
Tablets, both f/c, scored, metoprolol tartrate 50 mg (pink), net price 56-tab pack = £2.57; 100 mg (blue), 56-tab pack = £6.68. Label: 8

■ Modified release

Betaloc-SA® (AstraZeneca) [PoM]
Durules® (= tablets, m/r), metoprolol tartrate 200 mg, net price 28-tab pack = £4.56. Label: 8, 25
Dose: hypertension, angina, 200 mg daily in the morning, increased to 400 mg daily if necessary; migraine prophylaxis, 200 mg daily

Lopresor SR® (Novartis) [PoM]
Tablets, m/r, yellow, f/c, metoprolol tartrate 200 mg, net price 28-tab pack = £9.80. Label: 8, 25
Dose: hypertension, 200 mg daily; angina, 200-400 mg daily; migraine prophylaxis, 200 mg daily

■ With diuretic

Co-Betaloc® (Searle) [PoM]
Tablets, scored, metoprolol tartrate 100 mg, hydrochlorothiazide 12.5 mg, net price 28-tab pack = £5.59. Label: 8
Dose: hypertension, 1–3 tablets daily in single or divided doses

Co-Betaloc SA® (Searle) [PoM]
Tablets, yellow, f/c, metoprolol tartrate (m/r) 200 mg, hydrochlorothiazide 25 mg, net price 28-tab pack = £6.89. Label: 8, 25
Dose: hypertension, 1 tablet daily

NADOLOL

Indications: see under Dose

Cautions: see under Propranolol Hydrochloride; reduce dose in renal impairment

Contra-indications: see under Propranolol Hydrochloride

Side-effects: see under Propranolol Hydrochloride

Dose: hypertension, 80 mg daily, increased at weekly intervals if required; max. 240 mg daily
Angina, 40 mg daily, increased at weekly intervals if required; usual max. 160 mg daily
Arrhythmias, initially 40 mg daily, increased to 160 mg if required; reduce to 40 mg if bradycardia occurs
Migraine prophylaxis, initially 40 mg daily, increased by 40 mg at weekly intervals; usual maintenance dose 80–160 mg daily
Thyrotoxicosis (adjunct), 80–160 mg daily

Corgard® (Sanofi-Synthelabo) [PoM]
Tablets, both blue, nadolol 40 mg, net price 28-tab pack = £3.76; 80 mg, 28-tab pack = £5.20. Label: 8

■ With diuretic

Corgaretic® (Sanofi-Synthelabo) [PoM]
Tablets, scored, nadolol 40 mg, bendroflumethiazide 5 mg (*Corgaretic 40*®), net price 28-tab pack = £5.92; nadolol 80 mg, bendroflumethiazide 5 mg (*Corgaretic 80*®), 28-tab pack = £8.47. Label: 8
Dose: hypertension, 1–2 tablets daily

NEBIVOLOL

Indications: essential hypertension

Cautions: see under Propranolol Hydrochloride; reduce dose in renal impairment (Appendix 3); elderly

Contra-indications: see under Propranolol Hydrochloride; hepatic impairment

Side-effects: see under Propranolol Hydrochloride; oedema, headache, depression, visual disturbances, paraesthesia, impotence

Dose: 5 mg daily; ELDERLY initially 2.5 mg daily, increased if necessary to 5 mg daily

Nebilet® (Menarini) [PoM]
Tablets, scored, nebivolol (as hydrochloride) 5 mg, net price 28-tab pack = £9.80

OXPRENOLOL HYDROCHLORIDE

Indications: see under Dose

Cautions: see under Propranolol Hydrochloride

Contra-indications: see under Propranolol Hydrochloride

Side-effects: see under Propranolol Hydrochloride

Dose: hypertension, 80–160 mg daily in 2–3 divided doses, increased as required; max. 320 mg daily
Angina, 80–160 mg daily in 2–3 divided doses; max. 320 mg daily
Arrhythmias, 40–240 mg daily in 2–3 divided doses; max. 240 mg daily
Anxiety symptoms (short-term use), 40–80 mg daily in 1–2 divided doses

Oxprenolol (Non-proprietary) [PoM]
Tablets, all coated, oxprenolol hydrochloride 20 mg, net price 20 = 55p; 40 mg, 20 = £1.11; 80 mg, 20 = £2.21; 160 mg, 20 = £2.36. Label: 8
Available from Hillcross, IVAX

Trasicor® (Novartis) [PoM]
Tablets, all f/c, oxprenolol hydrochloride 20 mg (contain gluten), net price 56-tab pack = £1.55; 40 mg (contain gluten), 56-tab pack = £3.11; 80 mg (yellow), 56-tab pack = £6.20. Label: 8

■ Modified release

Slow-Trasicor® (Novartis) [PoM]
Tablets, m/r, f/c, oxprenolol hydrochloride 160 mg. Net price 28-tab pack = £6.63. Label: 8, 25
Dose: hypertension, angina, initially 160 mg once daily; if necessary may be increased to max. 320 mg daily
NOTE. Modified-release tablets containing oxprenolol hydrochloride 160 mg also available from IVAX

- With diuretic

Trasidrex® (Novartis) PoM

Tablets, red, s/c, co-prenozide 160/0.25 (oxprenolol hydrochloride 160 mg (m/r), cyclopenthiazide 250 micrograms). Net price 28-tab pack = £8.88. Label: 8, 25

Dose: hypertension, 1 tablet daily, increased if necessary to 2 daily as a single dose

PINDOLOL •

Indications: see under Dose

Cautions: see under Propranolol Hydrochloride; reduce dose in renal impairment

Contra-indications: see under Propranolol Hydrochloride

Side-effects: see under Propranolol Hydrochloride

Dose: hypertension, initially 5 mg 2–3 times daily *or* 15 mg once daily, increased as required at weekly intervals; usual maintenance 15–30 mg daily; max. 45 mg daily

Angina, 2.5–5 mg up to 3 times daily

Visken® (Novartis) PoM

Tablets, both scored, pindolol 5 mg, net price 56-tab pack = £4.88; 15 mg, 28-tab pack = £7.33. Label: 8

- With diuretic

Viskaldix® (Novartis) PoM

Tablets, scored, pindolol 10 mg, clopamide 5 mg. Net price 28-tab pack = £6.70. Label: 8

Dose: hypertension, 1 tablet daily in the morning, increased if necessary to 2 daily; max. 3 daily

SOTALOL HYDROCHLORIDE

Indications: *Tablets and injection:* life-threatening arrhythmias including ventricular tachyarrhythmias, symptomatic non-sustained ventricular tachyarrhythmias

Tablets only: prophylaxis of paroxysmal atrial tachycardia or fibrillation, paroxysmal AV re-entrant tachycardias (both nodal and involving accessory pathways), paroxysmal supraventricular tachycardia after cardiac surgery, maintenance of sinus rhythm following cardioversion of atrial fibrillation or flutter

Injection only: electrophysiological study of inducible ventricular and supraventricular arrhythmias; temporary substitution for tablets

CSM advice. The use of sotalol should be limited to the treatment of ventricular arrhythmias or prophylaxis of supraventricular arrhythmias (see above). It should no longer be used for angina, hypertension, thyrotoxicosis or for secondary prevention after myocardial infarction; when stopping sotalol for these indications, the dose should be reduced gradually

Cautions: see under Propranolol Hydrochloride; reduce dose in renal impairment (avoid if severe); correct hypokalaemia, hypomagnesaemia, or other electrolyte disturbances; severe or prolonged diarrhoea; **interactions:** Appendix 1 (beta-blockers), **important:** verapamil interaction see also p. 106

Contra-indications: see under Propranolol Hydrochloride; congenital or acquired long QT syndrome; torsades de pointes; renal failure

Side-effects: see under Propranolol Hydrochloride; arrhythmogenic (pro-arrhythmic) effect (torsades de pointes—increased risk in women)

Dose: *by mouth* with ECG monitoring and measurement of corrected QT interval, arrhythmias, initially 80 mg daily in 1–2 divided doses increased gradually at intervals of 2–3 days to usual dose of 160–320 mg daily in 2 divided doses; higher doses of 480–640 mg daily for life-threatening ventricular arrhythmias under specialist supervision

By intravenous injection over 10 minutes, acute arrhythmias, 20–120 mg with ECG monitoring, repeated if necessary with 6-hour intervals between injections

Diagnostic use, see product literature

NOTE. Excessive bradycardia can be countered with intravenous injection of atropine sulphate 0.6–2.4 mg in divided doses of 600 micrograms; for **overdosage** see Emergency Treatment of Poisoning, p. 25

Sotalol (Non-proprietary) PoM

Tablet, sotalol hydrochloride 40 mg, net price 20 = 79p; 80 mg, 28-tab pack = £1.64; 160 mg, 28-tab pack = £6.20. Label: 8

Available from Generics, Hillcross, Taro, Tillomed

Beta-Cardone® (Celltech) PoM

Tablets, all scored, sotalol hydrochloride 40 mg (green), net price 56-tab pack = £2.22; 80 mg (pink), 56-tab pack = £3.29; 200 mg, 28-tab pack = £4.15. Label: 8

Sotacor® (Bristol-Myers Squibb) PoM

Tablets, sotalol hydrochloride 80 mg, net price 28-tab pack = £3.49; 160 mg, 28-tab pack = £6.89. Label: 8

Injection, sotalol hydrochloride 10 mg/mL. Net price 4-mL amp = £1.76

TIMOLOL MALEATE

Indications: see under Dose; glaucoma (section 11.6)

Cautions: see under Propranolol Hydrochloride

Contra-indications: see under Propranolol Hydrochloride

Side-effects: see under Propranolol Hydrochloride

Dose: hypertension, initially 5 mg twice daily *or* 10 mg once daily; gradually increased if necessary to max. 60 mg daily (given in divided doses above 20 mg daily)

Angina, initially 5 mg 2–3 times daily, usual maintenance 35–45 mg daily (range 15–45 mg daily)

Prophylaxis after myocardial infarction, initially 5 mg twice daily, increased after 2 days to 10 mg twice daily, starting 7 to 28 days after infarction

Migraine prophylaxis, 10–20 mg once daily

Betim® (ICN) PoM

Tablets, scored, timolol maleate 10 mg. Net price 30-tab pack = £2.45. Label: 8

- With diuretic

Moducren® (MSD) PoM

Tablets, blue, scored, timolol maleate 10 mg, co-amilozide 2.5/25 (amiloride hydrochloride 2.5 mg, hydrochlorothiazide 25 mg). Net price 28-tab pack = £8.00. Label: 8

Dose: hypertension, 1–2 tablets daily as a single dose

Prestim® (ICN) PoM

Tablets, scored, timolol maleate 10 mg, bendroflumethiazide 2.5 mg. Net price 30-tab pack = £4.11. Label: 8

Dose: hypertension, 1–2 tablets daily; max. 4 daily

2.5 Drugs affecting the renin-angiotensin system and some other antihypertensive drugs

Lowering raised blood pressure decreases the frequency of stroke, coronary events, heart failure, and renal failure. Advice on antihypertensive therapy in this section reflects the recommendations of the British Hypertension Society (Guidelines for management of hypertension: report of the third working party of the British Hypertension Society. *J Hum Hypertens* 1999; **13**: 569–92).

Possible causes of hypertension (e.g. renal disease, endocrine causes), contributory factors, risk factors, and the presence of any complications of hypertension, such as left ventricular hypertrophy, should be established. Patients should be given advice on lifestyle changes to reduce blood pressure or cardiovascular risk; these include smoking cessation, weight reduction, reduction of excessive intake of alcohol, reduction of dietary salt, reduction of total and saturated fat, increasing exercise, and increasing fruit and vegetable intake.

THRESHOLDS AND TARGETS FOR TREATMENT. The following thresholds for treatment are recommended:

- Accelerated (malignant) hypertension (with papilloedema or fundal haemorrhages and exudates) *or* impending cardiovascular complications, admit for **immediate treatment**;
- Where the initial blood pressure is systolic ≥ 220 mmHg *or* diastolic ≥ 120 mmHg, **treat immediately**;
- Where the initial blood pressure is systolic 200–219 mmHg *or* diastolic 110–119 mmHg, confirm over 1–2 weeks then **treat** if these values are sustained;
- Where the initial blood pressure is systolic 160–199 mmHg *or* diastolic 100–109 mmHg, *and* the patient has cardiovascular complications, end-organ damage (e.g. left ventricular hypertrophy, renal impairment) or diabetes mellitus (type 1 or 2), confirm over 3–4 weeks then **treat** if these values are sustained;
- Where the initial blood pressure is systolic 160–199 mmHg *or* diastolic 100–109 mmHg, but the patient has *no* cardiovascular complications, end-organ damage or diabetes, advise lifestyle changes, reassess weekly initially and **treat** if these values are sustained on repeat measurements over 4–12 weeks;

- Where the initial blood pressure is systolic 140–159 mmHg *or* diastolic 90–99 mmHg *and the* patient has cardiovascular complications, end-organ damage or diabetes, confirm within 4–12 weeks and **treat** if these values are sustained;
- Where the initial blood pressure is systolic 140–159 mmHg *or* diastolic 90–99 mmHg and *no* cardiovascular complications, end-organ damage or diabetes, advise lifestyle changes and **reassess** monthly; if mild hypertension persists, **treat** if coronary heart disease risk[1] is ≥ 15% over 10 years.

An optimal target systolic blood pressure < 140 mmHg *and* diastolic blood pressure < 85 mmHg is suggested.[2]

DRUG TREATMENT OF HYPERTENSION. Low-dose *thiazides* (section 2.2.1) reduce coronary events, cardiovascular mortality and all-cause mortality. A thiazide is first-line treatment for hypertension unless there is a contra-indication or a specific indication for another drug (see below). A low dose is adequate and higher doses (e.g. more than 2.5 mg bendroflumethiazide (bendrofluazide) or 25 mg hydrochlorthiazide) have no additional antihypertensive effect and increase metabolic side-effects.

A beta-blocker is sometimes preferred as alternative first-line therapy, but in some individuals there may be contra-indications to these drugs or indications for other antihypertensive drugs (see below). No consistent or important differences have been found between the major classes of antihypertensive drugs in terms of antihypertensive efficacy, side-effects or changes to quality of life (although there have been differences in average response related to age and ethnic group). The choice of antihypertensive drug will depend on the relevant indications or contra-indications for the individual patient; where there are no special considerations, the least expensive drug should be selected. *Some* indications and contra-indications for various antihypertensive drugs are shown below (see also under individual drug entries for details):

- **Thiazides** (section 2.2.1)—particularly indicated for hypertension in the elderly (see below); a contra-indication is gout;
- **Beta-blockers** (section 2.4)—indications include myocardial infarction, angina; compelling contra-indications include asthma, heart block;
- **ACE inhibitors** (section 2.5.5.1)—indications include heart failure, left ventricular dysfunction and diabetic nephropathy; contra-indications include renovascular disease (but see section 2.5.5.1) and pregnancy;

---

1. Coronary heart disease risk may be formally estimated using the Joint British Societies' 'Cardiac Risk Assessor' computer program or chart (British Cardiac Society, British Hyperlipidaemia Association, British Hypertension Society. *Heart* 1998; **80**(suppl 2): S1–29)

See inside back cover

2. A lower target for blood pressure should be considered for the secondary prevention of stroke, and for patients with diabetes and renal disease

- **Calcium-channel blockers**. There are important differences between calcium-channel blockers (section 2.6.2). **Dihydropyridine calcium-channel blockers** are valuable in isolated systolic hypertension in the elderly when a low-dose thiazide is contra-indicated or not tolerated (see below). **'Rate-limiting' calcium-channel blockers** (e.g. diltiazem, verapamil) may be valuable in angina; contra-indications include heart failure and heart block;
- **Alpha-blockers** (section 2.5.4)—a possible indication is prostatism; a contra-indication is urinary incontinence;
- **Angiotensin-II receptor antagonists** (section 2.5.5.2) are alternatives for those who cannot tolerate ACE inhibitors because of persistent dry cough, but they have the same contra-indications as ACE inhibitors.

A single antihypertensive drug is often not adequate and other antihypertensive drugs are usually added in a step-wise manner until control is achieved. Unless it is necessary to lower the blood pressure urgently, an interval of at least 4 weeks should be allowed to determine response. In uncomplicated mild hypertension (systolic blood pressure < 160 mmHg and diastolic < 100 mmHg), drugs may be substituted rather than added.

Response to drug treatment for hypertension may be affected by the patient's ethnic background; in Afro-Caribbean subjects the response to beta-blockers and to ACE inhibitors may be reduced.

OTHER MEASURES TO REDUCE CARDIOVASCULAR RISK. **Aspirin** (section 2.9) in a dose of 75 mg daily reduces the risk of cardiovascular events and myocardial infarction; however, concerns about an increased risk of bleeding need to be considered. Unless it is contra-indicated, aspirin is recommended for *secondary prevention* in patients with cardiovascular complications (myocardial infarction, angina, non-haemorrhagic cerebrovascular disease, peripheral vascular disease, or atherosclerotic renovascular disease), and for *primary prevention* in patients aged over 50 years with controlled blood pressure (systolic pressure < 150 mmHg and diastolic pressure < 90 mmHg) who have end-organ damage, type 2 diabetes, or a coronary heart disease risk[1] ≥ 15% over 10 years.

A **statin** can be of benefit in those at high risk of coronary heart disease and stroke and in those with hypercholesterolaemia (see section 2.12 for details).

HYPERTENSION IN THE ELDERLY. Benefit from antihypertensive therapy is evident up to at least 85 years of age, but it is probably inappropriate to apply a strict age limit when deciding on drug therapy. Elderly individuals who have a good outlook for longevity should have their blood pressure lowered if they are hypertensive. The thresholds for treatment are diastolic pressure averaging ≥ 90 mmHg *or* systolic pressure averaging ≥ 160 mmHg over 3 to 6 months' observation (despite appropriate non-drug

treatment). A low dose of a thiazide is the clear drug of first choice, with addition of a beta-blocker when necessary.

ISOLATED SYSTOLIC HYPERTENSION. Isolated systolic hypertension (systolic pressure ≥ 160 mmHg, diastolic pressure < 90 mmHg) is associated with an increased risk of stroke and coronary events, particularly in those aged over 60 years. Systolic blood pressure averaging 160 mmHg or higher over 3 to 6 months (despite appropriate non-drug treatment) should be lowered in those over 60 years, even if diastolic hypertension is absent. Treatment with a low dose of a thiazide, with addition of a beta-blocker when necessary is effective; a long-acting dihydropyridine calcium-channel blocker is recommended when a thiazide is contra-indicated or not tolerated. Patients with severe postural hypotension should not receive blood pressure lowering drugs.

Isolated systolic hypertension in younger patients is uncommon but treatment may be indicated in those with a threshold systolic pressure of 160 mmHg (or less if at increased risk of coronary heart disease, see above).

HYPERTENSION IN DIABETES. Hypertension is common in type 2 (non-insulin-dependent) diabetes and treatment prevents both macrovascular and microvascular complications. Systolic blood pressure ≥ 140 mmHg *or* diastolic pressure ≥ 90 mmHg should be lowered to a target systolic blood pressure < 140 mmHg and a diastolic pressure < 80 mmHg. Low-dose thiazides, beta-blockers, ACE inhibitors and dihydropyridine calcium-channel blockers have all shown benefit in type 2 diabetes.

In type 1 (insulin-dependent) diabetes, hypertension usually indicates the presence of diabetic nephropathy and ACE inhibitors and angiotensin-II receptor antagonists have a specific role in this condition (section 6.1.5). The threshold for treatment of hypertension in type 1 diabetes is the same as that for type 2 diabetes, and the target for patients without nephropathy is a systolic blood pressure < 140 mmHg and a diastolic pressure < 80 mmHg; if nephropathy is present the target is a systolic blood pressure < 130 mmHg and a diastolic pressure < 80 mmHg, or even lower if proteinuria exceeds 1 g in 24 hours.

HYPERTENSION IN RENAL DISEASE. The threshold for antihypertensive treatment in patients with renal impairment or persistent proteinuria is a systolic blood pressure ≥ 140 mmHg *or* a diastolic blood pressure ≥ 90 mmHg. Optimal blood pressure is a systolic blood pressure < 130 mmHg and a diastolic pressure < 85 mmHg, or lower if proteinuria exceeds 1 g in 24 hours. Thiazides may be ineffective and high doses of loop diuretics may be required. Specific cautions apply to the use of ACE inhibitors in renal impairment, see section 2.5.5.1.

HYPERTENSION IN PREGNANCY. High blood pressure in pregnancy may usually be due to pre-existing essential hypertension or to pre-eclampsia. Methyldopa (section 2.5.2) is safe in pregnancy. Beta-blockers are effective and safe in the third trimester. Modified-release preparations of nifedipine [unlicensed] are also used for hypertension in pregnancy. Intravenous administration of labetalol (section 2.4) can be used to control hypertensive

---

1. Coronary heart disease risk may be formally estimated using the Joint British Societies' 'Cardiac Risk Assessor' computer program or chart (British Cardiac Society, British Hyperlipidaemia Association, British Hypertension Society. *Heart* 1998; **80**(suppl 2): S1–29)

See inside back cover

crises; alternatively hydralazine (section 2.5.1) may be used by the intravenous route. For use of magnesium sulphate in eclampsia, see section 9.5.1.3.

ACCELERATED OR VERY SEVERE HYPERTENSION. Accelerated (or malignant) hypertension or very severe hypertension (e.g. diastolic blood pressure > 140 mmHg) requires urgent treatment in hospital, but it is not an indication for parenteral antihypertensive therapy. Normally treatment should be by mouth with a beta-blocker (atenolol or labetalol) or a long-acting calcium-channel blocker (e.g. amlodipine or modified-release nifedipine). Within the first 24 hours the diastolic blood pressure should be reduced to 100–110 mmHg. Over the next 2 or 3 days blood pressure should be normalised by using beta-blockers, calcium-channel blockers, diuretics, vasodilators, or ACE inhibitors. Very rapid reduction in blood pressure can reduce organ perfusion leading to cerebral infarction and blindness, deterioration in renal function, and myocardial ischaemia. Parenteral antihypertensive drugs are rarely necessary; sodium nitroprusside by infusion is the drug of choice on the rare occasions when parenteral treatment is necessary.

For advice on short-term management of hypertensive episodes in phaeochromocytoma, see under Phaeochromocytoma, section 2.5.4.

2.5.1 Vasodilator antihypertensive drugs

These are potent drugs, especially when used in combination with a beta-blocker and a thiazide.

Important: for a warning on the hazards of a very rapid fall in blood pressure, see section 2.5.

Diazoxide has been used by intravenous injection in hypertensive emergencies.

Hydralazine given by mouth is a useful adjunct to other treatment, but when used alone causes tachycardia and fluid retention. Side-effects can be few if the dose is kept below 100 mg daily, but systemic lupus erythematosus should be suspected if there is unexplained weight loss, arthritis, or any other unexplained ill health.

Sodium nitroprusside is given by intravenous infusion to control severe hypertensive crises on the rare occasions when parenteral treatment is necessary.

Minoxidil should be reserved for the treatment of severe hypertension resistant to other drugs. Vasodilatation is accompanied by increased cardiac output and tachycardia and the patients develop fluid retention. For this reason the addition of a beta-blocker and a diuretic (usually furosemide, in high dosage) are mandatory. Hypertrichosis is troublesome and renders this drug unsuitable for women.

Prazosin, doxazosin, and **terazosin** (section 2.5.4) have alpha-blocking and vasodilator properties.

Bosentan is licensed for the treatment of pulmonary arterial hypertension.

BOSENTAN

Indications: pulmonary arterial hypertension

Cautions: not to be initiated if systemic systolic blood pressure is below 85 mmHg; monitor liver function before and during treatment (reduce dose or suspend treatement if liver enzymes raised significantly)—discontinue if symptoms of liver impairment; monitor haemoglobin; **interactions:** Appendix 1 (bosentan)

Contra-indications: hepatic impairment (Appendix 2); **avoid** pregnancy **during** and for **3 months after** treatment; breast feeding

Side-effects: dyspepsia, flushing, hypotension, palpitations, fatigue, oedema, anaemia, pruritus, nasopharyngitis, hepatic impairment (see Cautions above)

Dose: initially 62.5 mg twice daily increased after 4 weeks to 125 mg twice daily; max. 250 mg twice daily

Tracleer® (Actelion) ▼ PoM
Tablets, f/c, orange, bosentan (as monohydrate) 62.5 mg, net price 56-tab pack = £1615.00; 125 mg, 56-tab pack = £1615.00

DIAZOXIDE

Indications: severe hypertension associated with renal disease (but see section 2.5); hypoglycaemia (section 6.1.4)

Cautions: ischaemic heart disease, pregnancy, labour, impaired renal function; **interactions:** Appendix 1 (diazoxide)

Side-effects: tachycardia, hyperglycaemia, sodium and water retention

Dose: *by rapid intravenous injection* (less than 30 seconds), 1–3 mg/kg to max. single dose of 150 mg (see below); may be repeated after 5–15 minutes if required
NOTE. Single doses of 300 mg have been associated with angina and with myocardial and cerebral infarction

Eudemine® (Goldshield) PoM
Injection, diazoxide 15 mg/mL. Net price 20-mL amp = £30.00

HYDRALAZINE HYDROCHLORIDE

Indications: moderate to severe hypertension (adjunct); heart failure (with long-acting nitrate, but see section 2.5.5); hypertensive crisis (including during pregnancy) (but see section 2.5)

Cautions: hepatic impairment (Appendix 2), renal impairment (Appendix 3); coronary artery disease (may provoke angina, avoid after myocardial infarction until stabilised), cerebrovascular disease; occasionally blood pressure reduction too rapid even with low parenteral doses; pregnancy (Appendix 4), breast-feeding; manufacturer advises test for antinuclear factor and for proteinuria every 6 months and check acetylator status before increasing dose above 100 mg daily, but evidence of clinical value unsatisfactory; **interactions:** Appendix 1 (hydralazine)

Contra-indications: idiopathic systemic lupus erythematosus, severe tachycardia, high output heart failure, myocardial insufficiency due to mechanical obstruction, cor pulmonale, dissecting aortic aneurysm; porphyria (section 9.8.2)

Side-effects: tachycardia, palpitations, flushing, hypotension, fluid retention, gastro-intestinal disturbances; headache, dizziness; systemic lupus erythematosus-like syndrome after long-term therapy with over 100 mg daily (or less in women and in slow acetylator individuals) (see also notes

PERINDOPRIL

Indications: essential and renovascular hypertension (but see notes above); congestive heart failure (adjunct—see section 2.5.5)

Cautions: see notes above

Contra-indications: see notes above

Side-effects: see notes above; asthenia, flushing, mood and sleep disturbances

Dose: hypertension, initially 2 mg daily (before food); usual maintenance dose 4 mg once daily; max. 8 mg daily; if used in addition to diuretic see notes above

Heart failure (adjunct), initial dose 2 mg in the morning under close medical supervision (see notes above); usual maintenance 4 mg once daily (before food)

Coversyl® (Servier) PoM
Tablets, perindopril erbumine (= tert-butylamine) 2 mg, net price 30-tab pack = £10.68; 4 mg (scored), 30-tab pack = £10.68; 8 mg, 30-tab pack = £14.97

■ With diuretic
NOTE. For hypertension not adequately controlled by perindopril alone

Coversyl® **Plus** (Servier) ▼ PoM
Tablets, perindopril erbumine (= tert-butylamine) 4 mg, indapamide 1.25 mg, net price 30-tab pack = £14.97

QUINAPRIL

Indications: essential hypertension; congestive heart failure (adjunct—see section 2.5.5)

Cautions: see notes above

Contra-indications: see notes above

Side-effects: see notes above; asthenia, chest pain, oedema, flatulence, nervousness, depression, insomnia, blurred vision, impotence, back pain and myalgia

Dose: hypertension, initially 10 mg once daily; with a diuretic, in elderly, or in renal impairment initially 2.5 mg daily; usual maintenance dose 20–40 mg daily in single or 2 divided doses; up to 80 mg daily has been given

Heart failure (adjunct), initial dose 2.5 mg under close medical supervision (see notes above); usual maintenance 10–20 mg daily in single or 2 divided doses; up to 40 mg daily has been given

Accupro® (Parke-Davis) PoM
Tablets, all brown, f/c, quinapril (as hydrochloride) 5 mg, net price 28-tab pack = £7.17; 10 mg, 28-tab pack = £7.17; 20 mg, 28-tab pack = £8.99; 40 mg, 28-tab pack = £9.75

■ With diuretic
NOTE. For hypertension in patients stabilised on the individual components in the same proportions

Accuretic® (Parke-Davis) PoM
Tablets, pink, f/c, scored, quinapril (as hydrochloride) 10 mg, hydrochlorothiazide 12.5 mg. Net price 28-tab pack = £9.79

RAMIPRIL

Indications: mild to moderate hypertension; congestive heart failure (adjunct—see section 2.5.5); following myocardial infarction in patients with clinical evidence of heart failure; susceptible

patients over 55 years, prevention of myocardial infarction, stroke, cardiovascular death or need of revascularisation procedures (consult product literature)

Cautions: see notes above

Contra-indications: see notes above

Side-effects: see notes above; arrhythmias, angina, chest pain, syncope, cerebrovascular accident, myocardial infarction, loss of appetite, stomatitis, dry mouth, skin reactions including erythema multiforme and pemphigoid exanthema; precipitation or exacerbation of Raynaud's syndrome; conjunctivitis, onycholysis, confusion, nervousness, depression, anxiety, impotence, decreased libido, alopecia, bronchitis and muscle cramps

Dose: hypertension, initially 1.25 mg once daily, increased at intervals of 1–2 weeks; usual range 2.5–5 mg once daily; max. 10 mg once daily; if used in addition to diuretic see notes above

Heart failure (adjunct), initially 1.25 mg once daily under close medical supervision (see notes above), increased if necessary at intervals of 1–2 weeks; max. 10 mg daily (daily doses of 2.5 mg or more may be taken in 1–2 divided doses) (see also section 2.5.5)

Prophylaxis after myocardial infarction (started in hospital 3 to 10 days after infarction), initially 2.5 mg twice daily, increased after 2 days to 5 mg twice daily; maintenance 2.5–5 mg twice daily
NOTE. If initial 2.5-mg dose not tolerated, give 1.25 mg twice daily for 2 days before increasing to 2.5 mg twice daily, then 5 mg twice daily; withdraw if 2.5 mg twice daily not tolerated

Prophylaxis of cardiovascular events or stroke, initially 2.5 mg once daily, increased after 1 week to 5 mg once daily, then increased after a further 3 weeks to 10 mg once daily

Tritace® (Aventis Pharma) PoM
Capsules, ramipril 1.25 mg (yellow/white), net price 28-cap pack = £5.30; 2.5 mg (orange/white), 7-cap pack = £1.88, 28-cap pack = £7.51; 5 mg (red/white), 28-cap pack = £10.46; 10 mg (blue/white), 28-cap pack = £14.24; 35-day starter pack of 7 × 2.5 mg with 21 × 5 mg, and 7 × 10 mg = £13.00

■ With calcium-channel blocker
NOTE. For hypertension in patients stabilised on the individual components in the same proportions, but combination with calcium-channel blocker not first-line treatment. For cautions, contra-indications and side-effects of felodipine, see section 2.6.2

Triapin® (Aventis Pharma) ▼ PoM ▱
Triapin® *tablets*, f/c, brown, ramipril 5 mg, felodipine 5 mg (m/r), net price 28-tab pack = £24.46. Label: 25
Triapin mite® *tablets*, f/c, orange, ramipril 2.5 mg, felodipine 2.5 mg (m/r), net price 28-tab pack = £19.37. Label: 25

TRANDOLAPRIL

Indications: mild to moderate hypertension; following myocardial infarction in patients with left ventricular dysfunction; heart failure [unlicensed] see section 2.5.5

Cautions: see notes above

Contra-indications: see notes above

Side-effects: see notes above; tachycardia, arrhythmias, angina, transient ischaemic attacks, cerebral haemorrhage, myocardial infarction; ileus, dry mouth; skin reactions including Stevens-Johnson syndrome, toxic epidermal necrolysis, psoriasislike efflorescence; asthenia, alopecia, dyspnoea and bronchitis

Dose: hypertension, initially 500 micrograms once daily, increased at intervals of 2–4 weeks; usual range 1–2 mg once daily; max. 4 mg daily; if used in addition to diuretic see notes above

Prophylaxis after myocardial infarction (starting as early as 3 days after infarction), initially 500 micrograms daily, gradually increased to max. 4 mg once daily

NOTE. If symptomatic hypotension develops during titration, do not increase dose further; if possible, reduce dose of any adjunctive treatment and if this is not effective or feasible, reduce dose of trandolapril

Gopten® (Abbott) PoM
Capsules, trandolapril 500 micrograms (red/yellow), net price 14-cap pack = £2.65; 1 mg (red/orange), 28-cap pack = £12.28; 2 mg (red/red), 28-cap pack = £8.39

Odrik® (Hoechst Marion Roussel) PoM
Capsules, trandolapril 500 micrograms (red/yellow), net price 28-cap pack = £8.19; 1 mg (red/orange), 28-cap pack = £10.34; 2 mg (red/red), 28-cap pack = £12.29

■ With calcium-channel blocker
NOTE. For hypertension in patients stabilised on the individual components in the same proportions, but combination with calcium-channel blocker not first-line treatment. For cautions, contra-indications and side-effects of verapamil, see section 2.6.2

Tarka® (Abbott) ▼ PoM ▭
Capsules, pink, trandolapril 2 mg, verapamil hydrochloride 180 mg (m/r). Net price 28 cap-pack = £17.85. Label: 25

2.5.5.2 Angiotensin-II receptor antagonists

Candesartan, **irbesartan**, **losartan**, and **valsartan** are specific angiotensin-II receptor antagonists with many properties similar to those of the ACE inhibitors; **eprosartan**, **olmesartan**, and **telmisartan** have been introduced more recently. However, unlike ACE inhibitors, they do not inhibit the breakdown of bradykinin and other kinins, and thus do not appear to cause the persistent dry cough which commonly complicates ACE inhibitor therapy. They are therefore a useful alternative for patients who have to discontinue an ACE inhibitor because of persistent cough.

An angiotensin-II receptor antagonist may be used as an alternative to an ACE inhibitor in the management of heart failure [unlicensed indication] (section 2.5.5) or diabetic nephropathy (section 6.1.5).

CAUTIONS. Angiotensin-II receptor antagonists should be used with caution in renal artery stenosis (see also Renal Effects under ACE Inhibitors, section 2.5.5.1). Monitoring of plasma-potassium concentration is advised, particularly in the elderly and in patients with renal impairment; lower initial doses may be appropriate in these patients. Angiotensin-II receptor antagonists should be used with caution in

aortic or mitral valve stenosis and in obstructive hypertrophic cardiomyopathy. **Interactions:** Appendix 1 (as for ACE inhibitors).

CONTRA-INDICATIONS. Angiotensin-II receptor antagonists, like the ACE inhibitors, should be avoided in pregnancy (see also Appendix 4).

SIDE-EFFECTS. Side-effects are usually mild. Symptomatic hypotension may occur, particularly in patients with intravascular volume depletion (e.g. those taking high-dose diuretics). Hyperkalaemia occurs occasionally; angioedema has also been reported with some angiotensin-II receptor antagonists.

CANDESARTAN CILEXETIL

Indications: hypertension (see also notes above)

Cautions: see notes above; hepatic and renal impairment (Appendixes 2 and 3)

Contra-indications: see notes above; breast-feeding (Appendix 5), cholestasis

Side-effects: see notes above; also upper respiratory-tract and influenza-like symptoms including rhinitis and pharyngitis; abdominal pain, back pain, arthralgia, myalgia, nausea, headache, dizziness, peripheral oedema, rash also reported; rarely urticaria, pruritus, blood disorders reported

Dose: initially 4 mg (2 mg in hepatic and renal impairment) once daily adjusted according to response; usual maintenance dose 8 mg once daily; max. 16 mg once daily

Amias® (AstraZeneca, Takeda) PoM
Tablets, candesartan cilexetil 2 mg, net price 7-tab pack = £2.99; 4 mg (scored), 7-tab pack = £3.24; 28-tab pack = £12.95; 8 mg (pink, scored), 28-tab pack = £14.95; 16 mg (pink, scored), 28-tab pack = £17.75

EPROSARTAN

Indications: hypertension (see also notes above)

Cautions: see notes above; also renal impairment (Appendix 3); breast-feeding (Appendix 5)

Contra-indications: see notes above; also severe hepatic impairment (Appendix 2)

Side-effects: see notes above; also flatulence, dizziness, arthralgia, rhinitis; hypertriglyceridaemia, rarely anaemia

Dose: 600 mg once daily (elderly over 75 years, mild to moderate hepatic impairment, renal impairment, initially 300 mg once daily); if necessary increased after 2–3 weeks to 800 mg once daily

Teveten® (Solvay) PoM
Tablets, f/c, eprosartan (as mesilate) 300 mg, net price 28-tab pack = £12.50; 400 mg, 56-tab pack = £16.96; 600 mg, 28-tab pack = £14.75. Label: 21

IRBESARTAN

Indications: hypertension; renal disease in hypertensive type 2 diabetes mellitus (see also notes above)

Cautions: see notes above

Contra-indications: see notes above; breast-feeding (Appendix 5)

Nimodipine is related to nifedipine but the smooth muscle relaxant effect preferentially acts on cerebral arteries. Its use is confined to prevention of *vascular spasm following aneurysmal subarachnoid haemorrhage.*

Diltiazem is effective in most forms of *angina* (section 2.6); the longer-acting formulation is also used for *hypertension.* It may be used in patients for whom beta-blockers are contra-indicated or ineffective. It has a less negative inotropic effect than verapamil and significant myocardial depression occurs rarely. Nevertheless because of the risk of bradycardia it should be used with caution in association with beta-blockers.

UNSTABLE ANGINA. Calcium-channel blockers do not reduce the risk of myocardial infarction in unstable angina. The use of diltiazem or verapamil should be reserved for patients resistant to treatment with beta-blockers.

WITHDRAWAL. There is some evidence that sudden withdrawal of calcium-channel blockers may be associated with an exacerbation of angina.

AMLODIPINE BESILATE

Indications: hypertension, prophylaxis of angina

Cautions: hepatic impairment; **interactions:** Appendix 1 (calcium-channel blockers)

Contra-indications: cardiogenic shock, unstable angina, significant aortic stenosis; pregnancy and breast-feeding

Side-effects: headache, oedema, fatigue, nausea, flushing, dizziness, gum hyperplasia, rashes (including rarely pruritus and very rarely erythema multiforme); rarely gastro-intestinal disturbances, dry mouth, sweating, palpitations, dyspnoea, drowsiness, mood changes, myalgia, arthralgia, asthenia, peripheral neuropathy, impotence, increased urinary frequency, visual disturbances; also reported, jaundice, pancreatitis, hyperglycaemia, thrombocytopenia, vasculitis, angioedema, alopecia, gynaecomastia

Dose: hypertension or angina, initially 5 mg once daily; max. 10 mg once daily

Istin※ (Pfizer) [PoM]
Tablets, amlodipine (as besilate) 5 mg. Net price 28-tab pack = £11.85; 10 mg, 28-tab pack = £17.70

DILTIAZEM HYDROCHLORIDE

Indications: prophylaxis and treatment of angina; hypertension

Cautions: reduce dose in hepatic and renal impairment; heart failure or significantly impaired left ventricular function, bradycardia (avoid if severe), first degree AV block, or prolonged PR interval; **interactions:** Appendix 1 (calcium-channel blockers)

Contra-indications: severe bradycardia, left ventricular failure with pulmonary congestion, second- or third-degree AV block (unless pacemaker fitted), sick sinus syndrome; pregnancy and breast-feeding (see Appendixes 4 and 5)

Side-effects: bradycardia, sino-atrial block, AV block, palpitations, dizziness, hypotension, malaise, asthenia, headache, hot flushes, gastrointestinal disturbances, oedema (notably of ankles); rarely rashes (including erythema multi-

forme and exfoliative dermatitis), photosensitivity; hepatitis, gynaecomastia, gum hyperplasia, extrapyramidal symptoms, depression reported

Dose: angina, 60 mg 3 times daily (elderly initially twice daily); increased if necessary to 360 mg daily
Longer-acting formulations, see under preparations below

■ Standard formulations
NOTE. These formulations are licensed as generics and there is no requirement for brand name dispensing. Although their means of formulation has called for the strict designation 'modified-release' their duration of action corresponds to that of tablets requiring administration 3 times daily

Diltiazem (Non-proprietary) [PoM]
Tablets, m/r (but see note above), diltiazem hydrochloride 60 mg. Net price 100 = £5.25. Label: 25
Available from Alpharma, APS, Ashbourne (*Angiozem*※), Hillcross, IVAX, Niche, Opus (*Optil*※), Sterwin

Tildiem※ (Sanofi-Synthelabo) [PoM]
Tablets, m/r (but see note above), off-white, diltiazem hydrochloride 60 mg. Net price 90-tab pack = £8.28. Label: 25

■ Longer-acting formulations
NOTE. Different versions of modified-release preparations may not have the same clinical effect. To avoid confusion between these different formulations of diltiazem, prescribers should specify the brand to be dispensed

Adizem-SR※ (Napp) [PoM]
Capsules, m/r, diltiazem hydrochloride 90 mg (white), net price 56-cap pack = £10.56; 120 mg (brown/white), 56-cap pack = £11.74; 180 mg (brown/white), 56-cap pack = £17.60. Label: 25
Tablets, m/r, f/c, scored, diltiazem hydrochloride 120 mg. Net price 56-tab pack = £17.32. Label: 25
Dose: mild to moderate hypertension, usually 120 mg twice daily (dose form not appropriate for initial dose titration)
Angina, initially 90 mg twice daily (elderly, dose form not appropriate for initial dose titration); increased to 180 mg twice daily if required

Adizem-XL※ (Napp) [PoM]
Capsules, m/r, diltiazem hydrochloride 120 mg (pink/blue), net price 28-cap pack = £10.24; 180 mg (dark pink/blue), 28-cap pack = £11.61; 240 mg (red/blue), 28-cap pack = £12.90; 300 mg (maroon/blue), 28-cap pack = £10.24. Label: 25
Dose: angina and mild to moderate hypertension, initially 240 mg once daily, increased if necessary to 300 mg once daily; in elderly and in hepatic or renal impairment, initially 120 mg daily

Angitil SR※ (Trinity) [PoM]
Capsules, m/r, diltiazem hydrochloride 90 mg (white), net price 56-cap pack = £8.45; 120 mg (brown), 56-cap pack = £9.39; 180 mg (brown), 56-cap pack = £14.08. Label: 25
Dose: angina and mild to moderate hypertension, initially 90 mg twice daily; increased if necessary to 120 mg or 180 mg twice daily
NOTE. Also available as *Disogram*※ *SR* (Ranbaxy)

Angitil XL※ (Trinity) [PoM]
Capsules, m/r, diltiazem hydrochloride 240 mg (white), net price 28-cap pack = £10.15; 300 mg (yellow), 28-cap pack = £9.22. Label: 25
Dose: angina and mild to moderate hypertension, initially 240 mg once daily (elderly and in hepatic and renal

impairment, dose form not appropriate for initial dose titration); increased if necessary to 300 mg once daily NOTE. Also available as *Disogram*® SR (Ranbaxy)

Calcicard CR® (IVAX) PoM
Tablets, m/r, both f/c, diltiazem hydrochloride 90 mg, net price 56-tab pack = £6.33; 120 mg, 56-tab pack = £7.04. Label: 25
Dose: mild to moderate hypertension, initially 90 mg or 120 mg twice daily; up to 360 mg daily may be required: ELDERLY and in hepatic and renal impairment, initially 120 mg once daily; up to 240 mg daily may be required
Angina, initially 90 mg or 120 mg twice daily; up to 480 mg daily in divided doses may be required; ELDERLY and in hepatic and renal impairment, dose form not appropriate for initial dose titration; up to 240 mg daily may be required
NOTE. Also available as *Angiozem CR*® (Ashbourne)

Dilcardia SR® (Generics) PoM
Capsules, m/r, diltiazem hydrochloride 60 mg (pink/white), net price 56-cap pack = £8.13; 90 mg (pink/yellow), 56-cap pack = £10.33; 120 mg (pink/orange), 56-cap pack = £11.49. Label: 25
Dose: angina and mild to moderate hypertension, initially 90 mg twice daily; increased if necessary to 180 mg twice daily; ELDERLY and in hepatic or renal impairment, initially 60 mg twice daily, max. 90 mg twice daily

Dilzem SR® (Elan) PoM
Capsules, m/r, all beige, diltiazem hydrochloride 60 mg, net price 56-cap pack = £8.32; 90 mg, 56-cap pack = £11.23; 120 mg, 56-cap pack = £12.47. Label: 25
Dose: angina and mild to moderate hypertension, initially 90 mg twice daily (elderly 60 mg twice daily); up to 180 mg twice daily may be required

Dilzem XL® (Elan) PoM
Capsules, m/r, diltiazem hydrochloride 120 mg, net price 28-cap pack = £8.32; 180 mg, 28-cap pack = £11.40; 240 mg, 28-cap pack = £11.70. Label: 25
Dose: angina and mild to moderate hypertension, initially 180 mg once daily (elderly and in hepatic and renal impairment, 120 mg once daily); if necessary may be increased to 360 mg once daily

Slozem® (Merck) PoM
Capsules, m/r, diltiazem hydrochloride 120 mg (pink/clear), net price 28-cap pack = £7.00; 180 mg (pink/clear), 28-cap pack = £7.80; 240 mg (red/clear), 28-cap pack = £8.20; 300 mg (red/white), 28-cap pack = £8.50. Label: 25
Dose: angina and mild to moderate hypertension, initially 240 mg once daily (elderly and in hepatic and renal impairment, 120 mg once daily); if necessary may be increased to 360 mg once daily

Tildiem LA® (Sanofi-Synthelabo) PoM
Capsules, m/r, diltiazem hydrochloride 200 mg (pink/grey, containing white pellets), net price 28-cap pack = £11.61; 300 mg (white/yellow, containing white pellets), 28-cap pack = £12.80. Label: 25
Dose: angina and mild to moderate hypertension, initially 200 mg once daily before or with food, increased if necessary to 300–400 mg daily, max. 500 mg daily; ELDERLY and in hepatic or renal impairment, initially 200 mg daily, increased if necessary to 300 mg daily

Tildiem Retard® (Sanofi-Synthelabo) PoM
Tablets, m/r, diltiazem hydrochloride 90 mg, net price 56-tab pack = £9.95; 120 mg, 56-tab pack = £11.06. Label: 25
COUNSELLING. Tablet membrane may pass through gastro-intestinal tract unchanged, but being porous has no effect on efficacy
Dose: mild to moderate hypertension, initially 90 mg or 120 mg twice daily; increased if necessary to 360 mg daily in divided doses; ELDERLY and in hepatic or renal impairment, initially 120 mg once daily; increased if necessary to 120 mg twice daily
Angina, initially 90 mg or 120 mg twice daily; increased if necessary to 480 mg daily in divided doses; ELDERLY and in hepatic or renal impairment, dose form not appropriate for initial titration; up to 120 mg twice daily may be required

Viazem XL® (Genus) PoM
Capsules, m/r, diltiazem hydrochloride 120 mg (lavender), net price 28-cap pack = £6.95; 180 mg (white/blue-green), 28-cap pack = £7.75; 240 mg (blue-green/lavender), 28-cap pack = £8.15; 300 mg (white/lavender), 28-cap pack = £8.45; 360 mg (blue-green), 28-cap pack = £14.95. Label: 25
Dose: angina and mild to moderate hypertension, initially 180 mg once daily, adjusted according to response to 240 mg once daily; max. 360 mg once daily; ELDERLY and in hepatic or renal impairment, initially 120 mg once daily, adjusted according to response

Zemtard® (Galen) PoM
Zemtard 120XL capsules, m/r, brown/orange, diltiazem hydrochloride 120 mg, net price 28-cap pack = £7.65. Label: 25
Zemtard 180XL capsules, m/r, grey/pink, diltiazem hydrochloride 180 mg, net price 28-cap pack = £7.80. Label: 25
Zemtard 240XL capsules, m/r, blue, diltiazem hydrochloride 240 mg, net price 28-cap pack = £8.20. Label: 25
Zemtard 300XL capsules, m/r, white/blue, diltiazem hydrochloride 300 mg, net price 28-cap pack = £8.50. Label: 25
Dose: angina and mild to moderate hypertension, 180–300 mg once daily, increased if necessary to 360 mg once daily in hypertension and to 480 mg once daily in angina; ELDERLY and in hepatic or renal impairment, initially 120 mg once daily

FELODIPINE

Indications: hypertension, prophylaxis of angina
Cautions: withdraw if ischaemic pain occurs or existing pain worsens shortly after initiating treatment or if cardiogenic shock develops; severe left ventricular dysfunction; hepatic impairment; breast-feeding; avoid grapefruit juice (may affect metabolism); **interactions:** Appendix 1 (calcium-channel blockers)
Contra-indications: pregnancy; unstable angina, uncontrolled heart failure; significant aortic stenosis; within 1 month of myocardial infarction
Side-effects: flushing, headache, palpitations, dizziness, fatigue, gravitational oedema; rarely rash, pruritus, cutaneous vasculitis, gum hyperplasia, urinary frequency, impotence, fever
Dose: hypertension, initially 5 mg (elderly 2.5 mg) daily in the morning; usual maintenance 5–10 mg once daily; doses above 20 mg daily rarely needed
Angina, initially 5 mg daily in the morning, increased if necessary to 10 mg once daily

dilator treatment, which is most often successful in primary Raynaud's syndrome. **Nifedipine** (section 2.6.2) is useful for reducing the frequency and severity of vasospastic attacks. Alternatively, **naftidrofuryl** may produce symptomatic improvement; **inositol nicotinate** (a nicotinic acid derivative) may also be considered. Cinnarizine, pentoxifylline, prazosin and moxisylyte (thymoxamine) are not established as being effective.

Vasodilator therapy is not established as being effective for *chilblains* (section 13.14).

CILOSTAZOL

Indications: intermittent claudication in patients without rest pain and no peripheral tissue necrosis

Cautions: atrial or ventricular ectopy, atrial fibrillation, atrial flutter; diabetes mellitus (higher risk of intra-ocular bleeding); **interactions:** Appendix 1 (cilostazol)

Contra-indications: predisposition to bleeding (e.g. active peptic ulcer, haemorrhagic stroke in previous 6 months, surgery in previous 3 months, proliferative diabetic retinopathy, poorly controlled hypertension); history of ventricular tachycardia, of ventricular fibrillation and of multifocal ventricular ectopics, prolongation of QT interval, congestive heart failure; moderate or severe hepatic impairment (Appendix 2), renal impairment (Appendix 3); pregnancy (Appendix 4) and breast-feeding (Appendix 5)

Side-effects: diarrhoea, abnormal stools, and headache are very common; nausea, vomiting, dyspepsia, flatulence, abdominal pain; tachycardia, palpitation, angina, arrhythmia, chest pain; rhinitis; dizziness; ecchymosis; rash, pruritus; oedema, asthenia; less commonly, gastritis, myocardial infarction, congestive heart failure, postural hypotension, insomnia, anxiety, abnormal dreams, dyspnoea, pneumonia, cough, hypersensitivity reactions, diabetes mellitus, anaemia, haemorrhage, thrombocythaemia, myalgia, renal impairment

Dose: 100 mg twice daily (30 minutes before or 2 hours after food)

Pletal (Otsuka) ▼ PoM
Tablets, cilostazol 100 mg, net price 56-tab pack = £35.31

CINNARIZINE

Indications: peripheral vascular disease, Raynaud's syndrome

Cautions: see section 4.6

Contra-indications: see section 4.6

Side-effects: see section 4.6

Dose: initially, 75 mg 3 times daily; maintenance, 75 mg 2–3 times daily

Stugeron Forte (Janssen-Cilag)
Capsules, orange/ivory, cinnarizine 75 mg. Net price 100-cap pack = £5.50. Label: 2

Stugeron
See section 4.6

MOXISYLYTE/THYMOXAMINE

Indications: primary Raynaud's syndrome (short-term treatment)

Cautions: diabetes mellitus

Contra-indications: active liver disease

Side-effects: nausea, diarrhoea, flushing, headache, dizziness; hepatic reactions including cholestatic jaundice and hepatitis reported to CSM

Dose: initially 40 mg 4 times daily, increased to 80 mg 4 times daily if poor initial response; discontinue after 2 weeks if no response

Opilon (Hansam) PoM
Tablets, yellow, f/c, moxisylyte 40 mg (as hydrochloride). Net price 112-tab pack = £79.98. Label: 21

NAFTIDROFURYL OXALATE

Indications: see under Dose

Side-effects: nausea, epigastric pain, rash, hepatitis, hepatic failure

Dose: peripheral vascular disease (see notes above), 100–200 mg 3 times daily; cerebral vascular disease, 100 mg 3 times daily

Naftidrofuryl (Non-proprietary) PoM
Capsules, naftidrofuryl oxalate 100 mg. Net price 84-cap pack = £7.63. Label: 25, 27
Available from Alpharma

Praxilene (Merck) PoM
Capsules, pink, naftidrofuryl oxalate 100 mg. Net price 84-cap pack = £8.60. Label: 25, 27

NICOTINIC ACID DERIVATIVES

Indications: peripheral vascular disease; hyperlipidaemia (section 2.12)

Side-effects: flushing, dizziness, nausea, vomiting, hypotension (more frequent with nicotinic acid than derivatives); occasional diabetogenic effect reported with nicotinic acid and nicotinyl alcohol; rarely associated with nodular changes to liver (monitor on prolonged high dosage)

Hexopal (Sanofi-Synthelabo)
Tablets, scored, inositol nicotinate 500 mg. Net price 20 = £4.10
Dose: 1 g 3 times daily, increased to 4 g daily if required
Tablets forte, scored, inositol nicotinate 750 mg. Net price 112-tab pack = £34.02
Dose: 1.5 g twice daily

PENTOXIFYLLINE/OXPENTIFYLLINE

Indications: peripheral vascular disease; venous leg ulcers [unlicensed indication] (Appendix A8.2.5)

Cautions: hypotension, coronary artery disease; renal impairment (Appendix 3), severe hepatic impairment; avoid in porphyria (section 9.8.2); **interactions:** Appendix 1 (pentoxifylline)

Contra-indications: cerebral haemorrhage, extensive retinal haemorrhage, acute myocardial infarction; pregnancy and breast-feeding

Side-effects: gastro-intestinal disturbances, dizziness, agitation, sleep disturbances, headache; rarely flushing, tachycardia, angina, hypotension, thrombocytopenia, intrahepatic cholestasis, hypersensitivity reactions including rash, pruritus and bronchospasm

Dose: 400 mg 2–3 times daily

Trental (Aventis Pharma) PoM
Tablets, m/r, pink, s/c, pentoxifylline 400 mg. Net price 90-tab pack = £23.81. Label: 21, 25

Contra-indications: hypertension (monitor blood pressure and rate of flow frequently), pregnancy
Side-effects: hypertension, headache, bradycardia, arrhythmias, peripheral ischaemia
Dose: acute hypotension, *by intravenous infusion*, via central venous catheter, of a solution containing noradrenaline acid tartrate 80 micrograms/mL (equivalent to noradrenaline base 40 micrograms/mL) at an initial rate of 0.16–0.33 mL/minute, adjusted according to response
Cardiac arrest, *by rapid intravenous or intracardiac injection*, 0.5–0.75 mL of a solution containing noradrenaline acid tartrate 200 micrograms/mL (equivalent to noradrenaline base 100 micrograms/mL)

Noradrenaline/Norepinephrine (Non-proprietary) ▢PoM▢
Injection, noradrenaline acid tartrate 2 mg/mL (equivalent to noradrenaline base 1 mg/mL). For dilution before use. Net price 2-mL amp = £1.01, 20-mL amp = £6.35
Available from Abbott

PHENYLEPHRINE HYDROCHLORIDE

Indications: acute hypotension (see notes above)
Cautions: see under Noradrenaline Acid Tartrate; longer duration of action than noradrenaline (norepinephrine), see below; coronary disease
HYPERTENSIVE RESPONSE. Phenylephrine has a longer duration of action than noradrenaline, and an excessive vasopressor response may cause a prolonged rise in blood pressure
Contra-indications: see under Noradrenaline Acid Tartrate; severe hyperthyroidism
Side-effects: see under Noradrenaline Acid Tartrate; tachycardia and reflex bradycardia
Dose: *by subcutaneous or intramuscular injection*, 2–5 mg, followed if necessary by further doses of 1–10 mg
By slow intravenous injection of a 1 mg/mL solution, 100–500 micrograms repeated as necessary after at least 15 minutes
By intravenous infusion, initial rate up to 180 micrograms/minute reduced to 30–60 micrograms/minute according to response

Phenylephrine (Sovereign) ▢PoM▢
Injection, phenylephrine hydrochloride 10 mg/mL (1%). Net price 1-mL amp = £5.00

2.7.3 Cardiopulmonary resuscitation

The algorithm for cardiopulmonary resuscitation (see inside back cover) reflects the most recent recommendations of the Resuscitation Council (UK). In cardiac arrest **adrenaline (epinephrine)** 1 in 10 000 (100 micrograms/mL) is recommended in a dose of 10 mL by intravenous injection, preferably through a central line. If injected through a peripheral line, the drug must be flushed with at least 20 mL sodium chloride 0.9% injection (to aid entry into the central circulation). Intravenous injection of **amiodarone** 300 mg (from a prefilled syringe *or* diluted in glucose intravenous infusion 5%) should be considered after adrenaline to treat ventricular fibrillation or pulseless ventricular tachycardia in cardiac arrest refractory to defibrillation. **Atropine** 3 mg by

intravenous injection (section 15.1.3) as a single dose is also used in cardiopulmonary resuscitation to block vagal activity.
For the management of acute anaphylaxis see section 3.4.3.

ADRENALINE/EPINEPHRINE

Indications: see notes above
Cautions: heart disease, diabetes mellitus, hyperthyroidism, hypertension, arrhythmias, cerebrovascular disease, angle-closure glaucoma, avoid during second stage of labour; **interactions:** Appendix 1 (sympathomimetics)
Side-effects: anxiety, tremor, tachycardia, headache, cold extremities; in overdosage arrhythmias, cerebral haemorrhage, pulmonary oedema; nausea, vomiting, sweating, weakness, dizziness and hyperglycaemia also reported
Dose: see notes above

Adrenaline/Epinephrine I in 10 000, Dilute (Non-proprietary) ▢PoM▢
Injection, adrenaline (as acid tartrate) 100 micrograms/mL. 10-mL amp.
Available from Aurum, Martindale (special order); also from Aurum (1-mL and 10-mL prefilled syringe), Celltech (*Minijet® Adrenaline* 3- and 10-mL disposable syringes)

2.8 Anticoagulants and protamine

2.8.1	Parenteral anticoagulants
2.8.2	Oral anticoagulants
2.8.3	Protamine sulphate

The main use of anticoagulants is to prevent thrombus formation or extension of an existing thrombus in the slower-moving venous side of the circulation, where the thrombus consists of a fibrin web enmeshed with platelets and red cells. They are therefore widely used in the prevention and treatment of *deep-vein thrombosis in the legs*.
Anticoagulants are of less use in preventing thrombus formation in arteries, for in faster-flowing vessels thrombi are composed mainly of platelets with little fibrin. They are used to prevent thrombi forming on *prosthetic heart valves*.

2.8.1 Parenteral anticoagulants

Heparin

Heparin initiates anticoagulation rapidly but has a short duration of action. It is now often referred to as being **standard** or **unfractionated heparin** to distinguish it from the **low molecular weight heparins** (see p. 113), which have a longer duration of action.

TREATMENT. For the initial treatment of *deep-vein thrombosis and pulmonary embolism* heparin is given as an *intravenous loading dose,* followed by *continuous intravenous infusion* (using an infusion pump) or by *intermittent subcutaneous injection*; the

ABCIXIMAB

Indications: prevention of ischaemic cardiac complications in patients undergoing percutaneous coronary intervention; short-term prevention of myocardial infarction in patients with unstable angina not responding to conventional treatment and who are scheduled for percutaneous coronary intervention (use under specialist supervision)

Cautions: measure baseline prothrombin time, activated partial thromboplastin time, platelet count, haemoglobin and haematocrit; monitor haemoglobin and haematocrit 12 hours and 24 hours after start of treatment and platelet count 2–4 hours and 24 hours after start of treatment; concomitant use of drugs that increase risk of bleeding; discontinue if uncontrollable serious bleeding occurs or emergency cardiac surgery needed; consult product literature for details of procedures to minimise bleeding; pregnancy (Appendix 4)

Contra-indications: active internal bleeding, major surgery, intracranial or intraspinal surgery or trauma within last 2 months, stroke within last 2 years; intracranial neoplasm, arteriovenous malformation or aneurysm, severe hypertension, haemorrhagic diathesis, thrombocytopenia, vasculitis, hypertensive or diabetic retinopathy; severe hepatic or renal impairment (Appendixes 2 and 3); breast-feeding

Side-effects: bleeding manifestations; nausea, vomiting, hypotension, bradycardia, chest pain, back pain, headache, fever, puncture site pain, thrombocytopenia; rarely cardiac tamponade, adult respiratory distress, hypersensitivity reactions

Dose: ADULT initially *by intravenous injection* over 1 minute, 250 micrograms/kg, then *by intravenous infusion*, 125 nanograms/kg/minute (max. 10 micrograms/minute); for prevention of ischaemic complications start 10–60 minutes before percutaneous coronary intervention and continue infusion for 12 hours; for unstable angina start up to 24 hours before possible percutaneous coronary intervention and continue infusion for 12 hours after intervention

ReoProℝ (Lilly) [PoM]
Injection, abciximab 2 mg/mL, net price 5-mL vial = £280.00

ASPIRIN (antiplatelet)
(Acetylsalicylic Acid)

Indications: prophylaxis of cerebrovascular disease or myocardial infarction (see section 2.10.1 and notes above)

Cautions: asthma; uncontrolled hypertension; pregnancy (but see Appendix 4); **interactions:** Appendix 1 (aspirin)

Contra-indications: children under 16 years and in breast-feeding (Reye's syndrome, section 4.7.1); active peptic ulceration; haemophilia and other bleeding disorders

Side-effects: bronchospasm; gastro-intestinal haemorrhage (occasionally major), also other haemorrhage (e.g. subconjunctival)

Dose: see notes above

ᴵ**Aspirin** (Non-proprietary) [PoM]
Dispersible tablets, aspirin 75 mg, net price 20 = 13p; 300 mg, see section 4.7.1. Label: 13, 21, 32
Tablets, e/c, aspirin 75 mg, net price 56-tab pack = £3.03; 300 mg, see section 4.7.1. Label: 5, 25, 32
Available from Dexcel (*Micropirin*ℝ), Galen, Genus (*Gencardia*ℝ), Lagap

Angettes 75ℝ (Bristol-Myers Squibb)
Tablets, aspirin 75 mg. Net price 28-tab pack = 94p. Label: 32

Caprinℝ (Sinclair) [PoM]
Tablets, e/c, pink, aspirin 75 mg, net price 56-tab pack = £3.08; 300 mg, see section 4.7.1. Label: 5, 25, 32

Nu-Sealsℝ **Aspirin** (Alliance) [PoM]
Tablets, e/c, aspirin 75 mg, net price 56-tab pack = £3.09; 300 mg, see section 4.7.1. Label: 5, 25, 32
NOTE. Tablets may be chewed at diagnosis for rapid absorption

■ With isosorbide mononitrate
Section 2.6.1

CLOPIDOGREL

Indications: prevention of atherosclerotic events in peripheral arterial disease, or within 35 days of myocardial infarction, or within 6 months of ischaemic stroke, or (given with aspirin—see notes above) in acute coronary syndrome without ST-segment-elevation

Cautions: avoid for first few days after myocardial infarction and for 7 days after ischaemic stroke; patients at risk of increased bleeding from trauma, surgery or other pathological conditions; discontinue 7 days before elective surgery if antiplatelet effect not desirable; liver impairment (Appendix 2), renal impairment (Appendix 4); pregnancy (Appendix 4); **interactions:** Appendix 1 (clopidogrel)

Contra-indications: active bleeding, breast-feeding

Side-effects: haemorrhage (including gastro-intestinal and intracranial); other side-effects reported include abdominal discomfort, nausea, vomiting, diarrhoea, constipation, gastric and duodenal ulceration; headache, dizziness, vertigo, paraesthesia; rash, pruritus; hepatic and biliary disorders, neutropenia, thrombotic thrombocytopenic purpura, isolated report of aplastic anaemia

Dose: 75 mg once daily
Acute coronary syndrome, initially 300 mg then 75 mg daily (with aspirin, but see notes above)

Plavixℝ (Bristol-Myers Squibb, Sanofi-Synthelabo) [PoM]
Tablets, pink, f/c, clopidogrel (as hydrogen sulphate) 75 mg, net price 28-tab pack = £35.31

DIPYRIDAMOLE

Indications: see notes above and under Dose

Cautions: rapidly worsening angina, aortic stenosis, recent myocardial infarction, heart failure; may exacerbate migraine; hypotension; **interactions:** Appendix 1 (dipyridamole)

1. Aspirin tablets 75 mg may be sold to the public in packs of up to 100 tablets; for details relating to other strengths see section 4.7.1 and *Medicines, Ethics and Practice*, No. 27, London, Pharmaceutical Press, 2003 (and subsequent editions as available)

Side-effects: gastro-intestinal effects, dizziness, myalgia, throbbing headache, hypotension, hot flushes and tachycardia; worsening symptoms of coronary heart disease; hypersensitivity reactions such as rash, urticaria, severe bronchospasm and angioedema; increased bleeding during or after surgery; thrombocytopenia reported

Dose: *by mouth*, 300–600 mg daily in 3–4 divided doses before food
Modified-release preparations, see under preparation below
By intravenous injection, diagnostic only, consult product literature

Dipyridamole (Non-proprietary) PoM
Tablets, coated, dipyridamole 25 mg, net price 20 = 40p; 100 mg, 20 = £1.09; 84 = £4.57. Label: 22
Available from Alpharma, Ashbourne (*Cerebrovase*®), Hillcross, IVAX
Oral suspension, dipyridamole 50 mg/5 ml, net price 150 mL = £34.00
Available from Rosemont (sugar-free)

Persantin® (Boehringer Ingelheim) PoM
Tablets, both s/c, dipyridamole 25 mg (orange), net price 84-tab pack = £1.70; 100 mg, 84-tab pack = £4.73. Label: 22
Injection, dipyridamole 5 mg/mL. Net price 2-mL amp = 11p

■ Modified release
Persantin® **Retard** (Boehringer Ingelheim) PoM
Capsules, m/r, red/orange containing yellow pellets, dipyridamole 200 mg. Net price 60-cap pack = £9.75. Label: 21, 25
Dose: secondary prevention of ischaemic stroke and transient ischaemic attacks (used alone or with aspirin), adjunct to oral anticoagulation for prophylaxis of thromboembolism associated with prosthetic heart valves, 200 mg twice daily preferably with food
NOTE. Dispense in original container (pack contains a desiccant) and discard any capsules remaining 6 weeks after opening

■ With aspirin
For cautions, contra-indications and side-effects of aspirin, see under Aspirin, above
Asasantin® **Retard** (Boehringer Ingelheim) PoM
Capsules, red/ivory, aspirin 25 mg, dipyridamole 200 mg (m/r), net price 60-cap pack = £9.75. Label: 21, 25
Dose: secondary prevention of ischaemic stroke and transient ischaemic attacks, 1 capsule twice daily
Note: Dispense in original container (pack contains a desiccant) and discard any capsules remaining 6 weeks after opening

EPTIFIBATIDE

Indications: prevention of early myocardial infarction in patients with unstable angina or non-ST-segment-elevation myocardial infarction and with last episode of chest pain within 24 hours (use under specialist supervision)

Cautions: renal impairment (Appendix 3); risk of bleeding, concomitant drugs that increase risk of bleeding—discontinue immediately if uncontrolled serious bleeding; measure baseline prothrombin time, activated partial thromboplastin time, platelet count, haemoglobin, haematocrit and serum creatinine; monitor haemoglobin, haematocrit and platelets within 6 hours after start of treatment then at least once daily; discontinue if thrombolytic therapy, intra-aortic balloon pump or emergency cardiac surgery necessary; pregnancy (Appendix 4)

Contra-indications: abnormal bleeding within 30 days, major surgery or severe trauma within 6 weeks, stroke within last 30 days or any history of haemorrhagic stroke, intracranial disease (aneurysm, neoplasm or arteriovenous malformation), severe hypertension, haemorrhagic diathesis, increased prothrombin time or INR, thrombocytopenia, significant hepatic impairment; breast-feeding

Side-effects: bleeding manifestations

Dose: initially *by intravenous injection*, 180 micrograms/kg, then *by intravenous infusion*, 2 micrograms/kg/minute for up to 72 hours (up to 96 hours if percutaneous coronary intervention during treatment)

Integrilin® (Schering-Plough) ▼ PoM
Injection, eptifibatide 2 mg/mL, net price 10-mL (20-mg) vial = £15.54
Infusion, eptifibatide 750 micrograms/mL, net price 100-mL (75-mg) vial = £48.84

TIROFIBAN

Indications: prevention of early myocardial infarction in patients with unstable angina or non-ST-segment-elevation myocardial infarction and with last episode of chest pain within 12 hours (use under specialist supervision)

Cautions: renal impairment (Appendix 3); hepatic impairment (avoid if severe; Appendix 2); major surgery or severe trauma within 3 months (avoid if within 6 weeks); traumatic or protracted cardio-pulmonary resuscitation, organ biopsy or lithotripsy within last 2 weeks; risk of bleeding including active peptic ulcer within 3 months; acute pericarditis, aortic dissection, haemorrhagic retinopathy, vasculitis, haematuria, faecal occult blood; severe heart failure, cardiogenic shock, anaemia; puncture of non-compressible vessel within 24 hours; concomitant drugs that increase risk of bleeding (including within 48 hours after thrombolytic); monitor platelet count, haemoglobin and haematocrit before treatment, 2–6 hours after start of treatment and then at least once daily; discontinue if thrombolytic therapy, intra-aortic balloon pump or emergency cardiac surgery necessary; discontinue immediately if serious bleeding uncontrolled by pressure occurs; pregnancy (Appendix 4)

Contra-indications: abnormal bleeding within 30 days, stroke within 30 days or any history of haemorrhagic stroke, intracranial disease (aneurysm, neoplasm or arteriovenous malformation), severe hypertension, haemorrhagic diathesis, increased prothrombin time or INR, thrombocytopenia; breast-feeding

Side-effects: bleeding manifestations; reversible thrombocytopenia

Dose: *by intravenous infusion*, initially 400 nanograms/kg/minute for 30 minutes, then 100 nanograms/kg/minute for at least 48 hours (continue during and for 12–24 hours after percutaneous coronary intervention); max. duration of treatment 108 hours

Aggrastat® (MSD) ▼ PoM
Concentrate for intravenous infusion, tirofiban (as hydrochloride) 250 micrograms/mL. For dilution before use, net price 50-mL (12.5-mg) vial = £146.11
Intravenous infusion, tirofiban (as hydrochloride) 50 micrograms/mL, net price 250-mL *Intravia*® bag = £160.72

2.10 Myocardial infarction and fibrinolysis

2.10.1   Management of myocardial infarction
2.10.2   Fibrinolytic drugs

2.10.1 Management of myocardial infarction

> Local guidelines for the management of myocardial infarction should be followed where they exist

These notes give an overview of the initial and long-term management of myocardial infarction. The aims of management are to provide supportive care and pain relief, to promote revascularisation and to reduce mortality. Oxygen, diamorphine and nitrates provide initial support and pain relief; aspirin and percutaneous coronary intervention or thrombolytics promote revascularisation; long-term use of aspirin, beta-blockers, ACE inhibitors and statins help to reduce mortality further.

INITIAL MANAGEMENT. **Oxygen** (section 3.6) is administered unless the patient has severe chronic obstructive pulmonary disease.

The pain (and anxiety) of myocardial infarction is managed with slow intravenous injection of **diamorphine** (section 4.7.2); an antiemetic such as metoclopramide (or, if left ventricular function is not compromised, cyclizine) by intravenous injection should also be given (section 4.6).

Aspirin (chewed or dispersed in water) is given for its antiplatelet effect (section 2.9); a dose of 150–300 mg is suitable. If aspirin is given before arrival at hospital, a note saying that it has been given should be sent with the patient.

Patency of the occluded artery can be restored by percutaneous coronary intervention or by giving a **thrombolytic drug** (section 2.10.2), unless contra-indicated. Alteplase, reteplase and streptokinase need to be given within 12 hours of a myocardial infarction, ideally within 1 hour; use after 12 hours requires specialist advice. Tenecteplase should be given within 6 hours of a myocardial infarction. Streptokinase remains the drug of choice but antibodies appear after 4 days and streptokinase should not therefore be used again after this time. **Heparin** is used as adjunctive therapy with alteplase, reteplase, and tenecteplase to prevent re-thrombosis; heparin treatment should be continued for at least 24 hours (consult product literature).

Nitrates (section 2.6.1) are used to relieve ischaemic pain. If sublingual glyceryl trinitrate is not effective, intravenous glyceryl trinitrate or isosorbide dinitrate is given.

Early intravenous administration of some **beta-blockers** (section 2.4) has been shown to be of benefit and patients without contra-indications should receive **atenolol** by intravenous injection at a dose of 5 mg over 5 minutes, and the dose repeated once after 10–15 minutes; **metoprolol** by intravenous injection is an alternative.

ACE inhibitors (section 2.5.5.1) are also of benefit to patients who have no contra-indications; in hypertensive and normotensive patients treatment with an ACE inhibitor can be started within 24 hours of the myocardial infarction and continued for at least 5–6 weeks (see below for long-term treatment).

All patients should be closely monitored for hyperglycaemia; those with diabetes or raised blood-glucose concentration should receive **insulin**.

LONG-TERM MANAGEMENT. Long-term management involves the use of several drugs which should ideally be started before the patient is discharged from hospital.

Aspirin (section 2.9) should be given to all patients, unless contra-indicated, at a dose of 75–150 mg daily. **Warfarin** (with or without aspirin) may confer greater benefit than aspirin alone, but the risk of bleeding is increased.

Beta-blockers (section 2.4) should be given to all patients in whom they are not contra-indicated and continued for at least 2–3 years. Acebutolol, metoprolol, propranolol and timolol are suitable; for patients with left ventricular dysfunction, carvedilol, bisoprolol or long-acting metoprolol may be appropriate (section 2.5.5).

Although other calcium-channel blockers (section 2.6.2) have no place in routine management, **verapamil** may be useful in patients in whom beta-blockers are inappropriate.

ACE inhibitors (section 2.5.5.1) are recommended for any patient with evidence of left ventricular dysfunction.

Nitrates (section 2.6.1) are used for patients with angina.

Statins are beneficial in preventing recurrent coronary events (section 2.12).

2.10.2 Fibrinolytic drugs

Fibrinolytic drugs act as thrombolytics by activating plasminogen to form plasmin, which degrades fibrin and so breaks up thrombi.

Streptokinase is used in the treatment of *life-threatening venous thrombosis*, and in *pulmonary embolism*, but treatment must be started promptly.

The value of thrombolytic drugs for the treatment of *myocardial infarction* has been established (section 2.10.1). **Streptokinase** and **alteplase** have been shown to reduce mortality. **Reteplase**, and more recently, **tenecteplase** are also licensed for acute myocardial infarction; they are given by intravenous injection (tenecteplase is given as a bolus injection). Thrombolytic drugs are indicated for any patient with acute myocardial infarction for whom the benefit is likely to outweigh the risk of treatment. Trials have shown that the benefit is greatest in those with ECG changes that include ST segment elevation (especially in those with anterior infarction) and in patients with bundle branch block. Patients should not be denied thrombolytic treatment on account of age alone because mortality in this group is high and the reduction in mortality is the same as in younger patients.

CAUTIONS. Risk of bleeding including that from venepuncture or invasive procedures, external chest compression, pregnancy (see Appendix 4), abdominal aneurysm or conditions in which thrombolysis might give rise to embolic complications such as enlarged left atrium with atrial fibrillation (risk of dissolution of clot and subsequent embolisation), diabetic retinopathy (very small risk of retinal bleeding), recent or concurrent anticoagulant therapy.

CONTRA-INDICATIONS. Recent haemorrhage, trauma, or surgery (including dental extraction), coagulation defects, bleeding diatheses, aortic dissection, coma, history of cerebrovascular disease especially recent events or with any residual disability, recent symptoms of possible peptic ulceration, heavy vaginal bleeding, severe hypertension, active pulmonary disease with cavitation, acute pancreatitis, severe liver disease, oesophageal varices; also in the case of streptokinase, previous allergic reactions to either streptokinase or anistreplase (no longer available).

Prolonged persistence of antibodies to streptokinase and anistreplase (no longer available) may reduce the effectiveness of subsequent treatment, therefore streptokinase should not be used again beyond 4 days of first administration of either streptokinase or anistreplase.

SIDE-EFFECTS. Side-effects of thrombolytics are mainly nausea and vomiting and bleeding. When thrombolytics are used in myocardial infarction, reperfusion arrhythmias may occur. Hypotension may also occur and can usually be controlled by elevating the patient's legs, or by reducing the rate of infusion or stopping it temporarily. Back pain has been reported. Bleeding is usually limited to the site of injection, but intracerebral haemorrhage or bleeding from other sites may occur. Serious bleeding calls for discontinuation of the thrombolytic and may require administration of coagulation factors and antifibrinolytic drugs (aprotinin or tranexamic acid). Streptokinase may cause allergic reactions (including rash, flushing and uveitis) and anaphylaxis has been reported (for details of management see Allergic Emergencies, section 3.4.3). Guillain-Barré syndrome has been reported rarely after streptokinase treatment.

ALTEPLASE

(rt-PA, tissue-type plasminogen activator)

Indications: acute myocardial infarction (see notes above and section 2.10.1); pulmonary embolism; acute ischaemic stroke (treatment under specialist neurology physician **only**)

Cautions: see notes above; *in acute stroke*, monitor for intracranial haemorrhage, monitor blood pressure (antihypertensive recommended if systolic above 180 mm Hg or diastolic above 105 mmHg)

Contra-indications: see notes above; *in acute stroke*, convulsion accompanying stroke, severe stroke, history of stroke in patients with diabetes, stroke in last 3 months, hypoglycaemia, hyperglycaemia

Side-effects: see notes above; also risk of cerebral bleeding increased in acute stroke

Dose: myocardial infarction, accelerated regimen (initiated within 6 hours), 15 mg *by intravenous injection*, followed *by intravenous infusion* of 50 mg over 30 minutes, then 35 mg over 60 minutes (total dose 100 mg over 90 minutes); lower doses in patients less than 65 kg

Myocardial infarction, initiated within 6–12 hours, 10 mg *by intravenous injection*, followed *by intravenous infusion* of 50 mg over 60 minutes, then 4 *infusions* each of 10 mg over 30 minutes (total dose 100 mg over 3 hours; max. 1.5 mg/kg in patients less than 65 kg)

Pulmonary embolism, 10 mg *by intravenous injection* over 1–2 minutes, followed *by intravenous infusion* of 90 mg over 2 hours; max. 1.5 mg/kg in patients less than 65 kg

Acute stroke (treatment **must** begin within 3 hours), *by intravenous administration* over 60 minutes, 900 micrograms/kg (max. 90 mg); initial 10% of dose by intravenous injection, remainder by intravenous infusion; ELDERLY over 80 years not recommended

Actilyse® (Boehringer Ingelheim) ▣PoM▣
Injection, powder for reconstitution, alteplase 10 mg (5.8 million units)/vial, net price per vial (with diluent) = £135.00; 20 mg (11.6 million units)/vial (with diluent and transfer device) = £180.00; 50 mg (29 million units)/vial (with diluent, transfer device, and infusion bag) = £300.00

RETEPLASE

Indications: acute myocardial infarction (see notes above and section 2.10.1)

Cautions: see notes above

Contra-indications: see notes above

Side-effects: see notes above

Dose: *by intravenous injection,* 10 units over not more than 2 minutes, followed after 30 minutes by a further 10 units

Rapilysin® (Roche) ▣PoM▣
Injection, powder for reconstitution, reteplase 10 units/vial, net price pack of 2 vials (with 2 prefilled syringes of diluent and transfer device) = £716.25

STREPTOKINASE

Indications: acute myocardial infarction (see notes above and section 2.10.1); deep-vein thrombosis, pulmonary embolism, acute arterial thromboembolism, and central retinal venous or arterial thrombosis; topical use (section 13.11.7)

Cautions: see notes above

Contra-indications: see notes above

Side-effects: see notes above

Dose: myocardial infarction, 1 500 000 units over 60 minutes

Deep-vein thrombosis, pulmonary embolism, acute arterial thromboembolism, central retinal venous or arterial thrombosis, *by intravenous infusion,* 250 000 units over 30 minutes, then 100 000 units every hour for up to 12–72 hours according to condition with monitoring of clotting parameters (consult product literature)

and a family history of premature coronary heart disease). Treatment with statins (see Statins, below) has been shown to reduce myocardial infarction, coronary deaths and overall mortality rate and they are the drugs of choice in patients with a high risk of coronary heart disease. Lipid-regulating drug therapy must be combined with advice on diet and lifestyle measures to reduce coronary risk including, if appropriate, reduction of blood pressure (section 2.5) and use of aspirin (section 2.9).

A number of conditions, some familial, are characterised by very high plasma concentrations of cholesterol, or triglycerides, or both. Statins are drugs of first choice for treating hypercholesterolaemia, fibrates for treating hypertriglyceridaemia, and statins or fibrates can be used, either alone or together, to treat mixed hyperlipidaemia.

Severe hyperlipidaemia often requires a combination of lipid-regulating drugs such as an anion-exchange resin with a fibrate, a statin, or nicotinic acid; such treatment should generally be under specialist supervision. Combinations of a statin with nicotinic acid or a fibrate carry an increased risk of side-effects (including rhabdomyolysis) and should be used with caution. In particular, concomitant administration of gemfibrozil with a statin may increase the risk of rhabdomyolysis considerably (see also below); gemfibrozil and statins should therefore **not** be used concomitantly.

Patients wth hypothyroidism should receive adequate thyroid replacement therapy before assessing their requirement for lipid-regulating treatment because correction of hypothyroidism itself may resolve the lipid abnormality. Untreated hypothyroidism increases the risk of myositis with lipid-regulating drugs.

CSM advice (muscle effects). The CSM has advised that rhabdomyolysis associated with lipid-regulating drugs such as the fibrates and statins appears to be rare (approx. 1 case in every 100 000 treatment years) but may be increased in those with renal impairment and possibly in those with hypothyroidism (see also notes above). Concomitant treatment with ciclosporin may increase plasma-statin concentration and the risk of muscle toxicity; concomitant treatment with a fibrate and a statin may also be associated with an increased risk of serious muscle toxicity.

Anion-exchange resins

Colestyramine (cholestyramine) and **colestipol** are anion-exchange resins used in the management of hypercholesterolaemia. They act by binding bile acids, preventing their reabsorption; this promotes hepatic conversion of cholesterol into bile acids; the resultant increased LDL-receptor activity of liver cells increases the breakdown of LDL-cholesterol. Thus both compounds effectively reduce LDL-cholesterol but can aggravate hypertriglyceridaemia.

CAUTIONS. Anion-exchange resins interfere with the absorption of fat-soluble vitamins; supplements of vitamins A, D and K may be required when treatment is prolonged. **Interactions:** Appendix 1 (colestyramine and colestipol).

SIDE-EFFECTS. As colestyramine and colestipol are not absorbed, gastro-intestinal side-effects predominate. Constipation is common, but diarrhoea has occurred, as have nausea, vomiting, and gastrointestinal discomfort. An increased bleeding tendency has been reported due to hypoprothrombinaemia associated with vitamin K deficiency.

COUNSELLING. Other drugs should be taken at least 1 hour (in the case of ezetemibe, at least 2 hours) before or 4–6 hours after colestyramine or colestipol to reduce possible interference with absorption.

COLESTYRAMINE
(Cholestyramine)

Indications: hyperlipidaemias, particularly type IIa, in patients who have not responded adequately to diet and other appropriate measures; primary prevention of coronary heart disease in men aged 35–59 years with primary hypercholesterolaemia who have not responded to diet and other appropriate measures; pruritus associated with partial biliary obstruction and primary biliary cirrhosis (section 1.9.2); diarrhoeal disorders (section 1.9.2)

Cautions: see notes above; pregnancy and breast-feeding

Contra-indications: complete biliary obstruction (not likely to be effective)

Side-effects: see notes above; hyperchloraemic acidosis reported on prolonged use

Dose: lipid reduction (after initial introduction over 3–4 weeks) 12–24 g daily in water (or other suitable liquid) in single or up to 4 divided doses; up to 36 g daily if necessary

Pruritus, see section 1.9.2

Diarrhoeal disorders, see section 1.9.2

CHILD 6–12 years, see product literature

Colestyramine (Non-proprietary) [PoM]
Powder, colestyramine (anhydrous) 4 g/sachet, net price 50-sachet pack = £17.55. Label: 13, counselling, avoid other drugs at same time (see notes above)
Excipients: include aspartame (section 9.4.1)
Available from Dominion

Questran (Bristol-Myers Squibb) [PoM]
Powder, colestyramine (anhydrous) 4 g/sachet. Net price 50-sachet pack = £17.55. Label: 13, counselling, avoid other drugs at same time (see notes above)
Excipients: include sucrose 3.79g/sachet

Questran Light (Bristol-Myers Squibb) [PoM]
Powder, sugar-free, colestyramine (anhydrous) 4 g/sachet, net price 50-sachet pack = £18.43. Label: 13, counselling, avoid other drugs at same time (see notes above)
Excipients: include aspartame (section 9.4.1)

COLESTIPOL HYDROCHLORIDE

Indications: hyperlipidaemias, particularly type IIa, in patients who have not responded adequately to diet and other appropriate measures

Cautions: see notes above; pregnancy

Side-effects: see notes above

Dose: 5 g 1–2 times daily in liquid increased if necessary at intervals of 1–2 months to max. of 30 g daily (in single or 2 divided doses)

Colestid® (Pharmacia) [PoM]
Granules, yellow, colestipol hydrochloride
5 g/sachet. Net price 30 sachets = £15.05. Label: 13, counselling, avoid other drugs at same time (see notes above)
Colestid Orange, granules, yellow/orange, colestipol hydrochloride 5 g/sachet, with aspartame. Net price 30 sachets = £15.05. Label: 13, counselling, avoid other drugs at same time (see notes above)

Ezetimibe

Ezetimibe inhibits the intestinal absorption of cholesterol. It is licensed as adjunctive therapy to dietary manipulation in patients with hypercholesterolaemia in combination with a statin or alone (if a statin is inappropriate), in patients with homozygous familial hypercholesterolaemia in combination with a statin, and in patients with homozygous familial sitosterolaemia (phytosterolaemia).

EZETIMIBE

Indications: adjunct to dietary measures and statin in primary and homozygous familial hypercholesterolaemia (statin omitted in primary hypercholesterolaemia if inappropriate or not tolerated); adjunct to dietary measures in homozygous sitosterolaemia
Cautions: liver impairment (avoid if moderate or severe; Appendix 2); **interactions:** Appendix 1 (ezetimibe)
Contra-indications: breast-feeding (Appendix 5)
Side-effects: diarrhoea, abdominal pain, headache
Dose: 10 mg once daily; CHILD under 10 years not recommended

Ezetrol (MSD, Schering-Plough) ▼ [PoM]
Tablets, ezetimibe 10 mg, net price 28–tab pack = £26.31

Fibrates

Bezafibrate, ciprofibrate, fenofibrate, and **gemfibrozil** act mainly by decreasing serum triglycerides; they have variable effects on LDL–cholesterol. Fibrates may reduce the risk of coronary heart disease events in those with low HDL–cholesterol or with raised triglycerides.

All can cause a myositis-like syndrome, especially in patients with impaired renal function. Also, combination of a fibrate with a statin increases the risk of muscle effects (especially rhabdomyolysis) and should be used with caution (see CSM advice in section 2.12).

BEZAFIBRATE

Indications: hyperlipidaemias of types IIa, IIb, III, IV and V in patients who have not responded adequately to diet and other appropriate measures
Cautions: renal impairment (Appendix 3—see also under Myotoxicity below); correct hypothyroidism before initiating treatment (see section 2.12); **interactions:** Appendix 1 (fibrates)
MYOTOXICITY. Special care needed in patients with renal disease, as progressive increases in serum creatinine concentration or failure to follow dosage guidelines may result in myotoxicity (rhabdomyolysis); discontinue if myotoxicity suspected or creatine kinase concentration increases significantly

Contra-indications: severe hepatic impairment, hypoalbuminaemia, primary biliary cirrhosis, gall bladder disease, nephrotic syndrome, pregnancy and breast-feeding
Side-effects: gastro-intestinal (e.g. nausea, anorexia, gastric pain), pruritus, urticaria, impotence; also headache, dizziness, vertigo, fatigue, hair loss; myotoxicity (with myasthenia or myalgia)—special risk in renal impairment (see Cautions); also reported, anaemia, leucopenia, thrombocytopenia
Dose: see preparations below

Bezafibrate (Non-proprietary) [PoM]
Tablets, bezafibrate 200 mg, net price 100-tab pack = £9.76. Label: 21
Dose: 200 mg 3 times daily after food
Available from Dominion, Generics

Bezalip® (Roche) [PoM]
Tablets, f/c, bezafibrate 200 mg. Net price 100-tab pack = £9.84. Label: 21
Dose: 200 mg 3 times daily with or after food

■ Modified release

Bezalip® **Mono** (Roche) [PoM]
Tablets, m/r, f/c, bezafibrate 400 mg. Net price 30-tab pack = £8.70. Label: 21, 25
Dose: 1 tablet daily after food (dose form not appropriate in renal impairment)
NOTE. Modified-release tablets containing bezafibrate 400 mg also available from Ashbourne (*Liparol*® *XL*), Generics (*Bezagen*® *XL*), Link (*Zimbacol*®*XL*)

CIPROFIBRATE

Indications: hyperlipidaemias of types IIa, IIb, III, and IV in patients who have not responded adequately to diet
Cautions: see under Bezafibrate
Contra-indications: see under Bezafibrate
Side-effects: see under Bezafibrate
Dose: 100 mg daily

Modalim® (Sanofi-Synthelabo) [PoM]
Tablets, scored, ciprofibrate 100 mg. Net price 28-tab pack = £14.72

FENOFIBRATE

Indications: hyperlipidaemias of types IIa, IIb, III, IV, and V in patients who have not responded adequately to diet and other appropriate measures
Cautions: see under Bezafibrate; renal impairment (Appendix 3); liver function tests recommended every 3 months for first year (discontinue treatment if significantly raised)
Contra-indications: severe renal or hepatic impairment, existing gall bladder disease; pregnancy (Appendix 4) and breast-feeding (Appendix 5); photosensitivity to ketoprofen
Side-effects: see under Bezafibrate; also reported rash, photosensitivity, raised serum transaminases, hepatitis
Dose: see preparations below

Fenofibrate (Non-proprietary) [PoM]
Capsules, fenofibrate 200 mg, net price 30-cap pack = £14.75. Label: 21
Dose: 1 capsule daily (dose form not appropriate for children or in renal impairment)
Available from Genus (*Fenogal*®)

ROSUVASTATIN

Indications: primary hypercholesterolaemia (type IIa including heterozygous familial hypercholesterolaemia), mixed dyslipidaemia (type IIb), or homozygous familial hypercholesterolaemia in patients who have not responded adequately to diet and other appropriate measures

Cautions: see notes above

Contra-indications: see notes above; also renal impairment (Appendix 3)

Side-effects: see notes above; also dizziness and asthenia; proteinuria

Dose: 10 mg once daily increased if necessary after not less than 4 weeks to 20 mg once daily, further increased to 40 mg in severe hypercholesterolaemia and high cardiovascular risk

Crestorᴿ (AstraZeneca) ▼ PoM
Tablets, all pink, f/c, rosuvastatin (as calcium salt) 10 mg, net price 28-tab pack = £18.03; 20 mg, 28-tab pack = £29.69; 40 mg, 28-tab pack = £29.69. Counselling, muscle effects, see notes above

SIMVASTATIN

Indications: primary hypercholesterolaemia, heterozygous familial hypercholesterolaemia, homozygous familial hypercholesterolaemia or combined (mixed) hyperlipidaemia in patients who have not responded adequately to diet and other appropriate measures; prevention of coronary events, need for revascularisation procedures, and to slow progression of coronary atherosclerosis in patients with coronary heart disease and total cholesterol concentration of 5.5 mmol/litre or greater (see notes above)

Cautions: see notes above; severe renal impairment (Appendix 3)

Contra-indications: see notes above; also porphyria (see section 9.8.2)

Side-effects: see notes above; also alopecia, anaemia, dizziness, peripheral neuropathy, hepatitis, jaundice, pancreatitis

Dose: primary hypercholesterolaemia, heterozygous familial hypercholesterolaemia, combined hyperlipidaemia, 10 mg daily at night, adjusted at intervals of not less than 4 weeks; usual range 10–80 mg once daily at night

Homozygous familial hypercholesterolaemia, 40 mg daily at night *or* 80 mg daily in 3 divided doses (with largest dose at night)

Coronary heart disease, initially 20 mg once daily at night, adjusted at intervals of not less than 4 weeks; max. 80 mg once daily
NOTE. Max. 10 mg daily with concomitant ciclosporin, fibrate or lipid-lowering dose of nicotinic acid

Simvastatin (Non-proprietary) PoM
Tablets, simvastatin 10 mg, net price 28-tab pack = £18.02, 20 mg, 28-tab pack = £29.68; 40 mg, 28-tab pack = £29.68; 80 mg, 28-tab pack = £29.68. Counselling, muscle effects, see notes above
Available from APS (*Simzal*ᴿ), Generics

Zocorᴿ (MSD) PoM
Tablets, all f/c, simvastatin 10 mg (peach), net price 28-tab pack = £18.03; 20 mg (tan), 28-tab pack = £29.69; 40 mg (red), 28-tab pack = £29.69; 80 mg (red), 28-tab pack = £29.69. Counselling, muscle effects, see notes above

Nicotinic acid group

The value of **nicotinic acid** is limited by its side-effects, especially vasodilatation. In doses of 1.5 to 3 g daily it lowers both cholesterol and triglyceride concentrations by inhibiting synthesis; it also increases HDL-cholesterol. **Acipimox** seems to have fewer side-effects but may be less effective in its lipid-modulating capabilities.

ACIPIMOX

Indications: hyperlipidaemias of types IIa, IIb, and IV in patients who have not responded adequately to diet and other appropriate measures

Cautions: renal impairment (Appendix 3)

Contra-indications: peptic ulcer; pregnancy and breast-feeding

Side-effects: vasodilatation, flushing, itching, rashes, urticaria, erythema; heartburn, epigastric pain, nausea, diarrhoea, headache, malaise, dry eyes; rarely angioedema, bronchospasm, anaphylaxis

Dose: usually 500–750 mg daily in divided doses

Olbetamᴿ (Pharmacia) PoM
Capsules, brown/pink, acipimox 250 mg. Net price 90-cap pack = £46.33. Label: 21

NICOTINIC ACID

Indications: see notes above

Cautions: diabetes mellitus, gout, liver disease, peptic ulcer; **interactions:** Appendix 1 (nicotinic acid)

Contra-indications: pregnancy, breast-feeding

Side-effects: flushing, dizziness, headache, palpitations, pruritus (prostaglandin-mediated symptoms can be reduced by low initial doses taken with meals, or by taking aspirin 75 mg 30 minutes before the dose); nausea, vomiting; rarely impaired liver function and rashes

Dose: initially 100–200 mg 3 times daily (see above), gradually increased over 2–4 weeks to 1–2 g 3 times daily

¹**Nicotinic Acid** PoM
Tablets, nicotinic acid 50 mg, net price 100 = £9.25. Label: 21

1. May be sold to the public unless max. daily dose exceeds 600 mg or if intended for treatment of hyperlipidaemia

Fish oils

A fish-oil preparation (*Maxepa*ᴿ), rich in **omega-3-marine triglycerides**, is useful in the treatment of severe hypertriglyceridaemia; however, it can sometimes aggravate hypercholesterolaemia.

The preparation *Omacor*ᴿ, which contains **omega-3-acid ethyl esters**, is licensed for hypertriglyceridaemia and secondary prevention after myocardial infarction.

OMEGA-3-ACID ETHYL ESTERS

Indications: adjunct in the reduction of plasma triglycerides in patients with hypertriglyceridaemia judged to be at special risk of ischaemic heart disease or pancreatitis; adjunct in secondary prevention after myocardial infarction

Cautions: haemorrhagic disorders, anticoagulant treatment

Side-effects: nausea, belching, diarrhoea, constipation; eczema and acne reported

Dose: see under preparation below

Omacor® (Solvay)
Capsules, 1 g of 90% omega-3-acid ethyl esters containing eicosapentaenoic acid 46% and decosahexaenoic acid 38%, alpha-tocopherol 4 mg, net price 28-cap pack = £13.89. Label: 21
Dose: hypertriglyceridaemia, 4 capsules daily in 1–2 divided doses with food
Secondary prevention after myocardial infarction 1 capsule daily with food

OMEGA-3-MARINE TRIGLYCERIDES

Indications: adjunct in the reduction of plasma triglycerides in patients with severe hypertriglyceridaemia judged to be at special risk of ischaemic heart disease or pancreatitis

Cautions: haemorrhagic disorders, anticoagulant treatment; aspirin-sensitive asthma; diabetes mellitus

Side-effects: occasional nausea and belching

Dose: see under preparations below

Maxepa® (Seven Seas)
Capsules, 1 g (approx. 1.1 mL) concentrated fish oils containing eicosapentaenoic acid 170 mg, docosahexaenoic acid 115 mg. Vitamin A content less than 100 units/g, vitamin D content less than 10 units/g, net price 200-cap pack = £27.28. Label: 21
Dose: 5 capsules twice daily with food
Liquid, golden-coloured, concentrated fish oils containing eicosapentaenoic acid 170 mg, docosahexaenoic acid 115 mg/g (1.1 mL). Vitamin A content less than 100 units/g, vitamin D content less than 10 units/g, net price 150 mL = £20.46. Label: 21
Dose: 5 mL twice daily with food

2.13 Local sclerosants

Ethanolamine oleate and sodium tetradecyl sulphate are used in sclerotherapy of varicose veins, and phenol is used in haemorrhoids (section 1.7.3).

ETHANOLAMINE OLEATE
(Monoethanolamine Oleate)

Indications: sclerotherapy of varicose veins

Cautions: extravasation may cause necrosis of tissues

Contra-indications: inability to walk, acute phlebitis, oral contraceptive use, obese legs

Side-effects: allergic reactions (including anaphylaxis)

Ethanolamine Oleate PoM
Injection, ethanolamine oleate 5%. Net price 5-mL amp = £2.22
Available from Celltech
Dose: by slow injection into empty isolated segment of vein, 2–5 mL divided between 3–4 sites; repeated at weekly intervals

SODIUM TETRADECYL SULPHATE

Indications: sclerotherapy of varicose veins

Cautions: see under Ethanolamine Oleate

Contra-indications: see under Ethanolamine Oleate

Side-effects: see under Ethanolamine Oleate

Fibro-Vein® (STD Pharmaceutical) PoM
Injection, sodium tetradecyl sulphate 0.2%, net price 5-mL amp = £3.15; 0.5%, 2-mL amp = £1.88; 1%, 2-mL amp = £2.05; 3%, 2-mL amp = £2.30, 5-mL vial = £4.48
Dose: by slow injection into empty isolated segment of vein, 0.1–1 mL according to site and condition being treated (consult product literature)

MANAGEMENT OF ACUTE SEVERE ASTHMA IN GENERAL PRACTICE

MANAGEMENT OF ACUTE SEVERE ASTHMA IN GENERAL PRACTICE

Moderate asthma exacerbation

— Peak flow >50–75% of predicted or best
— No features of acute severe asthma
— Increasing symptoms

Treat at home but response to treatment **must** be assessed before doctor leaves

Treatment:
High-flow oxygen if available
Salbutamol or terbutaline via large-volume spacer or nebuliser
Monitor response 15–30 minutes after nebulisation
Give oral prednisolone 40–50 mg daily for at least 5 days and step up usual treatment

Follow up
Monitor symptoms and peak flow
Set up asthma action plan
Review in surgery within 48 hours
Modify treatment at review according to guidelines for chronic asthma (see Management of Chronic Asthma in Adults and Children)

Important: regard each emergency consultation as being for **acute severe asthma** until shown otherwise.

Important: failure to respond adequately **at any time** requires immediate referral to hospital.

Acute severe asthma in adults

— Cannot complete sentences in one breath
— Pulse ≥ 110 beats/minute
— Respiration ≥25 breaths/minute
— Peak flow 33–50% of predicted or best

Seriously consider hospital admission if more than one of above features present

Treatment:
High-flow oxygen if available
Salbutamol or terbutaline via large-volume spacer or nebuliser (oxygen driven if available)
Oral prednisolone 40–50 mg daily for at least 5 days (or i/v hydrocortisone 400 mg daily in 4 divided doses)
Monitor response 15–30 minutes after nebulisation

If any signs of acute asthma persist:
Arrange hospital admission
While awaiting ambulance repeat nebulised beta$_2$ agonist and give with nebulised ipratropium 500 micrograms
Alternatively if symptoms have improved, respiration and pulse settling, and peak flow >50% of predicted or best:
Step up usual treatment *and* continue prednisolone

Follow up
Monitor symptoms and peak flow
Set up asthma action plan
Review in surgery within 24 hours
Modify treatment at review (see Management of Chronic Asthma)

Life-threatening asthma in adults

— Silent chest
— Cyanosis
— Feeble respiratory effort
— Bradycardia, exhaustion, arrhythmia, hypotension, confusion, or coma
— Peak flow <33% of predicted or best
— Arterial oxygen saturation <92%
Arrange **immediate** hospital admission

Treatment:
Oral prednisolone 40–50 mg daily for at least 5 days (or i/v hydrocortisone 400 mg daily in 4 divided doses) (immediately)
Oxygen-driven nebuliser in ambulance
Nebulised beta$_2$ agonist with nebulised ipratropium
Stay with patient until ambulance arrives

1. If nebuliser not available give 1 puff of beta$_2$ agonist using large-volume spacer and repeat 10–20 times

Important: patients with severe or life-threatening attacks may not be distressed and may not have all these abnormalities; the presence of any should alert doctor.

Acute episodes or exacerbations of asthma in young children in primary care

Mild/moderate episode in young children
— short-acting beta$_2$ agonist from metered dose inhaler *via* large-volume spacer (and face mask in very young), up to 10 puffs; alternatively give by nebuliser
— if favourable response (respiratory rate reduced, reduced use of accessory muscles, improved 'behaviour' pattern), repeat inhaled beta$_2$ agonist as needed

— start short course of oral prednisolone for 3 days (under 2 years 10 mg; 2–5 years 20 mg; over 5 years 30–40 mg daily; those already on prednisolone tablets 2 mg/kg up to max. 60 mg)
— consider i/v hydrocortisone in those who are unable to retain oral prednisolone

If unresponsive or relapse within 3–4 hours:
— immediately refer to hospital
— give nebulised beta$_2$ agonist with nebulised ipratropium 250 micrograms every 20–30 minutes
— give high-flow oxygen *via* face mask

Signs of acute asthma in children

Acute severe asthma:
— too breathless to talk
— too breathless to feed
— respiration >50 breaths/minute (>30/minute in children over 5 years)
— pulse >130 beats/minute (>120 beats/minute in children over 5 years)
— in younger children, use of accessory muscles of breathing
— in older children, peak flow ≤50% of predicted or best

Life-threatening features:
— cyanosis, silent chest, or poor respiratory effort
— exhaustion
— agitation, hypotension, confusion, reduced level of consciousness, or coma
— in older children, peak flow <33% of predicted or best

Severe exacerbations of asthma can have an adverse effect on pregnancy and should be treated promptly with conventional therapy, including oral or parenteral administration of a corticosteroid and nebulisation of a beta$_2$ agonist; prednisolone is the preferred corticosteroid for oral administration since very little of the drug reaches the fetus. Oxygen should be given immediately to maintain arterial oxygen saturation above 95% and prevent maternal and fetal hypoxia. Inhaled drugs, theophylline, and prednisolone can be taken as normal during breast-feeding.

Acute severe asthma

Severe asthma can be fatal and **must** be treated promptly and energetically. It is characterised by persistent dyspnoea poorly relieved by broncho-dilators, exhaustion, a high pulse rate (usually over 110/minute), and a very low peak expiratory flow. As asthma becomes more severe, wheezing may be absent. Such patients should be given **oxygen** (if available) and **salbutamol** or **terbutaline** by nebu-liser. This should be followed by a large dose of a **corticosteroid** (section 6.3.2)—for adults, predniso-lone 30–60 mg by mouth or hydrocortisone 200 mg (preferably as sodium succinate) intravenously; for children, prednisolone 1–2 mg/kg by mouth (1–4 years max. 20 mg, 5–15 years max. 40 mg) or hydrocortisone 100 mg (preferably as sodium succinate) intravenously; if vomiting occurs, the parenteral route may be preferred for the first dose. For a table outlining the management of acute severe asthma, see p. 132.

If there is little response **ipratropium** by nebuliser (section 3.1.2) should be considered. Most patients do not require and do not benefit from the addition of intravenous aminophylline or of a beta$_2$ agonist; both cause more adverse effects than nebulised beta$_2$ agonists. Nevertheless, an occasional patient who has not been taking theophylline, may benefit from a slow intravenous infusion of aminophylline. Intra-venous magnesium sulphate [unlicensed indication] (section 9.5.1.3) may benefit patients with very severe acute asthma whose peak flow is less than 20% of predicted. Magnesium sulphate should only be given on specialist advice.

Treatment of these patients is safer in hospital where resuscitation facilities are immediately avail-able. Treatment should **never** be delayed for inves-tigations, patients should **never** be sedated, and the possibility of a pneumothorax should be considered.

If the patient deteriorates despite appropriate phar-macological treatment, intermittent positive pressure ventilation may be needed.

Chronic obstructive pulmonary disease

Chronic obstructive pulmonary disease (chronic bronchitis and emphysema) may be helped by an inhaled **short-acting beta$_2$ agonist** (section 3.1.1.1) used as required *or* when the airways obstruction is more severe, by a regular inhaled **antimuscarinic bronchodilator** (section 3.1.2) *or* an inhaled **long-acting beta$_2$ agonist**. Although many patients are treated with an inhaled corticosteroid, long-term studies have shown no reduction in the decline in lung function in patients taking regular inhaled

corticosteroids (section 3.2). A limited trial of high-dose inhaled corticosteroid *or* an oral cortico-steroid is recommended for patients with moderate airflow obstruction to determine the extent of the airway reversibility and to ensure that asthma has not been overlooked.

Long-term **oxygen** therapy (section 3.6) prolongs survival in some patients with chronic obstructive pulmonary disease. For the management of infec-tions in bronchitis see Table 1, section 5.1.

Croup

Mild croup requires no specific treatment and can be managed in the community. More severe croup calls for hospital admission; a single dose of a cortico-steroid (e.g. dexamethasone 150 micrograms/kg by mouth) may be administered before transfer to hospital. In hospital, dexamethasone 150 micr-ograms/kg (by mouth or by injection) or budesonide 2 mg (by nebulisation) will often reduce symptoms. For severe croup not effectively controlled with corticosteroid treatment, nebulised adrenaline solu-tion 1 in 1000 (1 mg/mL) may be given with close clinical monitoring in a dose of 400 micrograms/kg (max. 5 mg) repeated after 30 minutes if necessary; the effects of nebulised adrenaline last 2–3 hours.

3.1.1   Adrenoceptor agonists
(Sympathomimetics)

3.1.1.1   Selective beta$_2$ agonists
3.1.1.2   Other adrenoceptor agonists

The selective beta$_2$ agonists (selective beta$_2$-adreno-ceptor agonists, selective beta$_2$ stimulants) (section 3.1.1.1) such as salbutamol or terbutaline are the safest and most effective beta agonists for asthma. They are recommended over the less selective beta agonists such as orciprenaline (section 3.1.1.2), which should be avoided whenever possible.

Adrenaline (epinephrine) (which has both alpha- and beta-adrenoceptor agonist properties) is used in the emergency management of allergic and anaphy-lactic reactions (section 3.4.3).

3.1.1.1   Selective beta$_2$ agonists

Mild to moderate symptoms of asthma respond rapidly to the inhalation of a selective short-acting beta$_2$ agonist such as **salbutamol** or **terbutaline**. If beta$_2$ agonist inhalation is needed more often than once daily, prophylactic treatment should be con-sidered, using a stepped approach as outlined on p. 131.

Salmeterol and **formoterol** (eformoterol) are longer-acting beta$_2$ agonists which are administered by inhalation. They should not be used for the relief of an acute asthma attack. Salmeterol and formoterol should be added to existing corticosteroid therapy and not replace it. They can be useful in nocturnal asthma. Formoterol is also licensed for short-term symptom relief.

REGULAR TREATMENT. Short-acting beta$_2$ agonists should not be prescribed for use on a regular basis in patients with mild or moderate asthma since regular

vulsions especially if given rapidly by intravenous injection; **overdosage:** see Emergency Treatment of Poisoning, p. 26

Dose: see below

NOTE. Plasma theophylline concentration for optimum response 10–20 mg/litre (55–110 micromol/litre); narrow margin between therapeutic and toxic dose, see also notes above

Nuelinⁿ (3M)

Tablets, scored, theophylline 125 mg. Net price 90-tab pack = £3.29. Label: 21

Dose: 125 mg 3–4 times daily after food, increased to 250 mg if required; CHILD 7–12 years 62.5–125 mg 3–4 times daily

Liquid, brown, theophylline hydrate (as sodium glycinate) 60 mg/5 mL. Net price 300 mL = £2.93. Label: 21

Dose: 120–240 mg 3–4 times daily after food; CHILD 2–6 years 60–90 mg, 7–12 years 90–120 mg, 3–4 times daily

■ Modified release

NOTE. The Council of the Royal Pharmaceutical Society of Great Britain advises pharmacists that if a general practitioner prescribes a modified-release oral theophylline preparation without specifying a brand name, the pharmacist should contact the prescriber and agree the brand to be dispensed. Additionally, it is essential that a patient discharged from hospital should be maintained on the brand on which that patient was stabilised as an in-patient.

Nuelin SAⁿ (3M)

SA tablets, m/r, theophylline 175 mg. Net price 60-tab pack = £3.43. Label: 25

Dose: 175–350 mg every 12 hours; CHILD over 6 years 175 mg every 12 hours

SA 250 tablets, m/r, scored, theophylline 250 mg. Net price 60-tab pack = £4.80. Label: 25

Dose: 250–500 mg every 12 hours; CHILD over 6 years 125–250 mg every 12 hours

Slo-Phyllinⁿ (Merck)

Capsules, all m/r, theophylline 60 mg (white/clear, enclosing white pellets), net price 56-cap pack = £2.11; 125 mg (brown/clear, enclosing white pellets), 56-cap pack = £2.66; 250 mg (blue/clear, enclosing white pellets), 56-cap pack = £3.32. Label: 25, or counselling, see below

Dose: 250–500 mg every 12 hours; CHILD, every 12 hours, 2–6 years 60–120 mg, 7–12 years 125–250 mg

COUNSELLING. Swallow whole with fluid *or* swallow enclosed granules with soft food (e.g. yoghurt)

Uniphyllin Continusⁿ (Napp)

Tablets, m/r, all scored, theophylline 200 mg, net price 56-tab pack = £4.12; 300 mg, 56-tab pack = £6.27; 400 mg, 56-tab pack = £7.44. Label: 25

Dose: 200 mg every 12 hours increased according to response to 400 mg every 12 hours

May be appropriate to give larger evening or morning dose to achieve optimum therapeutic effect when symptoms most severe; in patients whose night or daytime symptoms persist despite other therapy, who are not currently receiving theophylline, total daily requirement may be added as single evening or morning dose

CHILD 9 mg/kg twice daily; some children with chronic asthma may require 10–16 mg/kg every 12 hours

For a list of **cough and decongestant preparations on sale to the public**, including those containing theophylline, see section 3.9.2

AMINOPHYLLINE

NOTE. Aminophylline is a stable mixture or combination of theophylline and ethylenediamine; the ethylenediamine confers greater solubility in water

Indications: reversible airways obstruction, acute severe asthma

Cautions: see under Theophylline

Side-effects: see under Theophylline; also allergy to ethylenediamine can cause urticaria, erythema, and exfoliative dermatitis

Dose: see under preparations, below

NOTE. Plasma theophylline concentration for optimum response 10–20 mg/litre (55–110 micromol/litre); narrow margin between therapeutic and toxic dose, see also notes above

Aminophylline (Non-proprietary)

Tablets, aminophylline 100 mg, net price 20 = 80p. Label: 21

Dose: by mouth, 100–300 mg, 3–4 times daily, after food

Injection, aminophylline 25 mg/mL, net price 10-mL amp = 69p PoM

Available from Celltech (*Minijet*ⁿ), Phoenix

Dose: deteriorating acute severe asthma **not** previously treated with theophylline, *by slow intravenous injection* over at least 20 minutes (with close monitoring), 250–500 mg (5 mg/kg), then as for acute severe asthma; CHILD 5 mg/kg, then as for acute severe asthma

Acute severe asthma, *by intravenous infusion* (with close monitoring), 500 micrograms/kg/hour, adjusted according to plasma-theophylline concentration; CHILD 6 months–9 years 1 mg/kg/hour, 10–16 years 800 micrograms/kg/hour, adjusted according to plasma-theophylline concentration

NOTE. Patients taking oral theophylline or aminophylline should not normally receive intravenous aminophylline unless plasma-theophylline concentration is available to guide dosage

■ Modified release

NOTE. Advice about modified-release theophylline preparations above also applies to modified-release aminophylline preparations

Phyllocontin Continusⁿ (Napp)

Tablets, m/r, yellow, f/c, aminophylline hydrate 225 mg. Net price 56-tab pack = £3.34. Label: 25

Dose: 1 tablet twice daily initially, increased after 1 week to 2 tablets twice daily

NOTE. Modified-release tablets containing aminophylline 225 mg also available from Ashbourne (*Amnivent*ⁿ 225 *SR*), IVAX (*Norphyllin*ⁿ *SR*)

Forte tablets, m/r, yellow, f/c, aminophylline hydrate 350 mg. Net price 56-tab pack = £5.55. Label: 25

NOTE. *Forte* tablets are for smokers and other patients with decreased theophylline half-life (see notes above)

Paediatric tablets, m/r, peach, aminophylline hydrate 100 mg. Net price 56-tab pack = £2.15. Label: 25

Dose: CHILD over 3 years, 6 mg/kg twice daily initially, increased after 1 week to 12 mg/kg twice daily; some children with chronic asthma may require 13–20 mg/kg every 12 hours

3.1.4   Compound bronchodilator preparations

In general, patients are best treated with single-ingredient preparations, such as a selective beta₂ agonist (section 3.1.1.1) or ipratropium bromide (section 3.1.2), so that the dose of each drug can be adjusted. This flexibility is lost with combinations. However, a combination product may be appropriate for patients stabilised on individual components in the same proportion.

For **cautions, contra-indications** and **side-effects** see under individual drugs.

Combivent® (Boehringer Ingelheim) PoM ▭
Aerosol inhalation, ipratropium bromide
20 micrograms, salbutamol (as sulphate)
100 micrograms/metered inhalation. Net price 200-dose unit = £6.45. Counselling, dose
Excipients: include CFC propellants
Dose: bronchospasm associated with chronic obstructive pulmonary disease, 2 puffs 4 times daily; CHILD under 12 years not recommended

Nebuliser solution, isotonic, ipratropium bromide 500 micrograms, salbutamol (as sulphate) 2.5 mg/2.5-mL vial, net price 60 unit-dose vials = £31.35
Dose: bronchospasm in chronic obstructive pulmonary disease, *by inhalation of nebulised solution,* 1 vial 3–4 times daily; CHILD under 12 years not recommended
GLAUCOMA. In addition to other potential side-effects acute angle-closure glaucoma has been reported with nebulised ipratropium—for details, see p. 138

Duovent® (Boehringer Ingelheim) PoM ▭
Nebuliser solution, isotonic, fenoterol hydrobromide 1.25 mg, ipratropium bromide 500 micrograms/4-mL vial, net price 20 unit-dose vials = £11.00
Dose: acute severe asthma or acute exacerbation of chronic asthma, *by inhalation of nebulised solution,* 1 vial (4 mL); may be repeated up to max. 4 vials in 24 hours; CHILD under 14 years, not recommended
GLAUCOMA. In addition to other potential side-effects acute angle-closure glaucoma has been reported with nebulised ipratropium—for details, see p. 138

■ Preparations on sale to the public
For **compound bronchodilator preparations** on sale to the public, see p. 163

3.1.5 Peak flow meters, inhaler devices and nebulisers

Peak flow meters

Measurement of peak flow is particularly helpful for patients who are 'poor perceivers'and hence slow to detect deterioration in their asthma, and for those with moderate or severe asthma. Patients must be given clear guidelines as to the action they should take if their peak flow falls below a certain level. Patients can be encouraged to adjust some of their own treatment (within specified limits) according to changes in peak flow rate.

Asmaplan® (Vitalograph)
Peak flow meter, standard (50 to 750 litres/minute), net price = £6.65, low range (25 to 280 litres /minute) = £6.65, replacement mouthpiece = 40p (for adult or child)

Ferraris Pocketpeak® (Ferraris)
Peak flow meter, standard (90–710 litres/minute), net price = £6.53, low range (40–370 litres/minute) = £6.53, replacement mouthpiece = 38p (for adult or child)

Mini-Wright® (Clement Clarke)
Peak flow meter, standard (60 to 800 litres/minute), net price = £6.86, low range (30 to 400 litres/minute) = £6.90, replacement mouthpiece = 38p (for adult or child)

Drug delivery devices

INHALER DEVICES. These include *pressurised metered-dose inhalers, breath-actuated inhalers* and *dry powder inhalers.* Many patients can be taught to use a pressurised metered-dose inhaler effectively but some patients, particularly the elderly and small children, find it difficult to use them. *Spacer devices* (see below) can help such patients because they remove the need to co-ordinate actuation with inhalation and are effective even for children under 5 years. Alternatively, breath-actuated inhalers or dry powder inhalers (which are activated by patient's inhalation) may be used but they are less suitable for young children. On changing from a pressurised metered-dose inhaler to a dry powder inhaler patients may notice a lack of sensation in the mouth and throat previously associated with each actuation. Coughing may also occur.

The patient should be instructed carefully on the use of the inhaler and it is important to check that the inhaler continues to be used correctly because inadequate inhalation technique may be mistaken for a lack of response to the drug.

> **NICE Guidance (inhaler devices for children with chronic asthma)**
> The National Institute for Clinical Excellence has advised that the child's needs, ability to develop and maintain effective technique, and likelihood of good compliance should govern the choice of inhaler and spacer device; only then should cost be considered
> For children aged under 5 years:
>
> • corticosteroid and bronchodilator therapy should be routinely delivered by pressurised metered-dose inhaler and spacer device, with a facemask if necessary;
>
> • if this is not effective, and depending on the child's condition, nebulised therapy may be considered and, in children over 3 years, a dry powder inhaler may also be considered [but see notes above];
>
> For children aged 5–15 years:
>
> • corticosteroid therapy should be routinely delivered by a pressurised metered-dose inhaler and spacer device
>
> • children and their carers should be trained in the use of the chosen device; suitability of the device should be reviewed at least annually. Inhaler technique and compliance should be monitored

SPACER DEVICES. Spacer devices remove the need for co-ordination between actuation of a pressurised metered-dose inhaler and inhalation. The spacer device reduces the velocity of the aerosol and subsequent impaction on the oropharynx. In addition the device allows more time for evaporation of the propellant so that a larger proportion of the particles can be inhaled and deposited in the lungs. The size of the spacer is important, the larger spacers with a one-way valve (*Nebuhaler®, Volumatic®*) being most effective. Spacer devices are particularly useful for patients with poor inhalation technique, for children, for patients requiring higher doses, for nocturnal asthma, and for patients prone to candidiasis with inhaled corticosteroids. It is important to prescribe a spacer device that is compatible with the metered-dose inhaler.

USE AND CARE OF SPACER DEVICES. Patients should inhale from the spacer device as soon as possible after actuation since the drug aerosol is very short-lived; single-dose actuation is recommended. The device should be cleansed once a month by washing in mild detergent, rinsing and then allowing to dry in air (wiping should be avoided since any electrostatic charge may affect drug delivery). Spacer devices should be replaced every 6–12 months.

Able Spacer® (Clement Clarke)
Spacer device, small-volume device. For use with pressurised (aerosol) inhalers, net price standard device = £4.20; with infant, child or adult mask = £6.86

AeroChamber® **Plus** (3M)
Spacer device, medium-volume device. For use with *Airomir*®, *Atrovent*®, *Atrovent*® *Forte*, *Combivent*®, *Duovent*®, *Oxivent*®, *Salbulin*®, and *Qvar*® inhalers, net price standard device (blue) = £4.28, with mask (blue) = £7.14; infant device (orange) with mask = £7.14; child device (yellow) with mask = £7.14

Babyhaler® (A&H) NHS
Spacer device for paediatric use with *Becotide*®-*50* and *Ventolin*® inhalers. Net price = £11.34

E-Z Spacer® (Vitalograph) NHS
Spacer device, large-volume, collapsible device. For use with pressurised (aerosol) inhalers, price (direct from manufacturer) = £23.00

Haleraid® (A&H) NHS
Device to place over standard inhalers to aid when strength in hands is impaired (e.g. in arthritis). Available as *Haleraid*®-*120* for 120-dose inhalers and *Haleraid*®-*200* for 200-dose inhalers. Net price = 80p

Nebuhaler® (AstraZeneca)
Spacer inhaler, large-volume device. For use with *Bricanyl*® and *Pulmicort*® inhalers, net price = £4.28; with paediatric mask = £4.28

PARI Space Chamber® (Pari)
Spacer device, medium volume device. For use with a pressurised (aerosol) inhaler, net price = £4.25; with mask for infant, child 1–4 years or child 4–7 years = £6.85

Pocket Chamber® (Ferraris)
Spacer device, small-volume device. For use with a pressurised (aerosol) inhaler, net price = £4.18; with infant, small, medium, or large mask = £9.75

Spinhaler® (Rhône-Poulenc Rorer)
Breath-actuated device for use with *Intal Spincaps*®. Net price = £2.08

Volumatic® (A&H)
Spacer inhaler, large-volume device. For use with *Becloforte*®, *Becotide*®, *Flixotide*®, *Seretide*®, *Serevent*®, and *Ventolin*® inhalers, net price = £2.75; with paediatric mask = £2.75

Nebulisers

In England and Wales nebulisers and compressors are not available on the NHS (but they are free of VAT); some nebulisers (but not compressors) are available on form GP10A in Scotland (for details consult Scottish Drug Tariff).

A nebuliser converts a solution of a drug into an aerosol for inhalation. It is used to deliver higher doses of drug to the airways than is usual with standard inhalers. The main indications for use of a nebuliser are:

- to deliver a beta agonist or ipratropium to a patient with an *acute exacerbation* of asthma or of airways obstruction;
- to deliver a beta agonist or ipratropium on a *regular basis* to a patient with severe asthma or reversible airways obstruction who has been shown to benefit from regular treatment with higher doses;
- to deliver *prophylactic medication* such as cromoglicate or a corticosteroid to a patient unable to use other inhalational devices (particularly a young child);
- to deliver an antibiotic (such as colistin) to a patient with chronic purulent infection (as in cystic fibrosis or bronchiectasis);
- to deliver pentamidine for the prophylaxis and treatment of pneumocystis pneumonia to a patient with AIDS.

The proportion of a nebuliser solution that reaches the lungs depends on the type of nebuliser and although it can be as high as 30% it is more frequently close to 10% and sometimes below 10%. The remaining solution is left in the nebuliser as residual volume or it is deposited in the mouth-piece and tubing. The extent to which the nebulised solution is deposited in the airways or alveoli depends on particle size. Particles with a mass median diameter of 1–5 microns are deposited in the airways and are therefore appropriate for asthma whereas a particle size of 1–2 microns is needed for alveolar deposition of pentamidine to combat pneumocystis infection. The type of nebuliser is therefore chosen according to the deposition required and according to the viscosity of the solution (anti-biotic solutions usually being more viscous).

Some jet nebulisers are able to increase drug output during inspiration and hence increase efficiency.

The patient should be aware that the dose of a bronchodilator given by nebulisation is usually **much higher** than that from an aerosol inhaler; see below for British Thoracic Society guidelines.

The British Thoracic Society has advised that nebulised bronchodilators may be given to patients with chronic persistent asthma or those with sudden catastrophic severe asthma (brittle asthma). In chronic asthma, nebulised bronchodilators should only be used to relieve persistent daily wheeze (see Chronic Asthma table p. 131). The British Thoracic Society has further recommended that the use of nebulisers in chronic persistent asthma should only be considered:

- after a review of the diagnosis;
- if the airflow obstruction is significantly reversible by bronchodilators without unacceptable side-effects;
- after the patient has been using the usual hand-held inhaler correctly;
- after a larger dose of bronchodilator from a hand-held inhaler (with a spacer if necessary) has been tried for at least 2 weeks;
- if the patient is complying with the prescribed dose and frequency of anti-inflammatory treatment including regular use of high-dose inhaled corticosteroid.

Before prescribing a nebuliser, a home trial should preferably be undertaken to monitor peak flow for up to 2 weeks on standard treatment and up to 2 weeks on nebulised treatment. If prescribed, patients must:

- have clear instructions from doctor, specialist nurse or pharmacist on the use of the nebuliser and on peak-flow monitoring;

- be instructed not to treat acute attacks at home without also seeking help;
- receive an education program;
- have regular follow up including peak-flow monitoring and be seen by doctor, specialist nurse or physiotherapist.

■ Jet nebulisers

Jet nebulisers are more widely used than ultrasonic nebulisers. Most jet nebulisers require an optimum gas flow rate of 6–8 litres/minute and in hospital can be driven by piped air or oxygen. Domiciliary oxygen cylinders do not provide an adequate flow rate therefore an electrical compressor is required for domiciliary use.

For patients with *chronic obstructive pulmonary disease and hypercapnia*, oxygen can be dangerous and the nebuliser should be driven by air (see also p. 134).

> **Important:** the Department of Health has reminded users of the need to use the correct grade of tubing when connecting a nebuliser to a medical gas supply or compressor.

Medix All Nebuliser® (Medix) ▐NHS▌
Jet nebuliser, disposable; for use with bronchodilators, antimuscarinics, corticosteroids, and antibiotics, replacement recommended every 2–3 months if used 4 times a day. Compatible with **AC 2000 Hi Flo**® ▐NHS▌, **World Traveller Hi Flo**® ▐NHS▌, and **Econoneb**® ▐NHS▌, net price 5 = £1.50

Medix Antibiotic Circuit® (Medix) ▐NHS▌
Jet nebuliser, closed-system; for use with antibiotics and other respiratory drugs. Compatible with **AC 2000 Hi Flo**® ▐NHS▌, **Econoneb**® ▐NHS▌, and **Turboneb**® ▐NHS▌, net price = £7.30

Medix System® (Medix) ▐NHS▌
Jet nebuliser, consisting of mouthpiece, tubing, and nebuliser chamber, net price = £2.80; mask kits with tubing and nebuliser chamber also available, net price (adult)= £2.00; (child) = £2.10

Omron CX® (Omron) ▐NHS▌
Jet nebuliser, non-disposable, with **Omron VC**® nebuliser kit, net price = £56.25

PARI LC PLUS FILTER® (Pari) ▐NHS▌
Jet nebuliser, closed system, non-disposable, for hospital or home use; for use with bronchodilators, antibiotics and corticosteroids; replacement recommended yearly if used 4 times a day. Compatible with **PARI Turbo BOY'N'**® ▐NHS▌ and **PARI Junior BOY'N'**® ▐NHS▌ compressors, net price = £23.60, replacement filters 100 = £34.00

PARI LC PLUS® (Pari) ▐NHS▌
Jet nebuliser, non-disposable, for hospital or home use; for use with bronchodilators, antibiotics, and corticosteroids, replacement recommended yearly if used 4 times a day. Compatible with **PARI Turbo BOY'N'**® ▐NHS▌, **PARI Junior BOY'N'**® ▐NHS▌ and **PARI WALK BOY**® ▐NHS▌ compressors, net price = £15.45

PARI BABY® (Pari) ▐NHS▌
Jet nebuliser, non-disposable, for hospital or home use; for use with bronchodilators, antibiotics and corticosteroids; replacement recommended yearly if used 4 times a day. Compatible with **PARI Turbo BOY'N'**® ▐NHS▌, **PARI Junior BOY'N'**® ▐NHS▌, **PARI WALK BOY**® ▐NHS▌ compressors. Available separately for children aged less than 1 year, 1–4 years or 4–7 years, net price (with mask and connection tube) = £29.85

Sidestream Durable® (Medic-Aid) ▐NHS▌
Jet nebuliser, non-disposable, for home use; for use with bronchodilators; yearly replacement recommended if 4 six-minute treatments used per day. Compatible with **CR50**® ▐NHS▌, **Freeway Lite**® ▐NHS▌ and **Porta-Neb**

50® ▐NHS▌ (depending on nebulising solution), net price 10 pack = £94.50; patient pack with **CR50**® ▐NHS▌ compressor = £98.50. **Disposable Sidestream**® ▐NHS▌ nebuliser also available

Ventstream® (Medic-Aid) ▐NHS▌
Jet nebuliser, closed-system, for use with low flow compressors, compatible with **CR50**® ▐NHS▌, **Porta-Neb 50**® ▐NHS▌, and **Freeway Lite**® ▐NHS▌ compressors; for use with antibiotics, bronchodilators, and corticosteroids, replacement recommended yearly if used 3 times a day, net price with filter = £27.00; 10-pack with filter = £250.00; without filter = £23.00; 10-pack without filter = £215.00; patient pack with **CR50**® ▐NHS▌ compressor = £119.95

■ Home compressors with nebulisers

AC 2000 HI FLO® (Medix) ▐NHS▌
Portable, home use, containing 1 **Jet Nebuliser**® ▐NHS▌ set with mouthpiece, 1 adult or 1 child mask,1 spare inlet filter, filter spanner. Mains operated. Nebulises bronchodilators and antibiotics, net price = £117.00; carrying case available

Aquilon® (Henleys) ▐NHS▌
Portable, home use, with 1 adult or 1 child mask and tubing. Mains operated; for use with bronchodilators, corticosteroids and antibiotics, net price = £81.00

Econoneb® (Medix) ▐NHS▌
Home, clinic and hospital use, used with 1 **Jet Nebuliser**® ▐NHS▌ set with mouthpiece, 1 adult or 1 child mask, 1 spare inlet filter, filter spanner. Compatible with all types of jet nebuliser sets and also the **Micro Cirrus**® ▐NHS▌ nebuliser (recommended for alveolar deposition). Nebulises bronchodilators, corticosteroids, and antibiotics. Mains operated, net price = £99.00

Freeway Lite® (Medic-Aid) ▐NHS▌
Portable, containing 1 **Sidestream Durable**® ▐NHS▌ reusable nebuliser, 1 adult or 1 child mask, 1 mouthpiece, 1 Coiled Duratube®, 2 filters, net price = £149.00 with carrying case. **Freeway Lite Luxury**® ▐NHS▌ contains additional battery, net price = £198.00

Also compatible with **Ventstream**® ▐NHS▌ closed system nebuliser

M-Flo® (Medix) ▐NHS▌
Portable, home use, containing 1 **Jet Nebuliser**® ▐NHS▌ set with mouthpiece, spare inlet filter, filter spanner. Mains operated. Nebulises bronchodilators and corticosteroids, net price = £95.00

Medi-Neb® (Timesco) ▐NHS▌
Range of compressors all supplied with adult and child mask, vapourising chamber, and PVC tubing, including: **Medi-Neb Elite**® ▐NHS▌, *home use*. Mains operated, net price = £84.96. **Medi-Neb Companion**® ▐NHS▌, *portable*. Mains/car battery operated, net price = £104.95 (includes car battery adaptor and carrying case). **Medi-Neb Companion Plus**® ▐NHS▌, *portable*. Mains/battery operated, net price = £144.96 (includes rechargeable battery, car battery adaptor, and carrying case). **Medi-Neb Tempest**® ▐NHS▌, *home/hospital use*. Mains operated, net price = £94.96

All used for nebulising antibiotics and bronchodilators

PARI Turbo BOY'N'® (Pari) ▐NHS▌
Portable, for hospital or home use, containing **PARI LC PLUS** ▐NHS▌ nebuliser with adult mouthpiece, mask, connection tube and mains cable. Filter replacement recommended every 12 months. Compatible with **PARI LC PLUS**® ▐NHS▌, **PARI LC PLUS FILTER**® ▐NHS▌, and **PARI BABY**® ▐NHS▌ nebulisers, net price = £115.00

PARI Junior BOY'N'® (Pari) ▐NHS▌
Portable, for hospital or home use, containing **PARI LC PLUS Junior** ▐NHS▌ nebuliser with child mouthpiece, mask, connection tube, and mains cable. Filter replacement recommended every 12 months. Compatible with **PARI LC PLUS**® ▐NHS▌, **PARI LC PLUS Filter**® ▐NHS▌, and **PARI Baby**® ▐NHS▌ nebulisers, net price = £125.00

PARI WALK BOY[®] (Pari) [NHS]
Portable, containing **PARI LC PLUS**[®] [NHS] nebuliser with connection tube, mains cable, rechargeable battery and carrying bag. Compatible with **PARI LC PLUS**[®] [NHS] and **PARI BABY**[®] [NHS] nebulisers, net price = £225.00; car cigarette lighter adapter = £55.00

Porta-Neb[®] (Medic-Aid) [NHS]
Portable, containing 1 **Sidestream Durable**[®] [NHS] reusable nebuliser, 1 angled flow-through mouthpiece, 1 adult or 1 child mask, 1 Duratube[®] supply tubing, 4 spare filters. Mains operated; for use with bronchodilators, net price = £109.50; carrying case available
Also compatible with **Ventstream**[®] [NHS] closed-system nebuliser; for use with antibiotics, bronchodilators, and corticosteroids

Pulmo-Aide[®] (De Vilbiss) [NHS]
Home, clinic use, containing disposable nebuliser set, mouthpiece, mask, mains lead, tubing, thumb-valve. For use with bronchodilators, net price = £99.50. **Pulmo-Aide Escort**[®] [NHS], *portable*, containing disposable nebuliser set, transformer, rechargeable battery, AC to DC adapter charger, DC lead with car adapter, and carrying case. For use with bronchodilators, net price = £198.50. **Pulmo-Aide AP50**[®] [NHS], *home, clinic, hospital use*, net price = £180.00, with anti-pollution kit = £188.50. **Pulmo-Aide Sunmist**[®] [NHS], *home use*, containing nebuliser set, mouthpiece, face mask, mains lead, net price = £84.25

SunMist[®] (De Vilbiss) [NHS]
Home, clinic and hospital use, with mouthpiece. Mains operated, net price = £89.50. **SunMist Plus**[®] [NHS], *home, clinic and hospital use*, with mouthpiece, higher flow rate. Mains operated, net price = £107.50

Tourer[®] (Henleys) [NHS]
Portable, home use. Mains/car battery operated; for use with bronchodilators, corticosteroids and antibiotics, net price = £118.50, rechargeable battery pack = £54.00

Ultima[®] (Henleys) [NHS]
Portable, home use. Rechargable or mains/car battery operated. Nebulises bronchodilators and corticosteroids, net price = £184.00 (includes case)

World Traveller HI FLO[®] (Medix) [NHS]
Portable, containing 1 **Jet Nebuliser**[®] [NHS] set with mouthpiece, 1 adult or 1 child mask, 1 spare inlet filter, filter spanner. Battery/mains operated; rechargeable battery pack available. Nebulises bronchodilators, corticosteroids, and antibiotics, net price excluding battery = £145.00; with battery = £199.00; carrying case available

■ Compressors

Omron CX3[®] (Omron) [NHS]
Home and hospital use. Mains operated, net price = £48.75

System 22 CR50[®] (Medic-Aid) [NHS]
Home, clinic and hospital use. Mains operated, net price = £89.50. Also compatible with **Ventstream**[®] [NHS], and **Sidestream Durable**[®] [NHS]

System 22 CR60[®] (Medic-Aid) [NHS]
Hospital use, high flow compressor. Mains operated, net price = £199.90. Also compatible with **System 22 Antibiotic Tee**[®] [NHS] for nebulisation of high viscosity drugs such as antibiotics

Turboneb[®] (Medix) [NHS]
Hospital use, high flow compressor. Mains operated, net price = £125.00. Also compatible with **Medix Antibiotic Circuit**[®] [NHS] for nebulisation of respiratory drugs in particular viscous antibiotics

■ Ultrasonic nebulisers
Ultrasonic nebulisers produce an aerosol by ultrasonic vibration of the drug solution and therefore do not require a gas flow

AeroSonic[®] (De Vilbiss) [NHS]
Portable, containing 1 controlling unit, chamber assembly, carrying case, AC to DC adapter/charger, DC lead, 1 mouthpiece with check valve and adapter, net price = £250.00

F16 Wave[®] (Parkside) [NHS]
Portable, adjustable delivery rate. Mains/car battery operated or rechargeable battery pack (supplied), net price = £120.00

Omron U1[®] (Omron) [NHS]
Portable. Battery operated/mains adaptor, net price = £146.25

Omron NE U07[®] (Omron) [NHS]
Portable. Mains operated or rechargeable battery pack, net price = £146.25 (mains version), rechargeable battery pack = £95.00

Sonix 2000[®] (Medix) [NHS]
Portable, adjustable delivery rate. Supplied with carrying case and DC lead. Mains/car battery operated; rechargeable battery pack available, net price excluding battery = £150.00, with battery = £215.00

Syst'am[®] (Vitalograph) [NHS]
Home and clinic use, adjustable delivery rate, mains operated, carry cases available, net price *Model 230* = £137.00; *Model 260* (fitted with *Flovision*[®] system indicating inspiratory flow rate) = £174.00; *Model 290* = £154.00

Ultra Neb 2000[®] (De Vilbiss) [NHS]
Hospital, clinic and home use, delivery rate adjustable. Supplied with stand, net price = £1125.50

Nebuliser diluent

Nebulisation may be carried out using an undiluted nebuliser solution or it may require dilution beforehand. The usual diluent is sterile sodium chloride 0.9% (physiological saline).

Sodium Chloride (Non-proprietary) [PoM]
Nebuliser solution, sodium chloride 0.9%, net price 20 × 2.5 mL = £5.49
Available from Galen (*Saline Steripoule*[®]), IVAX (*Saline Steri-Neb*[®])

3.2 Corticosteroids

Corticosteroids are very effective in *asthma*; they reduce airway inflammation (and hence reduce oedema and secretion of mucus into the airway).

Patients with *chronic obstructive pulmonary disease* usually show little or no response to corticosteroids. Long-term studies have shown no reduction in the decline in lung function in chronic obstructive pulmonary disease in patients taking regular inhaled corticosteroids. Higher doses of inhaled corticosteroids may reduce symptoms and exacerbations slightly in patients with more severe chronic obstructive pulmonary disease. A trial of a corticosteroid can distinguish patients who in fact have asthma from those who have chronic obstructive pulmonary disease.

INHALATION. Inhaled corticosteroids are recommended for prophylactic treatment of asthma when patients are using a beta$_2$ agonist more than once daily (see Chronic Asthma table, p. 131). *Regular use* of inhaled corticosteroids reduces the risk of exacerbation of asthma.

Corticosteroid inhalers must be used regularly for maximum benefit; alleviation of symptoms usually occurs 3 to 7 days after initiation. **Beclometasone dipropionate** (beclomethasone dipropionate), **budesonide** and **fluticasone propionate** appear to be equally effective. Doses for CFC-free corticosteroid inhalers may be different from those that contain CFCs.

CFC-free inhalers. Chlorofluorocarbon (CFC) propellants in pressurised aerosol inhalers are being replaced by hydrofluoroalkane (HFA) propellants. Patients receiving CFC-free inhalers should be reassured about the efficacy of the new inhalers and counselled that the aerosol may feel and taste different; any difficulty with the new inhaler should be discussed with the doctor or pharmacist.

CSM advice. The CSM has requested doctors to report any adverse reaction to the new HFA-containing inhalers and to include the brand name of the inhaler on the yellow card.

If the inhaled corticosteroid causes coughing, the use of a beta$_2$ agonist beforehand may help.

Patients who have been taking long-term oral corticosteroids can often be transferred to an inhaled corticosteroid but the transfer must be slow, with gradual reduction in the dose of oral corticosteroid, and at a time when the asthma is well controlled.

High-dose inhalers are available for patients who respond only partially to standard-dose inhalers and long-acting beta$_2$ agonists or other long-acting bronchodilators (see Chronic Asthma, table, p. 131). High doses should be continued only if there is clear benefit over the lower dose. The recommended maximum doses of inhaled corticosteroids should not generally be exceeded. However, if higher doses are required (e.g. fluticasone in a dose above 500 micrograms twice daily in an adult or 200 micrograms twice daily in child 4–16 years), then they should be initiated by specialists.

Systemic therapy may be necessary during episodes of infection or if asthma is worsening, when higher doses are needed and access of inhaled drug to small airways may be reduced; patients may need a reserve supply of tablets.

CAUTIONS OF INHALED CORTICOSTEROIDS. Caution is required in active or quiescent tuberculosis; systemic therapy may be required during periods of stress or when airways obstruction or mucus prevent drug access to smaller airways; **interactions:** Appendix 1 (corticosteroids)

PARADOXICAL BRONCHOSPASM. The potential for paradoxical bronchospasm (calling for discontinuation and alternative therapy) should be borne in mind—if mild it may be prevented by inhalation of a beta$_2$-adrenoceptor stimulant (or by transfer from an aerosol inhalation to a dry powder inhalation)

SIDE-EFFECTS OF INHALED CORTICOSTEROIDS. Inhaled corticosteroids have considerably fewer systemic effects than oral corticosteroids, but adverse effects have been reported including a small increased risk of glaucoma with prolonged high doses of inhaled corticosteroids; cataracts have also been reported with inhaled corticosteroids. Hoarseness and candidiasis of the mouth or throat have been reported, usually only with large doses (see also below). Hypersensitivity reactions (including rash and angioedema) have been reported rarely.

CANDIDIASIS. Candidiasis can be reduced by using spacer, see notes above, and responds to antifungal lozenges (section 12.3.2) without discontinuation of therapy—rinsing the mouth with water (or cleaning child's teeth) after inhalation of a dose may also be helpful

Higher doses of inhaled corticosteroids also have the potential to induce adrenal suppression (section 6.3.2) and patients on high doses should be given a 'steroid card'; such patients may need corticosteroid cover during an episode of stress (e.g. an operation).

Bone mineral density is reduced following long-term inhalation of higher doses of corticosteroids, and this may predispose patients to osteoporosis (section 6.6). It is therefore sensible to ensure that the dose of inhaled corticosteroid is no higher than necessary to keep a patient's asthma under good control. The dose may therefore be reduced cautiously when the asthma has been well controlled for a few weeks as long as the patient knows that it is necessary to reinstate it should the asthma deteriorate or the peak flow rate fall.

In children, growth retardation associated with oral corticosteroid therapy does not seem to be a significant problem with recommended doses of inhaled therapy; although initial growth velocity may be reduced, there appears to be no effect on normal adult height. However, the CSM recommends that the height of children receiving prolonged treatment is monitored; if growth is slowed, referral to a paediatrician should be considered. Large-volume spacer devices should be used for administering inhaled corticosteroids in children under 5 years (see NICE guidance, section 3.1.5); they are also useful in older children and adults, particularly if high doses are required. Spacer devices increase airway deposition and reduce oropharyngeal deposition, resulting in a marked reduction in the incidence of candidiasis.

Budesonide and fluticasone propionate are both available as suspensions for nebulisation.

ORAL. Acute attacks of asthma should be treated with short courses of oral corticosteroids starting with a high dose, e.g. prednisolone 40–50 mg daily for a few days. Patients whose asthma has deteriorated rapidly usually respond quickly to corticosteroids. The dose can usually be stopped abruptly in a mild exacerbation of asthma (see also Withdrawal of Corticosteroids, section 6.3.2) but it should be reduced gradually in those with poorer asthma control, to reduce the possibility of serious relapse. For use of corticosteroids in the emergency treatment of acute severe asthma see table on p. 132.

In chronic continuing asthma, when the response to other anti-asthma drugs has been relatively small, longer term administration of oral corticosteroids may be necessary; in such cases high doses of an inhaled corticosteroid should be continued to minimise oral corticosteroid requirements. Oral corticosteroids should normally be taken as a single dose in the morning to reduce the disturbance to circadian cortisol secretion. Dosage should always be titrated to the lowest dose that controls symptoms. Regular peak flow measurements often help to optimise the dose.

Alternate-day administration has not been very successful in the management of asthma in adults because control can deteriorate during the second 24 hours. If alternate-day administration is introduced, pulmonary function should be monitored carefully over the 48 hours.

PARENTERAL. For the use of hydrocortisone injection in the emergency treatment of acute severe asthma, see Acute Severe Asthma table, p. 132.

fumarate 4.5 micrograms/metered inhalation, net price 120-dose unit = £33.00. Label: 8, counselling, dose, 10 steroid card

NOTE. Each metered inhalation of *Symbicort* 100/6 delivers the same quantity of budesonide as a 100-microgram metered inhalation of *Pulmicort Turbohaler* and of formoterol as a 6-microgram metered inhalation of *Oxis Turbohaler*

Dose: by inhalation of powder, asthma, ADULT and CHILD over 12 years, 1–2 puffs twice daily, CHILD over 6 years, 2 puffs twice daily; may be reduced in well-controlled asthma to once daily

Symbicort 200/6 Turbohaler (= dry powder inhaler), budesonide 160 micrograms, formoterol fumarate 4.5 micrograms/metered inhalation, net price 120-dose unit = £38.00. Label: 8, counselling, dose, 10 steroid card

NOTE. Each metered inhalation of *Symbicort* 200/6 delivers the same quantity of budesonide as a 200-microgram metered inhalation of *Pulmicort Turbohaler* and of formoterol as a 6-microgram metered inhalation of *Oxis Turbohaler*

Dose: by inhalation of powder, asthma, ADULT and CHILD over 12 years, 1–2 puffs twice daily, may be reduced in well-controlled asthma to 1–2 puffs once daily

Chronic obstructive pulmonary disease, 2 puffs twice daily; CHILD not recommended

Symbicort 400/12 Turbohaler (= dry powder inhaler), budesonide 320 micrograms, formoterol fumarate 9 micrograms/metered inhalation, net price 60-dose unit = £38.00. Label: 8, counselling, dose, 10 steroid card

NOTE. Each metered inhalation of *Symbicort* 400/12 delivers the same quantity of budesonide as a 400-microgram metered inhalation of *Pulmicort Turbohaler* and of formoterol as a 12-microgram metered inhalation of *Oxis Turbohaler*

Dose: by inhalation of powder, asthma, ADULT and CHILD over 12 years, 1 puff twice daily, may be reduced in well-controlled asthma to 1 puff once daily

Chronic obstructive pulmonary disease, 1 puff twice daily; CHILD not recommended

▪ Inhaler devices
Section 3.1.5

FLUTICASONE PROPIONATE

Indications: prophylactic treatment for asthma (see also Chronic Asthma table, p. 131)

Cautions: see notes above

Side-effects: see notes above

Dose: see preparations below

Flixotide (A&H) PoM

Accuhaler (dry powder for inhalation), disk containing 60 blisters of fluticasone propionate 50 micrograms/blister with *Accuhaler* device, net price = £6.86; 100 micrograms/blister with *Accuhaler* device = £9.60; 250 micrograms/blister with *Accuhaler* device = £22.86; 500 micrograms/blister with *Accuhaler* device = £38.86. Label: 8, counselling, dose; 250- and 500-microgram strengths also label 10 steroid card

NOTE. *Flixotide Accuhaler* 250 micrograms and 500 micrograms are not indicated for children

Dose: by inhalation of powder, ADULT and CHILD over 16 years, 100–250 micrograms twice daily, increased according to severity of asthma to 1 mg twice daily; CHILD 4–16 years, 50–100 micrograms twice daily adjusted as necessary; max. 200 micrograms twice daily

Aerosol inhalation, fluticasone propionate 25 micrograms/metered inhalation, net price 120-dose unit = £6.86. Label: 8, counselling, dose

Excipients: include CFC propellants

Dose: by aerosol inhalation, CHILD over 4 years, 50–100 micrograms twice daily adjusted as necessary; max. 200 micrograms twice daily

Diskhaler (dry powder for inhalation), fluticasone propionate 50 micrograms/blister, net price 15 disks of 4 blisters with *Diskhaler* device = £8.78, 15-disk refill = £8.21; 100 micrograms/blister, 15 disks of 4 blisters with *Diskhaler* device = £13.67, 15-disk refill = £13.10; 250 micrograms/blister, 15 disks of 4 blisters with *Diskhaler* device = £25.92, 15-disk refill = £25.35; 500 micrograms/blister, 15 disks of 4 blisters with *Diskhaler* device = £43.06, 15-disk refill = £42.49. Label: 8, counselling, dose; 250- and 500-microgram strengths also label 10 steroid card

NOTE. *Flixotide Diskhaler* 250 micrograms and 500 micrograms are not indicated for children

Dose: by inhalation of powder, ADULT and CHILD over 16 years, 100–250 micrograms twice daily, increased according to severity of asthma to 1 mg twice daily; CHILD 4–16 years, 50–100 micrograms twice daily adjusted as necessary; max. 200 micrograms twice daily

Evohaler ▼*aerosol inhalation*, fluticasone propionate 50 micrograms/metered inhalation, net price 120-dose unit = £5.85; 125 micrograms/metered inhalation, 120-dose unit = £22.86; 250 micrograms/metered inhalation, 120-dose unit = £38.86. Label: 8, counselling, dose, change to CFC-free inhaler; 250-microgram strength also label 10 steroid card

Excipients: include HFA-134a (a non-CFC propellant)

NOTE. *Flixotide Evohaler* 125 micrograms and 250 micrograms not indicated for children

Dose: by aerosol inhalation, ADULT and CHILD over 16 years, 100–250 micrograms twice daily, increased according to severity of asthma to 1 mg twice daily; CHILD 4–16 years, 50–100 micrograms twice daily adjusted as necessary; max. 200 micrograms twice daily

Nebules (= single-dose units for nebulisation) fluticasone propionate 250 micrograms/mL, net price 10 × 2-mL (500-microgram) unit = £10.04; 1 mg/mL, 10 × 2-mL (2-mg) unit = £40.16. May be diluted with sterile sodium chloride 0.9%. Label: 8, counselling, dose, 10 steroid card

Dose: by inhalation of nebulised suspension, ADULT and CHILD over 16 years, 0.5–2 mg twice daily

▪ Compound preparations

Seretide (A&H) PoM

Seretide 100 Accuhaler (dry powder for inhalation), disk containing 60 blisters of fluticasone propionate 100 micrograms, salmeterol (as xinafoate) 50 micrograms/blister with *Accuhaler* device, net price = £33.54. Label: 8, counselling, dose

Dose: by inhalation of powder, ADULT and CHILD over 4 years, 1 blister twice daily, reduced to 1 blister once daily if control maintained

Seretide 250 Accuhaler (dry powder for inhalation), disk containing 60 blisters of fluticasone propionate 250 micrograms, salmeterol (as xinafoate) 50 micrograms/blister with *Accuhaler* device, net price = £39.41. Label: 8, counselling, dose, 10 steroid card

Dose: by inhalation of powder, ADULT and CHILD over 12 years, 1 blister twice daily

Seretide 500 Accuhaler® (dry powder for inhalation), disk containing 60 blisters of fluticasone propionate 500 micrograms, salmeterol (as xinafoate) 50 micrograms/blister with *Accuhaler*® device, net price = £66.98. Label: 8, counselling, dose, 10 steroid card

Dose: by inhalation of powder, ADULT and CHILD over 12 years, 1 blister twice daily

Seretide 50 Evohaler® (aerosol inhalation), fluticasone propionate 50 micrograms, salmeterol (as xinafoate) 25 micrograms/metered inhalation, net price 120-dose unit = £19.50. Label: 8, counselling, dose, change to CFC-free inhaler

Excipients: include HFA-134a (a non-CFC propellant)

Dose: by aerosol inhalation, ADULT and CHILD over 12 years, 2 puffs twice daily, reduced to 2 puffs once daily if control maintained

Seretide 125 Evohaler® (aerosol inhalation), fluticasone propionate 125 micrograms, salmeterol (as xinafoate) 25 micrograms/metered inhalation, net price 120-dose unit = £39.41. Label: 8, counselling, dose, change to CFC-free inhaler, 10 steroid card

Excipients: include HFA-134a (a non-CFC propellant)

Dose: by aerosol inhalation, ADULT and CHILD over 12 years, 2 puffs twice daily

Seretide 250 Evohaler® (aerosol inhalation), fluticasone propionate 250 micrograms, salmeterol (as xinafoate) 25 micrograms/metered inhalation, net price 120-dose unit = £66.98. Label: 8, counselling, dose, change to CFC-free inhaler, 10 steroid card

Excipients: include HFA-134a (a non-CFC propellant)

Dose: by aerosol inhalation, ADULT and CHILD over 12 years, 2 puffs twice daily

MOMETASONE FUROATE

Indications: prophylactic treatment for asthma (see also Chronic Asthma table, p. 131)

Cautions: see notes above

Side-effects: see notes above; also pharyngitis

Dose: *by inhalation of powder*, 200–400 micrograms as a single dose in the evening or in 2 divided doses; dose increased to 400 micrograms twice daily if necessary; CHILD not recommended

Asmanex® (Schering-Plough) ▼ PoM
Twisthaler (= dry powder inhaler), mometasone furoate 200 micrograms/metered inhalation, net price 30-dose unit = £16.00, 60-dose unit = £24.00; 400 micrograms/metered inhalation, 30-dose unit = £22.20, 60-dose unit = £36.75. Label: 8, counselling, dose, 10 steroid card

---

3.3 Cromoglicate, related therapy and leukotriene receptor antagonists

3.3.1 Cromoglicate and related therapy
3.3.2 Leukotriene receptor antagonists

3.3.1 Cromoglicate and related therapy

The mode of action of **sodium cromoglicate** and **nedocromil** is not completely understood. They may be of value in asthma with an allergic basis, but, in practice, it is difficult to predict who will benefit; they could probably be given for 4 to 6 weeks to assess response. Dose frequency is adjusted according to response but is usually 3 or 4 times a day initially; this may subsequently be reduced.

In general, *prophylaxis* with sodium cromoglicate is less effective than prophylaxis with corticosteroid inhalations (see Chronic Asthma table, p. 131). There is evidence of efficacy of nedocromil sodium in children aged 5–12 years. Sodium cromoglicate is of no value in the treatment of acute attacks of asthma.

Sodium cromoglicate can prevent exercise-induced asthma. However, exercise-induced asthma may reflect poor overall control and the patient should be assessed.

If inhalation of the dry powder form of sodium cromoglicate causes bronchospasm a selective beta$_2$-adrenoceptor stimulant such as salbutamol or terbutaline should be inhaled a few minutes beforehand. The nebuliser solution is an alternative means of delivery for children who cannot manage the dry powder inhaler or the aerosol.

SODIUM CROMOGLICATE
(Sodium Cromoglycate)

Indications: prophylaxis of asthma; food allergy (section 1.5); allergic conjunctivitis (section 11.4.2); allergic rhinitis (section 12.2.1)

Side-effects: coughing, transient bronchospasm, and throat irritation due to inhalation of powder (see also notes above)

Dose: *by aerosol inhalation*, ADULT and CHILD, 10 mg (2 puffs) 4 times daily, increased in severe cases or during periods of risk to 6–8 times daily; additional doses may also be taken before exercise; maintenance 5 mg (1 puff) 4 times daily

By inhalation of powder (*Spincaps*®), ADULT and CHILD, 20 mg 4 times daily, increased in severe cases to 8 times daily; additional doses may also be taken before exercise

By inhalation of nebulised solution, ADULT and CHILD, 20 mg 4 times daily, increased in severe cases to 6 times daily

COUNSELLING. Regular use is necessary

Sodium Cromoglicate (Non-proprietary) PoM
Aerosol inhalation, sodium cromoglicate 5 mg/metered inhalation. Net price 112-dose unit = £15.30. Label: 8
Available from IVAX (*Cromogen*®)
Excipients: include CFC propellants

Nebuliser solution, sodium cromoglicate 10 mg/mL. Net price 60 × 2-mL unit-dose vials = £11.58
Available from IVAX (*Cromogen Steri-Neb*®)

Cromogen Easi-Breathe® (IVAX) PoM
Aerosol inhalation, sodium cromoglicate 5 mg/metered inhalation. Net price 112-dose breath-actuated unit = £13.91. Label: 8
Excipients: include CFC propellants

Intal® (Rhône-Poulenc Rorer) PoM
Aerosol inhalation, sodium cromoglicate 5 mg/metered inhalation. Net price 112-dose unit = £19.09; 2 × 112-dose unit with spacer device (*Syncroner*®) = £37.98; also available with large volume spacer inhaler (*Fisonair*®), complete unit = £22.06. Label: 8
Excipients: include CFC propellants

Side-effects: see notes above; incidence of sedation and antimuscarinic effects low

Dose: 8 mg 3 times daily; CHILD under 12 years, not recommended; ELDERLY not recommended

■ Preparations

Capsules can be sold to the public for the treatment of hayfever and allergic skin conditions in adults and children over 12 years provided packs do not contain over 10 days' supply (*Benadryl® Allergy Relief*)

CETIRIZINE HYDROCHLORIDE

Indications: symptomatic relief of allergy such as hay fever, urticaria

Cautions: see notes above

Contra-indications: see notes above; also pregnancy (Appendix 4) and breast-feeding (Appendix 5)

Side-effects: see notes above; incidence of sedation and antimuscarinic effects low

Dose: ADULT and CHILD over 6 years, 10 mg daily *or* 5 mg twice daily; CHILD 2–6 years, hayfever, 5 mg daily *or* 2.5 mg twice daily

Cetirizine (Non-proprietary)
Tablets, cetirizine hydrochloride 10 mg, net price 30-tab pack = £7.90. Counselling, driving
Available from Alpharma, APS (*Cetirocol®*), CP, Generics, Lagap, Sterwin
Oral solution, cetirizine hydrochloride 5 mg/5 mL, net price 200 mL = £10.50. Counselling, driving
Available from Lagap
Proprietary brands of cetirizine on sale to the public include *Benadryl® One A Day, Piriteze® Allergy, Zirtek® Allergy, Zirtek® Allergy Relief*

DESLORATADINE

NOTE. Desloratadine is a metabolite of loratadine

Indications: symptomatic relief of allergy such as hay fever, urticaria

Cautions: see notes above

Contra-indications: see notes above; also hypersensitivity to loratadine; pregnancy (Appendix 4) and breast-feeding (Appendix 5)

Side-effects: see notes above; also fatigue; incidence of sedation and antimuscarinic effects low

Dose: ADULT and ADOLESCENT over 12 years, 5 mg daily; CHILD 2–5 years 1.25 mg daily, 6–11 years 2.5 mg daily

Neoclarityn® (Schering-Plough) ▼ PoM
Tablets, blue, f/c, desloratadine 5 mg, net price 30-tab pack = £7.57. Counselling, driving
Syrup, desloratadine 2.5 mg/5 mL, net price 100 mL (bubblegum-flavour) = £7.57. Counselling, driving

FEXOFENADINE HYDROCHLORIDE

NOTE. Fexofenadine is a metabolite of terfenadine

Indications: see under preparations below

Cautions: see notes above; also pregnancy (Appendix 4)

Contra-indications: see notes above; also breast-feeding (Appendix 5)

Side-effects: see notes above; incidence of sedation and antimuscarinic effects low

Dose: see under preparations below

Telfast® 120 (Aventis Pharma) PoM
Tablets, f/c, peach, fexofenadine hydrochloride 120 mg. Net price 30-tab pack = £7.40. Counselling, driving
Dose: symptomatic relief of seasonal allergic rhinitis, 120 mg once daily; CHILD under 12 years, not recommended

Telfast® 180 (Aventis Pharma) PoM
Tablets, f/c, peach, fexofenadine hydrochloride 180 mg. Net price 30-tab pack = £9.63. Counselling, driving
Dose: symptomatic relief of chronic idiopathic urticaria, 180 mg once daily; CHILD under 12 years, not recommended

LEVOCETIRIZINE DIHYDROCHLORIDE

NOTE. Levocetirizine is an isomer of cetirizine

Indications: symptomatic relief of allergy such as hay fever, urticaria

Cautions: see notes above; also pregnancy (Appendix 4) and breast-feeding (Appendix 5)

Contra-indications: see notes above; also severe renal impairment

Side-effects: see notes above; incidence of sedation and antimuscarinic effects low

Dose: ADULT and CHILD over 6 years, 5 mg daily

Xyzal (UCB Pharma) ▼ PoM
Tablets, f/c, levocetirizine dihydrochloride 5 mg, net price 30-tab pack = £7.45. Counselling, driving

LORATADINE

Indications: symptomatic relief of allergy such as hay fever, urticaria

Cautions: see notes above

Contra-indications: see notes above; also pregnancy (Appendix 4) and breast-feeding (Appendix 5)

Side-effects: see notes above; incidence of sedation and antimuscarinic effects low

Dose: ADULT and CHILD over 6 years 10 mg daily; CHILD 2–5 years 5 mg daily

Loratadine (Non-proprietary)
Tablets, loratadine 10 mg, net price 30-tab pack = £7.19
Syrup, loratadine 5 mg/5 mL, net price 100 mL = £7.57. Counselling, driving
Proprietary brands of loratadine on sale to the public include *Boots Hayfever and Allergy Relief All Day®*, and *Clarityn Allergy®* NHS

MIZOLASTINE

Indications: symptomatic relief of allergy such as hay fever, urticaria

Cautions: see notes above

Contra-indications: see notes above; also susceptibility to QT-interval prolongation (including cardiac disease and hypokalaemia); significant hepatic impairment; pregnancy (Appendix 4) and breast-feeding (Appendix 5)

Side-effects: see notes above; also may cause weight gain; incidence of sedation and antimuscarinic effects low

Dose: 10 mg daily; CHILD under 12 years, not recommended

Intravenous adrenaline (epinephrine)

Where the patient is severely ill and there is real doubt about adequacy of the circulation and absorption from the intramuscular injection site, adrenaline (epinephrine) may be given by **slow** *intravenous injection* in a dose of 500 micrograms (5 mL of the dilute 1 in 10 000 adrenaline injection) given at a rate of 100 micrograms (1 mL of the dilute 1 in 10 000 adrenaline injection) per minute, *stopping when a response has been obtained*; children can be given a dose of 10 micrograms/kg (0.1 mL/kg of the dilute 1 in 10 000 adrenaline injection) by **slow** *intravenous injection* over several minutes. Great vigilance is needed to ensure that the *correct strength* is used; anaphylactic shock kits need to make a *very clear distinction* between the 1 in 10 000 strength and the 1 in 1000 strength. It is also important that, where intramuscular injection might still succeed, time should not be wasted seeking intravenous access.

For reference to the use of the intravenous route for *cardiac resuscitation*, see section 2.7.3.

Self-administration of adrenaline (epinephrine)

Individuals at considerable risk of anaphylaxis need to carry adrenaline (epinephrine) at all times and need to be *instructed in advance* how to inject it. In addition, the packs need to be labelled so that in the case of rapid collapse someone else is able to administer the adrenaline. It is important to ensure that an adequate supply is provided to treat symptoms until medical assistance is available.

Some patients may best cope with a pre-assembled syringe fitted with a needle suitable for very rapid administration (if necessary by a bystander). *Anapen*® and *EpiPen*® consist of a fully assembled syringe and needle delivering a dose of 300 micrograms of adrenaline by *intramuscular injection*; 150-microgram versions (*Anapen*® Junior, *EpiPen*® Jr) are also available for use in children. Other products for the immediate treatment of anaphylaxis are available but are not licensed for use in the UK. *Ana-Guard*® is a prefilled syringe that delivers two 300-microgram doses of adrenaline by *subcutaneous or intramuscular injection*; it can be adjusted to administer smaller doses for children. *Ana-Kit*® includes a prefilled adrenaline syringe, chewable tablets of chlorphenamine maleate (chlorphenamine maleate) 2 mg, 2 sterile pads impregnated with 70% isopropyl alcohol, and a tourniquet. *Ana-Guard*® and *Ana-Kit*® are available on a named-patient basis from IDIS.

ADRENALINE/EPINEPHRINE

Indications: emergency treatment of acute anaphylaxis; angioedema; cardiopulmonary resuscitation (section 2.7.3)

Cautions: hyperthyroidism, diabetes mellitus, heart disease, hypertension, arrhythmias, cerebrovascular disease, angle-closure glaucoma, second stage of labour, elderly patients

INTERACTIONS. Severe anaphylaxis in patients on non-cardioselective beta-blockers may not respond to adrenaline injection calling for intravenous injection of salbutamol (see p. 134); furthermore, adrenaline may cause severe hypertension in those receiving beta-blockers. Patients on tricyclic antidepressants are considerably more susceptible to arrhythmias, calling for a much reduced dose of adrenaline. Other **interactions**, see Appendix 1 (sympathomimetics).

Side-effects: anxiety, tremor, tachycardia, arrhythmias, headache, cold extremities; also hypertension (risk of cerebral haemorrhage) and pulmonary oedema (on excessive dosage or extreme sensitivity); nausea, vomiting, sweating, weakness, dizziness and hyperglycaemia also reported

Dose: acute anaphylaxis, *by intramuscular injection* (preferably midpoint in anterolateral thigh) (*or by subcutaneous injection*) of 1 in 1000 (1 mg/mL) solution, see notes and table above

Acute anaphylaxis when there is doubt as to the adequacy of the circulation, *by slow intravenous injection* of 1 in 10 000 (100 micrograms/mL) solution (extreme caution), see notes above

IMPORTANT. Intravenous route should be used with **extreme care**, see notes above

■ Intramuscular or subcutaneous

Adrenaline/Epinephrine 1 in 1000 (Non-proprietary) PoM

Injection, adrenaline (as acid tartrate) 1 mg/mL, net price 0.5-mL amp = 49p; 1-mL amp = 41p

Available from Antigen, BCM Specials, Hillcross, Martindale, Phoenix; also available from Aurum (1-mL prefilled syringe)

Excipients: include sulphites

Minijet® Adrenaline (Celltech) PoM

Injection, adrenaline (as acid tartrate) 1 in 1000 (1 mg/mL). Net price 1 mL (with 25 gauge × 0.25 inch needle for subcutaneous injection) = £8.11, 1 mL (with 21 gauge × 1.5 inch needle for intramuscular injection) = £4.40 (both disposable syringes)

Excipients: include sulphites

■ Intravenous

Extreme caution, see notes above

Adrenaline/Epinephrine 1 in 10 000, Dilute (Non-proprietary) PoM

Injection, adrenaline (as acid tartrate) 100 micrograms/mL, 10-mL amp

Available from Aurum, Martindale (special order); also from Aurum (1-mL and 10-mL prefilled syringe) and Celltech (Minijet® Adrenaline 3- and 10-mL disposable syringes)

Excipients: include sulphites

■ Intramuscular injection for self-administration

Anapen® (Celltech) PoM

Anapen® 0.3 mg solution for injection (delivering a single dose of adrenaline 300 micrograms), adrenaline 1 mg/mL (1 in 1000), net price 1.05-mL auto-injector device = £25.37

Excipients: include sulphites

NOTE. 0.75 mL of the solution remains in the auto-injector device after use

Dose: by intramuscular injection, ADULT and CHILD over 30 kg, 300 micrograms repeated after 10–15 minutes as necessary

Long-term oxygen therapy

Long-term administration of oxygen (at least 15 hours daily) prolongs survival in some patients with chronic obstructive pulmonary disease.

The Royal College of Physicians has produced guidelines for oxygen therapy (*Domiciliary oxygen therapy services: Clinical guidelines and advice for prescribers*; June 1999). Assessment for long-term oxygen therapy requires measurement of arterial blood gas tensions. Measurements should be taken on 2 occasions at least 3 weeks apart to demonstrate clinical stability, and not sooner than 4 weeks after an acute exacerbation of the disease. The guidelines recommend that long-term oxygen therapy should be considered for patients with:

- chronic obstructive pulmonary disease with $P_aO_2 < 7.3$ kPa when breathing air during a period of clinical stability;
- chronic obstructive pulmonary disease with P_aO_2 7.3–8 kPa in the presence of secondary polycythaemia, nocturnal hypoxaemia, peripheral oedema or evidence of pulmonary hypertension;
- interstitial lung disease with $P_aO_2 < 8$ kPa and in patients with $P_aO_2 > 8$ kPa with disabling dyspnoea;
- cystic fibrosis when $P_aO_2 < 7.3$ kPa *or* if P_aO_2 7.3–8 kPa in the presence of secondary polycythaemia, nocturnal hypoxaemia, pulmonary hypertension or peripheral oedema;
- pulmonary hypertension, without parenchymal lung involvement when $P_aO_2 < 8$ kPa;
- neuromuscular or skeletal disorders, after specialist assessment;
- obstructive sleep apnoea despite continuous positive airways pressure therapy, after specialist assessment;
- pulmonary malignancy or other terminal disease with disabling dyspnoea;
- heart failure with daytime $P_aO_2 < 7.3$ kPa (on air) or with nocturnal hypoxaemia;
- paediatric respiratory disease, after specialist assessment.

Increased respiratory depression is seldom a problem in patients with stable respiratory failure treated with low concentrations of oxygen although it may occur during exacerbations; patients and relatives should be warned to call for medical help if drowsiness or confusion occur.

Oxygen concentrators are more economical for patients requiring oxygen for long periods, and in England and Wales are prescribable on the NHS on a regional tendering basis (see below). A concentrator is cost-effective for a patient requiring oxygen for 8 hours a day (or 21 cylinders per month). Exceptionally if a higher concentration of oxygen is required the output of 2 oxygen concentrators can be combined using a 'Y' connection.

A nasal cannula is usually preferred for long-term oxygen therapy from an oxygen concentrator. It can, however, produce dermatitis and mucosal drying in sensitive individuals. Nasal cannulas are provided with oxygen concentrators but they are not prescribable on the NHS.

Prescribing arrangements for oxygen concentrators

Prescribe concentrator and accessories (face mask, nasal cannula, and humidifier) on form FP10. Specify amount of oxygen required (hours per day) and flow rate. If required, prescribe back-up oxygen set and cylinder at same time. Inform patient that the supplier will be in contact to make arrangements and that the prescription form is to be given to the person who installs the concentrator.

Inform supplier by telephone (see table below) that a concentrator has been prescribed. The supplier will send written confirmation of the order to the prescriber, the patient, and the Health Authority.

Follow the same procedure if a back-up oxygen set and cylinder are required later.

Health Authority regional group	Supplier
South Western London South (includes Kent, Surrey, and Sussex)	BOC Medical *to order*: Dial 0800 136 603
Eastern London North North Western and North Wales West Midlands	De Vilbiss Medequip Ltd *to order*: Dial 0800 020 202
Central and South Wales Northern Yorkshire (South and West) and Humberside	Oxygen Therapy Co Ltd *to order*: Dial 0800 373 580

In **Scotland** refer the patient for assessment by a respiratory consultant. If the need for a concentrator is confirmed the consultant will arrange for the provision of a concentrator through the Common Services Agency.

3.7   Mucolytics

Mucolytics are sometimes prescribed to facilitate expectoration by reducing sputum viscosity. Regular use of oral mucolytics may be of some benefit in patients with chronic obstructive pulmonary disease who suffer from particularly troublesome exacerbations. Steam inhalation with postural drainage, is good expectorant therapy in bronchiectasis and in some cases of chronic bronchitis.

For reference to dornase alfa, see below.

CARBOCISTEINE

Indications: reduction of sputum viscosity

Contra-indications: active peptic ulceration

Side-effects: occasional gastro-intestinal irritation, rashes

Dose: 750 mg 3 times daily initially, then 1.5 g daily in divided doses; CHILD 2–5 years 62.5–125 mg 4 times daily, 6–12 years 250 mg 3 times daily

Carbocisteine (Non-proprietary) PoM
Capsules, carbocisteine 375 mg. Net price 30-cap pack = £4.48
Available from Beacon (*Mucodyne*®)
Oral liquid, carbocisteine 125 mg/5 mL, net price 300 mL = £4.91; 250 mg/5 mL, 300 mL = £6.28
Available from Aventis Pharma (*Mucodyne*® Paediatric 125 mg/5 mL) and Beacon (*Mucodyne*® 250 mg/5 mL)

MECYSTEINE HYDROCHLORIDE
(Methyl Cysteine Hydrochloride)
Indications: reduction of sputum viscosity
Dose: 200 mg 4 times daily for 2 days, then 200 mg 3 times daily for 6 weeks, then 200 mg twice daily; CHILD over 5 years 100 mg 3 times daily

Visclair® (Sinclair)
Tablets, yellow, s/c, e/c, mecysteine hydrochloride 100 mg. Net price 20 = £3.66. Label: 5, 22, 25

Dornase alfa

Dornase alfa is a genetically engineered version of a naturally occurring enzyme which cleaves extracellular deoxyribonucleic acid (DNA). It is used in cystic fibrosis and is administered by inhalation using a jet nebuliser (section 3.1.5).

DORNASE ALFA
Phosphorylated glycosylated recombinant human deoxyribonuclease 1 (rhDNase)
Indications: management of cystic fibrosis patients with a forced vital capacity (FVC) of greater than 40% of predicted to improve pulmonary function
Cautions: pregnancy (Appendix 4); breast-feeding (Appendix 5)
Side-effects: pharyngitis, voice changes, chest pain; occasionally laryngitis, rashes, urticaria, conjunctivitis
Dose: *by inhalation of nebulised solution* (by jet nebuliser), 2500 units (2.5 mg) once daily (patients over 21 years may benefit from twice daily dosage); CHILD under 5 years not recommended

Pulmozyme® (Roche) [PoM]
Nebuliser solution, dornase alfa 1000 units (1 mg)/mL. Net price 2.5-mL (2500 units) vial = £19.47
NOTE. For use undiluted with jet nebulisers only; ultrasonic nebulisers are unsuitable

---

3.8 Aromatic inhalations

Inhalations containing volatile substances such as eucalyptus oil are traditionally used and although the vapour may contain little of the additive it encourages deliberate inspiration of warm moist air which is often comforting in bronchitis; boiling water should not be used owing to the risk of scalding. Inhalations are also used for the relief of nasal obstruction in acute rhinitis or sinusitis.

CHILDREN. The use of strong aromatic decongestants (applied as rubs or to pillows) is not advised for infants under the age of 3 months. Mothers with young infants in whom nasal obstruction with mucus is a problem can readily be taught appropriate techniques of suction aspiration.

Benzoin Tincture, Compound, BP
(Friars' Balsam)
Tincture, balsamic acids approx. 4.5%. Label: 15
Dose: add one teaspoonful to a pint of hot, **not** boiling, water and inhale the vapour

Menthol and Eucalyptus Inhalation, BP 1980
Inhalation, racementhol or levomenthol 2 g, eucalyptus oil 10 mL, light magnesium carbonate 7 g, water to 100 mL
Dose: add one teaspoonful to a pint of hot, **not** boiling, water and inhale the vapour

Karvol® (Crookes) [NHS]
Inhalation capsules, levomenthol 35.55 mg, with chlorobutanol, pine oils, terpineol, and thymol, net price 10-cap pack = £1.40; 20-cap pack = £2.52
Inhalation solution, levomenthol 7.9%, with chlorobutanol, pine oils, terpineol, and thymol, net price 12-mL dropper bottle = £1.84
Dose: express into handkerchief or add to a pint of hot, **not** boiling, water the contents of 1 capsule or 6 drops of solution; avoid in infants under 3 months

---

3.9 Cough preparations

3.9.1   Cough suppressants
3.9.2   Expectorant and demulcent cough preparations

3.9.1 Cough suppressants

Cough is usually a symptom of an underlying disorder e.g. asthma (section 3.1.1), gastro-oesophageal reflux disease (section 1.1), and 'post-nasal drip'; where there is no identifiable cause, cough suppressants may be useful, for example if sleep is disturbed. They may cause sputum retention and this may be harmful in patients with chronic bronchitis and bronchiectasis.

Codeine may be effective but it is constipating and can cause dependence; **dextromethorphan** and **pholcodine** have fewer side-effects.

Sedating antihistamines, such as diphenhydramine, are used as the cough suppressant component of many compound cough preparations on sale to the public; all tend to cause drowsiness which may reflect their main mode of action.

CHILDREN. The use of cough suppressants containing codeine or similar opioid analgesics is not generally recommended in children and should be avoided altogether in those under 1 year of age.

CODEINE PHOSPHATE
Indications: dry or painful cough; diarrhoea (section 1.4.2); pain (section 4.7.2)
Cautions: asthma; hepatic and renal impairment; history of drug abuse; see also notes above and section 4.7.2; **interactions:** Appendix 1 (opioid analgesics)
Contra-indications: liver disease, ventilatory failure
Side-effects: constipation, respiratory depression in sensitive patients or if given large doses

¹**Codeine Linctus, BP** [PoM]
Linctus (= oral solution), codeine phosphate 15 mg/5 mL. Net price 100 mL = 40p (diabetic, 73p)
Dose: 5–10 mL 3–4 times daily; CHILD (but not generally recommended) 5–12 years, 2.5–5 mL
Available from Alpharma, IVAX, Thornton & Ross (*Galcodine*®)
NOTE. BP directs that when Diabetic Codeine Linctus is prescribed, Codeine Linctus formulated with a vehicle appropriate for administration to diabetics, whether or not labelled 'Diabetic Codeine Linctus', shall be dispensed or supplied
1. Can be sold to the public provided the maximum single dose does not exceed 5 mL

systemic nasal decongestants can have unwanted sympathomimetic effects. **Pseudoephedrine** is available over-the-counter; it has few sympathomimetic effects.

Systemic decongestants should be used with **caution** in diabetes, hypertension, hyperthyroidism, raised intraocular pressure, prostate hypertrophy, hepatic impairment, renal impairment, and ischaemic heart disease and **avoided** in patients taking monoamine oxidase inhibitors; **interactions:** Appendix 1 (sympathomimetics). See below for CSM advice on phenylpropanolamine.

CSM advice. The CSM has advised that evidence of a link between phenylpropanolamine and an increased risk of haemorrhagic stroke is weak and is mainly associated with indications that are not licensed in the UK. The CSM has issued a reminder that:

- the maximum daily dose of phenylpropanolamine should not exceed 100 mg;

- patients with high blood pressure, hyperthyroidism, heart disease or who are receiving MAOIs should not take products containing phenylpropanolamine;

- phenylpropanolamine may aggravate conditions such as diabetes, glaucoma or prostatic enlargement.

The main ingredients in systemic nasal decongestant preparations are shown in the list of cough and decongestant preparations on sale to the public (section 3.9.2). Many preparations also contain antihistamines, which may cause drowsiness and affect the ability to drive or operate machinery.

PSEUDOEPHEDRINE HYDROCHLORIDE

Indications: see notes above
Cautions: see notes above
Side-effects: tachycardia, anxiety, restleness, insomnia; rarely hallucinations, rash; urinary retention also reported
Dose: see preparations below

Galpseud® (Thornton & Ross) ▭
Tablets, pseudoephedrine hydrochloride 60 mg. Net price 20 = 91p
Dose: 1 tablet 4 times daily
Linctus, orange, sugar-free, pseudoephedrine hydrochloride 30 mg/5 mL. Net price 140 mL = 96p
Dose: 10 mL 3 times daily; CHILD 2–6 years 2.5 mL, 6–12 years 5 mL

Sudafed® (Warner Lambert) ▭
Tablets, red, f/c, pseudoephedrine hydrochloride 60 mg. Net price 20 = 96p
Dose: 1 tablet every 4–6 hours (up to 4 times daily)
Elixir, red, pseudoephedrine hydrochloride 30 mg/5 mL. Net price 100 mL = 77p
Dose: 10 mL every 4–6 hours (up to 4 times daily); CHILD 2–5 years 2.5 mL, 6–12 years 5 mL

■ Preparations on sale to the public
For a list of **cough and decongestant preparations on sale to the public**, including those containing pseudoephedrine, see p. 163

4: Central nervous system

4.1   Hypnotics and anxiolytics

4.1.1   Hypnotics
4.1.2   Anxiolytics
4.1.3   Barbiturates

Most anxiolytics ('sedatives') will induce sleep when given at night and most hypnotics will sedate when given during the day. Prescribing of these drugs is widespread but dependence (both physical and psychological) and tolerance occurs. This may lead to difficulty in withdrawing the drug after the patient has been taking it regularly for more than a few weeks (see Dependence and Withdrawal, below). Hypnotics and anxiolytics should therefore be reserved for short courses to alleviate acute conditions after causal factors have been established.

Benzodiazepines are the most commonly used anxiolytics and hypnotics; they act at benzodiazepine receptors which are associated with gamma-aminobutyric acid (GABA) receptors. Older drugs such as meprobamate and barbiturates (section 4.1.3) are **not** recommended—they have more side-effects and interactions than benzodiazepines and are much more dangerous in overdosage.

PARADOXICAL EFFECTS. A paradoxical increase in hostility and aggression may be reported by patients taking benzodiazepines. The effects range from talkativeness and excitement, to aggressive and antisocial acts. Adjustment of the dose (up or down) usually attenuates the impulses. Increased anxiety and perceptual disorders are other paradoxical effects. Increased hostility and aggression after barbiturates and alcohol usually indicates intoxication.

DRIVING. Hypnotics and anxiolytics may impair judgement and increase reaction time, and so affect ability to drive or operate machinery; they increase the effects of alcohol. Moreover the hangover effects of a night dose may impair driving on the following day. See also Drugs and Driving under General Guidance, p. 2.

DEPENDENCE AND WITHDRAWAL. Withdrawal of a benzodiazepine should be gradual because abrupt withdrawal may produce confusion, toxic psychosis, convulsions, or a condition resembling delirium tremens. Abrupt withdrawal of a barbiturate (section 4.1.3) is even more likely to have serious effects.

The benzodiazepine withdrawal syndrome may develop at any time up to 3 weeks after stopping a long-acting benzodiazepine, but may occur within a few hours in the case of a short-acting one. It is characterised by insomnia, anxiety, loss of appetite and of body-weight, tremor, perspiration, tinnitus, and perceptual disturbances. These symptoms may be similar to the original complaint and encourage further prescribing; some symptoms may continue for weeks or months after stopping benzodiazepines.

Dose: 10 mg at bedtime or after going to bed if difficulty falling asleep; ELDERLY 5 mg; CHILD under 18 years not recommended
NOTE. Patients should be advised not to take a second dose during a single night

Sonata® (Wyeth) ▼ PoM
Capsules, zaleplon 5 mg (white/light brown), net price 14-cap pack = £3.36; 10 mg (white), 14-cap pack = £4.04. Label: 2

ZOLPIDEM TARTRATE

Indications: insomnia (short-term use)
Cautions: depression, history of drug or alcohol abuse, hepatic impairment (avoid if severe; Appendix 2); renal impairment; elderly; avoid prolonged use (and abrupt withdrawal thereafter); **interactions:** Appendix 1 (anxiolytics and hypnotics)
DRIVING. Drowsiness may persist the next day and affect performance of skilled tasks (e.g. driving); effects of alcohol enhanced
Contra-indications: obstructive sleep apnoea, acute pulmonary insufficiency, respiratory depression, myasthenia gravis, severe hepatic impairment, psychotic illness, pregnancy and breast-feeding
Side-effects: diarrhoea, nausea, vomiting, vertigo, dizziness, headache, drowsiness, asthenia; dependence, memory disturbances, nightmares, nocturnal restlessness, depression, confusion, perceptual disturbances or diplopia, tremor, ataxia, falls reported
Dose: 10 mg at bedtime; ELDERLY (or debilitated) 5 mg; CHILD not recommended

Zolpidem (Non-proprietary) PoM
Tablets, zolpidem tartrate 5 mg, net price 28-tab pack = £2.95; 10 mg, 28-tab pack = £4.28. Label: 19
Available from APS, Lagap

Stilnoct® (Sanofi-Synthelabo) PoM
Tablets, both f/c, zolpidem tartrate 5 mg, net price 28-tab pack = £3.08; 10 mg, 28-tab pack = £4.48. Label: 19

ZOPICLONE

Indications: insomnia (short-term use)
Cautions: hepatic (avoid if severe) and renal impairment (Appendixes 2 and 3); elderly; history of drug abuse, psychiatric illness; avoid prolonged use (and abrupt withdrawal thereafter); **interactions:** Appendix 1 (anxiolytics and hypnotics)
DRIVING. Drowsiness may persist the next day and affect performance of skilled tasks (e.g. driving); effects of alcohol enhanced
Contra-indications: myasthenia gravis, respiratory failure, severe sleep apnoea syndrome, severe hepatic impairment; pregnancy and breast-feeding
Side-effects: bitter or metallic taste; gastro-intestinal disturbances including nausea and vomiting, dry mouth; irritability, confusion, depressed mood; drowsiness, dizziness, lightheadedness, and incoordination, headache; dependence; hypersensitivity reactions reported (including urticaria and rashes); hallucinations, nightmares, amnesia, and behavioural disturbances (including aggression) reported
Dose: 7.5 mg at bedtime; ELDERLY initially 3.75 mg at bedtime increased if necessary; CHILD not recommended

Zopiclone (Non-proprietary) PoM
Tablets, zopiclone 3.75 mg, net price 28-tab pack = £3.07; 7.5 mg, 28-tab pack = £4.47. Label: 19
Available from Alpharma, APS, Arrow, CP, Dominon, Generics, IVAX, Opus (*Zileze*®)

Zimovane® (Rhône-Poulenc Rorer) PoM
Tablets, f/c, zopiclone 3.75 mg (*Zimovane*® LS , blue), net price 28-tab pack = £3.08; 7.5 mg, 28-tab pack = £4.48. Label: 19

Chloral and derivatives

Chloral hydrate and derivatives were formerly popular hypnotics for children (but the use of hypnotics in children is not usually justified). There is no convincing evidence that they are particularly useful in the elderly and their role as hypnotics is now very limited. **Triclofos** causes fewer gastrointestinal disturbances than chloral hydrate.

CHLORAL HYDRATE ▬

Indications: insomnia (short-term use)
Cautions: respiratory disease, history of drug or alcohol abuse, marked personality disorder; reduce dose in elderly and debilitated; avoid prolonged use (and abrupt withdrawal thereafter); avoid contact with skin and mucous membranes; **interactions:** Appendix 1 (anxiolytics and hypnotics)
DRIVING. Drowsiness may persist the next day and affect performance of skilled tasks (e.g. driving); effects of alcohol enhanced
Contra-indications: cardiac disease, gastritis, hepatic impairment (Appendix 2), renal impairment (Appendix 3); pregnancy and breast-feeding; porphyria
Side-effects: gastric irritation (nausea and vomiting reported), abdominal distention and flatulence; also vertigo, ataxia, staggering gait, rashes, headache, light headedness, malaise, ketonuria, excitement, nightmares, delirium (especially in the elderly), eosinophilia, reduction in white cell count; dependence (may be associated with gastritis and renal damage) on prolonged use
Dose: insomnia, 0.5–1 g (max. 2 g) with plenty of water at bedtime; CHILD 30–50 mg/kg up to a max. single dose of 1 g

Chloral Mixture, BP PoM ▬
(Chloral Oral Solution)
Mixture, chloral hydrate 500 mg/5 mL in a suitable vehicle. Extemporaneous preparations should be recently prepared according to the following formula: chloral hydrate 1 g, syrup 2 mL, water to 10 mL. Net price 100 mL = 44p. Label: 19, 27
Dose: 5–20 mL; CHILD 1–5 years 2.5–5 mL, 6–12 years 5–10 mL, taken well diluted with water at bedtime

Chloral Elixir, Paediatric, BP PoM ▬
(Chloral Oral Solution, Paediatric)
Elixir, chloral hydrate 4% in a suitable vehicle with a blackcurrant flavour. Extemporaneous preparations should be recently prepared according to the following formula: chloral hydrate 200 mg, water 0.1 mL, blackcurrant syrup 1 mL, syrup to 5 mL. Net price 100 mL = 95p. Label: 1, 27
Dose: up to 1 year 5 mL, taken well diluted with water at bedtime

Welldorm® (S&N Hlth.) PoM ▰
Tablets, blue-purple, f/c, cloral betaine 707 mg
(≡ chloral hydrate 414 mg). Net price 30-tab pack
= £2.43. Label: 19, 27
Dose: 1–2 tablets with water or milk at bedtime, max. 5
tablets (2 g chloral hydrate) daily
Elixir, red, chloral hydrate 143.3 mg/5 mL. Net
price 150-mL pack = £2.05. Label: 19, 27
Dose: 15–45 mL (0.4–1.3 g chloral hydrate) with water or
milk, at bedtime, max. 70 mL (2 g chloral hydrate) daily;
CHILD 1–1.75 mL/kg (30–50 mg/kg chloral hydrate),
max. 35 mL (1 g chloral hydrate) daily

TRICLOFOS SODIUM ▰

Indications: insomnia (short-term use)
Cautions: see Chloral Hydrate
Contra-indications: see Chloral Hydrate
Side-effects: see Chloral Hydrate but less gastric irritation
Dose: see under preparation below

Triclofos Oral Solution, BP PoM ▰
(Triclofos Elixir)
Oral solution, triclofos sodium 500 mg/5 mL. Net
price 300 mL = £35.13. Label: 19
Available from Celltech
Dose: 10–20 mL (1–2 g triclofos sodium) at bedtime;
CHILD up to 1 year 25–30 mg/kg, 1–5 years 2.5–5 mL
(250–500 mg triclofos sodium), 6–12 years 5–10 mL
(0.5–1 g triclofos sodium)

Clomethiazole

Clomethiazole (chlormethiazole) may be a useful
hypnotic for elderly patients because of its freedom
from hangover but, as with all hypnotics, routine
administration is undesirable and dependence
occurs. It is licensed for use as a hypnotic only in
the elderly (and for *very short-term use* in younger
adults to attenuate alcohol withdrawal symptoms,
see section 4.10).

CLOMETHIAZOLE
(Chlormethiazole)

Indications: see under Dose; alcohol withdrawal
(section 4.10)
Cautions: cardiac and respiratory disease (confu-
sional state may indicate hypoxia); history of drug
abuse; marked personality disorder; elderly; excessive sedation may occur (particularly with higher
doses); hepatic impairment (especially if severe
because sedation can mask hepatic coma); renal
impairment; avoid prolonged use (and abrupt
withdrawal thereafter); **interactions:** Appendix 1
(anxiolytics and hypnotics)
DRIVING. Drowsiness may persist the next day and affect
performance of skilled tasks (e.g. driving); effects of
alcohol enhanced

Contra-indications: acute pulmonary insufficiency; alcohol-dependent patients who continue
to drink
Side-effects: nasal congestion and irritation
(increased nasopharyngeal and bronchial secretions), conjunctival irritation, headache; rarely,
paradoxical excitement, confusion, dependence,
gastro-intestinal disturbances, rash, urticaria, bullous eruption, anaphylaxis, alterations in liver
enzymes

Dose: severe insomnia in the elderly (short-term
use), 1–2 capsules (*or* 5–10 mL syrup) at bedtime;
CHILD not recommended
Restlessness and agitation in the elderly, 1 capsule
(*or* 5 mL syrup) 3 times daily
Alcohol withdrawal, initially 2–4 capsules, if necessary repeated after some hours;
day 1 (first 24 hours), 9–12 capsules in 3–4 divided
doses;
day 2, 6–8 capsules in 3–4 divided doses;
day 3, 4–6 capsules in 3–4 divided doses; then
gradually reduced over days 4–6; total treatment
for not more than 9 days
NOTE. For an equivalent therapeutic effect 1 capsule ≡
5 mL syrup

Heminevrin® (AstraZeneca) PoM
Capsules, grey-brown, clomethiazole base 192 mg
in an oily basis. Net price 60-cap pack = £4.34.
Label: 19
Syrup, sugar-free, clomethiazole edisilate
250 mg/5 mL. Net price 300-mL pack = £3.63.
Label: 19

Antihistamines

Some **antihistamines** such as diphenhydramine
(section 3.4.1) and promethazine are on sale to the
public for occasional insomnia; their prolonged
duration of action may often lead to drowsiness the
following day. The sedative effect of antihistamines
may diminish after a few days of continued treatment; antihistamines are associated with headache,
psychomotor impairment and antimuscarinic effects.
Promethazine is also popular for use in children, but
the use of hypnotics in children is not usually
justified.

PROMETHAZINE HYDROCHLORIDE
▰

Indications: night sedation and insomnia (short-
term use); other indications (section 3.4.1, section
4.6)
Cautions: section 3.4.1
Contra-indications: section 3.4.1
Side-effects: section 3.4.1
Dose: *by mouth*, 25 mg at bedtime increased to
50 mg if necessary; CHILD under 2 years not
recommended, 2–5 years 15–20 mg, 5–10 years
20–25 mg, at bedtime

■ Preparations
Section 3.4.1

Alcohol

Alcohol is a poor hypnotic because its diuretic action
interferes with sleep during the latter part of the
night. With chronic use, alcohol disturbs sleep
patterns and causes insomnia; **interactions:** Appendix 1 (alcohol).

4.1.2 Anxiolytics

Benzodiazepine anxiolytics can be effective in
alleviating anxiety states. Although these drugs are
often prescribed to almost anyone with stress-related
symptoms, unhappiness, or minor physical disease,

BUSPIRONE HYDROCHLORIDE

Indications: anxiety (short-term use)

Cautions: does not alleviate benzodiazepine withdrawal (see notes above); **interactions:** Appendix 1 (anxiolytics and hypnotics)

DRIVING. May affect performance of skilled tasks (e.g. driving); effects of alcohol may be enhanced

Contra-indications: epilepsy, severe hepatic impairment, moderate to severe renal impairment, pregnancy and breast-feeding

Side-effects: nausea, dizziness, headache, nervousness, lightheadedness, excitement; rarely tachycardia, palpitations, chest pain, drowsiness, confusion, seizures, dry mouth, fatigue, and sweating

Dose: initially 5 mg 2–3 times daily, increased as necessary every 2–3 days; usual range 15–30 mg daily in divided doses; max. 45 mg daily; CHILD not recommended

Buspirone Hydrochloride (Non-proprietary) PoM
Tablets, buspirone hydrochloride 5 mg, net price 30-tab pack = £8.42; 10 mg, 30-tab pack = £11.64. Counselling, driving
Available from Alpharma, Galen

Buspar® (Bristol-Myers Squibb) PoM
Tablets, buspirone hydrochloride 5 mg, net price 90-tab pack = £28.08; 10 mg, 90-tab pack = £42.12. Counselling, driving

---

Beta-blockers

Beta-blockers (e.g. propranolol, oxprenolol) (section 2.4) do not affect psychological symptoms, such as worry, tension, and fear, but they do reduce autonomic symptoms, such as palpitations and tremor; they do not reduce non-autonomic symptoms, such as muscle tension. Beta-blockers are therefore indicated for patients with predominantly somatic symptoms; this, in turn, may prevent the onset of worry and fear. Patients with predominantly psychological symptoms may obtain no benefit.

Meprobamate

Meprobamate is **less effective** than the benzodiazepines, more hazardous in overdosage, and can also induce dependence. It is **not** recommended.

MEPROBAMATE

Indications: short-term use in anxiety, but see notes above

Cautions: respiratory disease, muscle weakness, epilepsy (may induce seizures), history of drug or alcohol abuse, marked personality disorder, pregnancy; elderly and debilitated; hepatic and renal impairment; avoid prolonged use, abrupt withdrawal may precipitate convulsions; **interactions:** Appendix 1 (anxiolytics and hypnotics)

DRIVING. Drowsiness may affect performance of skilled tasks (e.g. driving); effects of alcohol enhanced

Contra-indications: acute pulmonary insufficiency; respiratory depression; porphyria (section 9.8.2); breast-feeding

Side-effects: see under Diazepam, but incidence greater and drowsiness most common side-effect; also gastro-intestinal disturbances, hypotension,

paraesthesia, weakness, CNS effects including headache, paradoxical excitement, disturbances of vision; rarely agranulocytosis and rashes

Dose: 400 mg 3–4 times daily; elderly patients half adult dose or less; CHILD not recommended

Meprobamate (Non-proprietary) CD ▰
Tablets, scored, meprobamate 400 mg. Net price 84-tab pack = £19.95. Label: 2
Available from Genus

4.1.3   Barbiturates

The intermediate-acting **barbiturates** have a place only in the treatment of severe intractable insomnia in patients **already taking** barbiturates; they should be **avoided** in the elderly. The long-acting barbiturate, phenobarbital is still sometimes of value in epilepsy (section 4.8.1) but its use as a sedative is unjustified. The very short-acting barbiturate thiopental is used in anaesthesia (section 15.1.1).

BARBITURATES

Indications: severe intractable insomnia **only** in patients already taking barbiturates; see also notes above

Cautions: avoid use where possible; dependence and tolerance readily occur; abrupt withdrawal may precipitate serious withdrawal syndrome (rebound insomnia, anxiety, tremor, dizziness, nausea, convulsions, delirium, and death); repeated doses are cumulative and may lead to excessive sedation; respiratory disease, renal disease, hepatic impairment; **interactions:** Appendix 1 (barbiturates)

DRIVING. Drowsiness may persist the next day and affect performance of skilled tasks (e.g. driving); effects of alcohol enhanced

Contra-indications: insomnia caused by pain; porphyria (section 9.8.2), pregnancy, breast-feeding; children, young adults, elderly and debilitated patients, also patients with history of drug or alcohol abuse

Side-effects: include hangover with drowsiness, dizziness, ataxia, respiratory depression, hypersensitivity reactions, headache, particularly in elderly; paradoxical excitement and confusion occasionally precede sleep; **overdosage:** see Emergency Treatment of Poisoning, p. 25

Dose: see under preparations below

Amytal® (Flynn) CD ▰
Tablets, amobarbital (amylobarbitone) 50 mg, net price 20 = £1.84. Label: 19
Dose: 100–200 mg at bedtime (**important:** but see also contra-indications)

Sodium Amytal® (Flynn) CD ▰
Capsules, both blue, amobarbital (amylobarbitone) sodium 60 mg, net price 20 = £3.43; 200 mg, 20 = £6.75. Label: 19
Dose: 60–200 mg at bedtime (**important:** but see also contra-indications)

Soneryl® (Concord) CD ▰
Tablets, pink, scored, butobarbital (butobarbitone) 100 mg. Net price 56-tab pack = £10.65. Label: 19
Dose: 100–200 mg at bedtime (**important:** but see also contra-indications)

■ Preparations containing secobarbital (quinalbarbitone)

NOTE. Secobarbital (quinalbarbitone) is in schedule 2 of the Misuse of Drugs Regulations 2001; receipt and supply must therefore be recorded in the CD register.

Seconal Sodium® (Flynn) CD ▬
Capsules, both orange, secobarbital (quinalbarbitone) sodium 50 mg, net price 20 = £5.30; 100 mg, 20 = £6.96. Label: 19

Dose: 100 mg at bedtime (**important:** but see also contra-indications)

Tuinal® (Flynn) CD ▬
Capsules, orange/blue, a mixture of amobarbital (amylobarbitone) sodium 50 mg, secobarbital (quinalbarbitone) sodium 50 mg. Net price 20 = £3.88. Label: 19

Dose: 1–2 capsules at bedtime (**important:** but see also contra-indications)

NOTE. Prescriptions need only specify 'Tuinal capsules'

4.2 Drugs used in psychoses and related disorders

4.2.1	Antipsychotic drugs
4.2.2	Antipsychotic depot injections
4.2.3	Antimanic drugs

Advice of Royal College of Psychiatrists on doses above BNF upper limit. Unless otherwise stated, doses in the BNF are licensed doses—any higher dose is therefore **unlicensed** (for an explanation of the significance of this, see p. 1).

1. Consider alternative approaches including adjuvant therapy and newer or atypical neuroleptics such as clozapine.
2. Bear in mind risk factors, including obesity—particular caution is indicated in older patients especially those over 70.
3. Consider potential for drug interactions—see **interactions:** Appendix 1 (antipsychotics).
4. Carry out ECG to exclude untoward abnormalities such as prolonged QT interval; repeat ECG periodically and reduce dose if prolonged QT interval or other adverse abnormality develops.
5. Increase dose slowly and not more often than once weekly.
6. Carry out regular pulse, blood pressure, and temperature checks; ensure that patient maintains adequate fluid intake.
7. Consider high-dose therapy to be for limited period and review regularly; abandon if no improvement after 3 months (return to standard dosage).

Important: When prescribing an antipsychotic for administration on an emergency basis, the intramuscular dose should be **lower** than the corresponding oral dose (owing to absence of first-pass effect), particularly if the patient is very active (increased blood flow to muscle considerably increases the rate of absorption). The prescription should specify the dose for **each route** and should **not** imply that the same dose can be given by mouth or by intramuscular injection. The dose of antipsychotic for emergency use should be reviewed at least **daily**.

Antipsychotic drugs are also known as 'neuroleptics' and (misleadingly) as 'major tranquillisers'. Antipsychotic drugs generally tranquillise without impairing consciousness and without causing paradoxical excitement but they should not be regarded merely as tranquillisers. For conditions such as schizophrenia the tranquillising effect is of secondary importance.

In the short term they are used to quieten disturbed patients whatever the underlying psychopathology, which may be schizophrenia, brain damage, mania, toxic delirium, or agitated depression. Antipsychotic drugs are used to alleviate severe anxiety but this too should be a short-term measure.

SCHIZOPHRENIA. Antipsychotic drugs relieve florid psychotic symptoms such as thought disorder, hallucinations, and delusions, and prevent relapse. Although they are usually less effective in apathetic withdrawn patients, they sometimes appear to have an activating influence. Patients with acute schizophrenia generally respond better than those with chronic symptoms.

Long-term treatment of a patient with a definite diagnosis of schizophrenia may be necessary even after the first episode of illness in order to prevent the manifest illness from becoming chronic. Withdrawal of drug treatment requires careful surveillance because the patient who appears well on medication may suffer a disastrous relapse if treatment is withdrawn inappropriately. In addition the need for continuation of treatment may not become immediately evident because relapse is often delayed for several weeks after cessation of treatment.

Antipsychotic drugs are considered to act by interfering with dopaminergic transmission in the brain by blocking dopamine D_2 receptors, which may give rise to the extrapyramidal effects described below, and also to hyperprolactinaemia. Antipsychotic drugs may also affect cholinergic, alpha-adrenergic, histaminergic, and serotonergic receptors.

CAUTIONS AND CONTRA-INDICATIONS. Antipsychotics should be used with **caution** in patients with hepatic impairment (Appendix 2), renal impairment (Appendix 3), cardiovascular disease, Parkinson's disease (may be exacerbated by antipsychotics), epilepsy (and conditions predisposing to epilepsy), depression, myasthenia gravis, prostatic hypertrophy, or a personal or family history of angle-closure glaucoma (avoid chlorpromazine, pericyazine and prochlorperazine in these conditions). Caution is also required in severe respiratory disease and in patients with a history of jaundice or who have blood dyscrasias (perform blood counts if unexplained infection or fever develops). Antipsychotics should be used with caution in the elderly, who are particularly susceptible to postural hypotension and to hyper- or hypothermia in very hot or cold weather. Serious consideration should be given before prescribing these drugs for elderly patients. As photosensitisation may occur with higher dosages, patients should avoid direct sunlight.

Antipsychotic drugs may be **contra-indicated** in comatose states, CNS depression, and phaeochromocytoma. Most antipsychotics are best avoided during pregnancy, unless essential (Appendix 4) and it is

Chlorpromazine (Non-proprietary) PoM
Tablets, coated, chlorpromazine hydrochloride
10 mg, net price 56-tab pack = 71p; 25 mg, 28-tab
pack = 96p; 50 mg, 28-tab pack = 95p; 100 mg, 28-
tab pack = £1.16. Label: 2, 11
Available from Antigen, APS, Arrow, DDSA (*Chlor-actil*®), Hillcross, IVAX
Oral solution, chlorpromazine hydrochloride
25 mg/5 mL, net price 150 mL = £1.35,
100 mg/5 mL, 150 mL = £3.76. Label: 2, 11
Available from Hillcross, Rosemont
Injection, chlorpromazine hydrochloride
25 mg/mL, net price 1-mL amp = 60p; 2-mL amp
= 67p
Available from Antigen
Suppositories, chlorpromazine 100 mg. Label: 2, 11
'Special order' [unlicensed] product; contact Martindale or
regional hospital manufacturing unit

Largactil® (Hawgreen) PoM
Tablets, all off-white, f/c, chlorpromazine
hydrochloride 10 mg. Net price 56-tab pack= 71p;
25 mg, 56-tab pack = 98p; 50 mg, 56-tab pack =
£2.05; 100 mg, 56-tab pack = £3.81. Label: 2, 11
Syrup, brown, chlorpromazine hydrochloride
25 mg/5 mL. Net price 100-mL pack = £1.11.
Label: 2, 11
Suspension forte, orange, sugar-free, chlorpromazine hydrochloride 100 mg (as embonate)/5 mL.
Net price 100-mL pack = £2.56. Label: 2, 11
Injection, chlorpromazine hydrochloride
25 mg/mL. Net price 2-mL amp = 67p

FLUPENTIXOL
(Flupenthixol)
Indications: schizophrenia and other psychoses,
particularly with apathy and withdrawal but not
mania or psychomotor hyperactivity; depression
(section 4.3.4)
Cautions: see notes above; avoid in porphyria
(section 9.8.2)
Contra-indications: see notes above; also excita-
ble and overactive patients
Side-effects: see notes above; less sedating but
extrapyramidal symptoms frequent
Dose: psychosis, initially 3–9 mg twice daily
adjusted according to the response; max. 18 mg
daily; ELDERLY (or debilitated) initially quarter to
half adult dose; CHILD not recommended

Depixol® (Lundbeck) PoM
Tablets, yellow, s/c, flupentixol 3 mg (as
dihydrochloride). Net price 20 = £2.99. Label: 2
Depot injection (flupentixol decanoate): section
4.2.2

FLUPHENAZINE HYDROCHLORIDE
Indications: see under Dose
Cautions: see notes above
Contra-indications: see notes above
Side-effects: see notes above; less sedating and
fewer antimuscarinic or hypotensive symptoms,
but extrapyramidal symptoms, particularly dystonic reactions and akathisia, more frequent; systemic lupus erythematosus
Dose: schizophrenia and other psychoses, mania,
initially 2.5–10 mg daily in 2–3 divided doses,
adjusted according to response to 20 mg daily;
doses above 20 mg daily (10 mg in elderly) only
with special caution; CHILD not recommended

Short-term adjunctive management of severe
anxiety, psychomotor agitation, excitement, and
violent or dangerously impulsive behaviour, initially 1 mg twice daily, increased as necessary to
2 mg twice daily; CHILD not recommended

Moditen® (Sanofi-Synthelabo) PoM
Tablets, all s/c, fluphenazine hydrochloride 1 mg
(pink), net price 20 = £1.06; 2.5 mg (yellow), 20 =
£1.33; 5 mg, 20 = £1.77. Label: 2
Modecate® PoM Section 4.2.2

HALOPERIDOL
Indications: see under Dose; motor tics (section
4.9.3)
Cautions: see notes above; also subarachnoid
haemorrhage and metabolic disturbances such as
hypokalaemia, hypocalcaemia, or hypomagnesaemia
Contra-indications: see notes above
Side-effects: see notes above, but less sedating and
fewer antimuscarinic or hypotensive symptoms;
pigmentation and photosensitivity reactions rare;
extrapyramidal symptoms, particularly dystonic
reactions and akathisia especially in thyrotoxic
patients; rarely weight loss; hypoglycaemia; inappropriate antidiuretic hormone secretion
Dose: *by mouth*, schizophrenia and other psychoses,
mania, short-term adjunctive management of psychomotor agitation, excitement, and violent or
dangerously impulsive behaviour, initially 1.5–
3 mg 2–3 times daily *or* 3–5 mg 2–3 times daily in
severely affected or resistant patients; in resistant
schizophrenia up to 30 mg daily may be needed;
adjusted according to response to lowest effective
maintenance dose (as low as 5–10 mg daily);
ELDERLY (or debilitated) initially half adult dose;
CHILD initially 25–50 micrograms/kg daily (in 2
divided doses) to max. 10 mg
Agitation and restlessness in the elderly, initially
0.5–1.5 mg once or twice daily
Short-term adjunctive management of severe
anxiety, 500 micrograms twice daily; CHILD not
recommended
Intractable hiccup, 1.5 mg 3 times daily adjusted
according to response; CHILD not recommended
Nausea and vomiting, 1 mg daily (see also Prescribing in Palliative Care, p. 15)
By intramuscular or by intravenous injection, initially 2–10 mg, then every 4–8 hours according to
response to total max. 18 mg daily; severely
disturbed patients may require initial dose of up
to 18 mg; ELDERLY (or debilitated) initially half
adult dose; CHILD not recommended
Nausea and vomiting, 0.5–2 mg

Haloperidol (Non-proprietary) PoM
Tablets, haloperidol 500 micrograms, net price 28-
tab pack = 91p; 1.5 mg, 20 = £1.02; 5 mg, 20 =
£1.78; 10 mg, 20 = £3.27; 20 mg, 20 = £8.47.
Label: 2

Dozic® (Rosemont) PoM
Oral liquid, sugar-free, haloperidol 1 mg/mL. Net
price 100-mL pack = £7.30. Label: 2

Haldol® (Janssen-Cilag) PoM
Tablets, both scored, haloperidol 5 mg (blue), net
price 20 = £1.65; 10 mg (yellow), 20 = £3.21.
Label: 2

Oral liquid, sugar-free, haloperidol 2 mg/mL. Net price 100-mL pack (with pipette) = £5.08. Label: 2
Injection, haloperidol 5 mg/mL. Net price 1-mL amp = 33p
Depot injection (haloperidol decanoate): section 4.2.2

Serenace® (IVAX) PoM
Capsules, green, haloperidol 500 micrograms, net price 30-cap pack = 98p. Label: 2
Tablets, haloperidol 1.5 mg, net price 30-tab pack = £1.73; 5 mg (pink), 30-tab pack = £4.90; 10 mg (pale pink), 30-tab pack = £8.81. Label: 2
Oral liquid, sugar-free, haloperidol 2 mg/mL, net price 500-mL pack = £43.85. Label: 2
Injection, haloperidol 5 mg/mL, net price 1-mL amp = 59p; 10 mg/mL, 2-mL amp = £2.03

LEVOMEPROMAZINE/ METHOTRIMEPRAZINE

Indications: see under Dose

Cautions: see notes above; patients receiving large initial doses should remain supine
ELDERLY. Risk of postural hypotension; not recommended for ambulant patients over 50 years unless risk of hypotensive reaction assessed

Contra-indications: see notes above

Side-effects: see notes above; occasionally raised erythrocyte sedimentation rate occurs

Dose: *by mouth*, schizophrenia, initially 25–50 mg daily in divided doses increased as necessary; bedpatients initially 100–200 mg daily usually in 3 divided doses, increased if necessary to 1 g daily; ELDERLY, see Cautions
Adjunctive treatment in palliative care (including management of pain and associated restlessness, distress, or vomiting), 12.5–50 mg every 4–8 hours, but see also Prescribing in Palliative Care, p. 14

By intramuscular injection or by intravenous injection (by intravenous injection after dilution with an equal volume of sodium chloride 0.9% injection), adjunct in palliative care, 12.5–25 mg (severe agitation up to 50 mg) every 6–8 hours if necessary

By continuous subcutaneous infusion, adjunct in palliative care (via syringe driver), diluted in a suitable volume of sodium chloride 0.9% injection, see Prescribing in Palliative Care, p. 16; CHILD (experience limited), 0.35–3 mg/kg daily

Nozinan® (Link) PoM
Tablets, scored, levomepromazine maleate 25 mg, net price 84-tab pack = £21.42. Label: 2
Injection, levomepromazine hydrochloride 25 mg/mL, net price 1-mL amp = £2.13

PERICYAZINE
(Periciazine)

Indications: see under Dose

Cautions: see notes above

Contra-indications: see notes above

Side-effects: see notes above; more sedating; hypotension common when treatment initiated; respiratory depression

Dose: schizophrenia and other psychoses, initially 75 mg daily in divided doses increased at weekly intervals by steps of 25 mg according to response; usual max. 300 mg daily (elderly initially 15–30 mg daily)

Short-term adjunctive management of severe anxiety, psychomotor agitation, and violent or dangerously impulsive behaviour, initially 15–30 mg (elderly 5–10 mg) daily divided into 2 doses, taking the larger dose at bedtime, adjusted according to response
CHILD (severe mental or behavioural disorders only), initially, 500 micrograms daily for 10-kg child, increased by 1 mg for each additional 5 kg to max. total daily dose of 10 mg; dose may be gradually increased according to response but maintenance should not exceed twice initial dose
INFANT under 1 year not recommended

Neulactil® (JHC) PoM
Tablets, all yellow, scored, pericyazine 2.5 mg, net price 84-tab pack = £7.69; 10 mg, 84-tab pack = £20.79. Label: 2
Syrup forte, brown, pericyazine 10 mg/5 mL. Net price 100-mL pack =£10.07. Label: 2

PERPHENAZINE

Indications: see under Dose; anti-emetic (section 4.6)

Cautions: see notes above

Contra-indications: see notes above; also agitation and restlessness in the elderly

Side-effects: see notes above; less sedating; extrapyramidal symptoms, especially dystonia, more frequent, particularly at high dosage; rarely systemic lupus erythematosus

Dose: schizophrenia and other psychoses, mania, short-term adjunctive management of anxiety, severe psychomotor agitation, excitement, and violent or dangerously impulsive behaviour, initially 4 mg 3 times daily adjusted according to the response; max. 24 mg daily; ELDERLY quarter to half adult dose (but see Cautions); CHILD under 14 years not recommended

Fentazin® (Goldshield) PoM
Tablets, both s/c, perphenazine 2 mg, net price 20 = £3.73; 4 mg, 20 = £4.39. Label: 2

PIMOZIDE

Indications: see under Dose

Cautions: see notes above
CSM WARNING. Following reports of sudden unexplained death, the CSM recommends ECG before treatment. The CSM also recommends that patients on pimozide should have an annual ECG (if the QT interval is prolonged, treatment should be reviewed and either withdrawn or dose reduced under close supervision) and that pimozide should **not** be given with other antipsychotic drugs (including depot preparations), tricyclic antidepressants or other drugs which prolong the QT interval, such as certain antimalarials, anti-arrhythmic drugs and certain antihistamines and should **not** be given with drugs which cause electrolyte disturbances (especially diuretics)

Contra-indications: see notes above; history of arrhythmias or congenital QT prolongation

Side-effects: see notes above; less sedating; serious arrhythmias reported; glycosuria and, rarely, hyponatraemia reported

Dose: schizophrenia, initially 2 mg daily, increased according to response in steps of 2–4 mg at intervals of not less than 1 week; usual dose range 2–20 mg daily; ELDERLY half usual starting dose; CHILD not recommended
Monosymptomatic hypochondriacal psychosis, paranoid psychosis, initially 4 mg daily, increased according to response in steps of 2–4 mg at

other antipsychotics, a reduction in prolactin may increase fertility.

Clozapine is licensed for the treatment of schizophrenia only in patients unresponsive to, or intolerant of, conventional antipsychotic drugs. It can cause agranulocytosis and its use is restricted to patients registered with the Clozaril Patient Monitoring Service (see under Clozapine, below).

Sertindole has been reintroduced following an earlier suspension of the drug because of concerns about arrhythmias; its use is restricted to patients who are enrolled in clinical studies and who are intolerant of at least one other antipsychotic.

NICE guidance (atypical antipsychotics for schizophrenia)

NICE has recommended (June 2002) that:

- the atypical antipsychotics (amisulpride, olanzapine, quetiapine, risperidone, and zotepine) should be considered when choosing first-line treatment of *newly diagnosed schizophrenia*;

- an atypical antipsychotic is considered the treatment option of choice for managing an *acute schizophrenic episode* when discussion with the individual is not possible;

- an atypical antipsychotic should be considered for an individual who is suffering unacceptable side-effects from a conventional antipsychotic;

- an atypical antipsychotic should be considered for an individual in relapse whose symptoms were previously inadequately controlled;

- changing to an atypical antipsychotic is not necessary if a conventional antipsychotic controls symptoms adequately and the individual does not suffer unacceptable side-effects;

- clozapine should be introduced if schizophrenia is inadequately controlled despite the sequential use of two or more antipsychotics (one of which should be an atypical antipsychotic) each for at least 6–8 weeks.

CAUTIONS AND CONTRA-INDICATIONS. While atypical antipsychotics have not generally been associated with clinically significant prolongation of the QT interval, they should be used with care if prescribed with other drugs that increase the QT interval. Atypical antipsychotics should be used with caution in patients with cardiovascular disease, or a history of epilepsy; they should be used with caution in the elderly; **interactions:** Appendix 1 (antipsychotics).

DRIVING. Atypical antipsychotics may affect performance of skilled tasks (e.g. driving); effects of alcohol are enhanced.

WITHDRAWAL. Withdrawal of antipsychotic drugs after long-term therapy should always be gradual and closely monitored to avoid the risk of acute withdrawal syndromes or rapid relapse.

SIDE-EFFECTS. Side-effects of the atypical antipsychotics include weight gain, dizziness, postural hypotension (especially during initial dose titration) which may be associated with syncope or reflex tachycardia in some patients, extrapyramidal symptoms (usually mild and transient and which respond to dose reduction or to an antimuscarinic drug), and occasionally tardive dyskinesia on long-term admin-istration (discontinue drug on appearance of early signs). Hyperglycaemia and sometimes diabetes can occur, particularly with clozapine and olanzapine; monitoring weight and plasma glucose may identify the development of hyperglycaemia. Neuroleptic malignant syndrome has been reported rarely.

AMISULPRIDE

Indications: schizophrenia

Cautions: see notes above; also renal impairment (Appendix 3); Parkinson's disease; elderly (risk of hypotension or sedation)

Contra-indications: see notes above; also pregnancy (Appendix 4) and breast-feeding (Appendix 5), phaeochromocytoma, prolactin-dependent tumours

Side-effects: see notes above; also insomnia, anxiety, agitation, drowsiness, gastro-intestinal disorders such as constipation, nausea, vomiting, and dry mouth; hyperprolactinaemia (with galactorrhoea, amenorrhoea, gynaecomastia, breast pain, sexual dysfunction), occasionally bradycardia

Dose: acute psychotic episode, 400–800 mg daily in divided doses, adjusted according to response; max. 1.2 g daily

Predominantly negative symptoms, 50–300 mg daily; CHILD under 15 years, not recommended

NOTE. Doses up to 300 mg may be administered once daily

Solian® (Sanofi-Synthelabo) PoM

Tablets, scored, amisulpride 50 mg, net price 60-tab pack = £19.74; 100 mg, 60-tab pack = £39.48; 200 mg, 60-tab pack = £66.00, 400 mg, 60-tab pack = £132.00. Label: 2

Solution, 100 mg/mL, net price 60 mL (caramel flavour) = £33.00. Label: 2

CLOZAPINE

Indications: schizophrenia (including psychosis in Parkinson's disease) in patients unresponsive to, or intolerant of, conventional antipsychotic drugs

Cautions: see notes above; monitor leucocyte and differential blood counts (see Agranulocytosis, below); taper off conventional neuroleptic before starting; hepatic impairment (Appendix 2); renal impairment (Appendix 3); prostatic hypertrophy, angle-closure glaucoma

WITHDRAWAL. On planned withdrawal reduce dose over 1–2 weeks to avoid risk of rebound psychosis. If abrupt withdrawal necessary observe patient carefully

AGRANULOCYTOSIS. Neutropenia and potentially fatal agranulocytosis reported. Leucocyte and differential blood counts must be normal before starting; monitor counts every week for 18 weeks then at least every 2 weeks and if clozapine continued and blood count stable after 1 year at least every 4 weeks (and 4 weeks after discontinuation); if leucocyte count below 3000/mm³ or if absolute neutrophil count below 1500/mm³ discontinue permanently and refer to haematologist. Avoid drugs which depress leucopoiesis; patients should report immediately symptoms of infection, especially influenza-like illness

MYOCARDITIS AND CARDIOMYOPATHY. Fatal myocarditis (most commonly in first 2 months) and cardiomyopathy reported. The CSM has advised:

- physical examination and medical history before starting clozapine;

- specialist examination if cardiac abnormalities or history of heart disease found—clozapine initiated only in absence of severe heart disease and if benefit outweighs risk;

- persistent tachycardia especially in first 2 months should prompt observation for other indicators for myocarditis or cardiomyopathy;
- if myocarditis or cardiomyopathy suspected clozapine should be stopped and patient evaluated urgently by cardiologist;
- discontinue permanently in clozapine-induced myocarditis or cardiomyopathy

GASTRO-INTESTINAL OBSTRUCTION. Reactions resembling gastro-intestinal obstruction reported. Clozapine should be used cautiously with drugs which cause constipation (e.g. antimuscarinic drugs) or in history of colonic disease or bowel surgery. Monitor for constipation and prescribe laxative if required

Contra-indications: severe cardiac disorders (e.g. myocarditis; see Myocarditis and Cardiomyopathy, above); active liver disease (Appendix 2), severe renal impairment (Appendix 3); history of neutropenia or agranulocytosis; bone-marrow disorders; paralytic ileus (see Gastro-intestinal Obstruction, above); alcoholic and toxic psychoses; history of circulatory collapse; drug intoxication; coma or severe CNS depression; uncontrolled epilepsy; pregnancy (Appendix 4) and breast-feeding (Appendix 5)

Side-effects: see notes above; also constipation (see Gastro-intestinal Obstruction, above), hypersalivation, nausea, vomiting; tachycardia, ECG changes, hypertension; drowsiness, blurred vision, headache, tremor, rigidity, extrapyramidal symptoms, convulsions, fatigue, impaired temperature regulation, fever; hepatitis, cholestatic jaundice, pancreatitis; urinary incontinence and retention; agranulocytosis (**important:** see Agranulocytosis, above), leucopenia, eosinophilia, leucocytosis; rarely dysphagia, circulatory collapse, arrhythmias, myocarditis (**important:** see Myocarditis and Cardiomyopathy, above), pericarditis, thromboembolism, confusion, delirium, restlessness, agitation, diabetes mellitus; also reported, intestinal obstruction, paralytic ileus (see Gastro-intestinal Obstruction, above), enlarged parotid gland, fulminant hepatic necrosis, thrombocytopenia, hypertriglyceridaemia, cardiomyopathy, cardiac arrest, respiratory arrest, interstitial nephritis, priapism, skin reactions

Dose: schizophrenia, ADULT over 16 years (close medical supervision on initiation—risk of collapse due to hypotension) 12.5 mg once or twice on first day then 25–50 mg on second day then increased gradually (if well tolerated) in steps of 25–50 mg daily over 14–21 days up to 300 mg daily in divided doses (larger dose at night, up to 200 mg daily may be taken as a single dose at bedtime); if necessary may be further increased in steps of 50–100 mg once (preferably) or twice weekly; usual dose 200–450 mg daily (max. 900 mg daily)
NOTE. *Restarting* after *interval of more than 2 days,* 12.5 mg once or twice on first day (but may be feasible to increase more quickly than on initiation)—extreme caution if previous respiratory or cardiac arrest with initial dosing
ELDERLY AND SPECIAL RISK GROUPS. In *elderly,* 12.5 mg once on first day—subsequent adjustments restricted to 25 mg daily

Psychosis in Parkinson's disease, ADULT over 16 years, 12.5 mg at bedtime then increased in steps of 12.5 mg up to twice weekly to 50 mg at bedtime; usual dose range 25–37.5 mg at bedtime; excep-

tionally, dose may be increased further in steps of 12.5 mg weekly to max. 100 mg daily in 1–2 divided doses

Clozaril® (Novartis) PoM
Tablets, both yellow, clozapine 25 mg (scored), net price 28-tab pack = £12.33, 84-tab pack (hosp. only) = £36.97; 100 mg, 28-tab pack = £49.28, 84-tab pack (hosp. only) = £147.84. Label: 2, 10, patient information leaflet
NOTE. Patient, prescriber, and supplying pharmacist must be registered with the Clozaril Patient Monitoring Service—takes several days to do this

OLANZAPINE

Indications: schizophrenia, treatment of moderate to severe episodes of mania

Cautions: see notes above; also pregnancy (Appendix 4), prostatic hypertrophy, paralytic ileus, hepatic impairment (Appendix 2), renal impairment (Appendix 3), diabetes mellitus (risk of exacerbation or ketoacidosis), low leucocyte or neutrophil count, bone-marrow depression, hypereosinophilic disorders, myeloproliferative disease, Parkinson's disease

Contra-indications: angle-closure glaucoma; breast-feeding

Side-effects: see notes above; also mild, transient antimuscarinic effects; drowsiness, speech difficulty, exacerbation of Parkinson's disease, akathisia, asthenia, increased appetite, raised triglyceride concentration, oedema, hyperprolactinaemia (but clinical manifestations rare), occasionally blood dyscrasias, rarely bradycardia, rash, photosensitivity, diabetes mellitus, priapism, hepatitis, pancreatitis, and elevated creatine kinase concentration

Dose: schizophrenia, combination therapy for mania, ADULT over 18 years, 10 mg daily adjusted to usual range of 5–20 mg daily; doses greater than 10 mg daily only after reassessment

Monotherapy for mania, ADULT over 18 years, 15 mg daily adjusted to usual range of 5–20 mg daily; doses greater than 15 mg daily only after reassessment
NOTE. When one or more factors present that might result in slower metabolism (e.g. female gender, elderly, non-smoker) consider lower initial dose and more gradual dose increase

Zyprexa® (Lilly) PoM
Tablets, f/c, olanzapine 2.5 mg, net price 28-tab pack = £31.70; 5 mg, 28-tab pack = £48.78; 7.5 mg, 56-tab pack = £146.34; 10 mg, 28-tab pack = £97.56, 56-tab pack = £195.11; 15 mg (blue), 28-tab pack = £146.34. Label: 2
Orodispersible tablet (Velotab®), olanzapine 5 mg, net price 28-tab pack = £56.10; 10 mg, 28-tab pack = £112.19; 15 mg, 28-tab pack = £168.29. Label: 2, counselling, administration
Excipients: include aspartame (section 9.4.1)
COUNSELLING. *Velotab®* may be placed on the tongue and allowed to dissolve or dispersed in water, orange juice, apple juice, milk, or coffee

QUETIAPINE

Indications: schizophrenia

Cautions: see notes above; also pregnancy, hepatic impairment (Appendix 2), renal impairment (Appendix 3), cerebrovascular disease

Contra-indications: breast-feeding (Appendix 5)

ANXIETY. Management of *acute anxiety* generally involves the use of a benzodiazepine or buspirone (section 4.1.2). For *chronic anxiety* (of longer than 4 weeks' duration), it may be appropriate to use an antidepressant before a benzodiazepine. *Generalised anxiety disorder* which does not respond to buspirone or to a benzodiazepine is treated with an antidepressant. Antidepressants such as SSRIs and venlafaxine may be effective in specific anxiety disorders.

Compound preparations of an antidepressant and an anxiolytic are not recommended because it is not possible to adjust the dosage of the individual components separately. Whereas antidepressants are given continuously over several months, anxiolytics are prescribed on a short-term basis.

PANIC DISORDERS. Antidepressants are generally used for *panic disorders* and *phobias*; clomipramine (section 4.3.1) is licensed for *obsessional and phobic states*; paroxetine (section 4.3.3) and moclobemide (section 4.3.2) are licensed for the management of social phobia. However, in panic disorders (with or without agarophobia) resistant to antidepressant therapy, a benzodiazepine may be considered (section 4.1.2).

4.3.1 Tricyclic and related antidepressant drugs

This section covers tricyclic antidepressants and also 1-, 2-, and 4-ring structured drugs with broadly similar properties.

These drugs are most effective for treating moderate to severe *endogenous depression* associated with psychomotor and physiological changes such as loss of appetite and sleep disturbances; improvement in sleep is usually the first benefit of therapy. Since there may be an interval of 2 weeks before the antidepressant action takes place electroconvulsive treatment may be required in severe depression when delay is hazardous or intolerable.

Some tricyclic antidepressants are also effective in the management of *panic disorder*.

For reference to the role of some tricyclic antidepressants in some forms of *neuralgia*, see section 4.7.3, and in *nocturnal enuresis* in children, see section 7.4.2.

DOSAGE. About 10 to 20% of patients fail to respond to tricyclic and related antidepressant drugs and inadequate dosage may account for some of these failures. It is important to use doses that are sufficiently high for effective treatment but not so high as to cause toxic effects. Low doses should be used for initial treatment in the **elderly** (see under Side-effects, below).

In most patients the long half-life of tricyclic antidepressant drugs allows **once-daily** administration, usually at night; the use of modified-release preparations is therefore unnecessary.

CHOICE. Tricyclic and related antidepressant drugs can be roughly divided into those with additional sedative properties and those which are less so. Agitated and anxious patients tend to respond best to the sedative compounds whereas withdrawn and apathetic patients will often obtain most benefit from the less sedating ones. Those with **sedative** properties include amitriptyline, clomipramine, dosulepin (dothiepin), doxepin, maprotiline, mianserin, trazodone, and trimipramine. Those with **less sedative** properties include amoxapine, imipramine, lofepramine, and nortriptyline.

Imipramine and **amitriptyline** are well established and relatively safe and effective, but they have more marked antimuscarinic and cardiac side-effects than compounds such as **doxepin**, **mianserin**, and **trazodone**; this may be important in individual patients. **Lofepramine** also has a lower incidence of antimuscarinic and sedative side-effects and is less dangerous in overdosage; it is, however, infrequently associated with hepatic toxicity. **Amoxapine** is related to the antipsychotic loxapine and its side-effects include tardive dyskinesia.

For a comparison of tricyclic and related antidepressants with SSRIs and related antidepressants and MAOIs, see section 4.3.

SIDE-EFFECTS. *Arrhythmias* and *heart block* occasionally follow the use of tricyclic antidepressants, particularly amitriptyline, and may be a factor in the sudden death of patients with cardiac disease. They are also sometimes associated with *convulsions* (and should be prescribed with special caution in epilepsy as they lower the convulsive threshold); maprotiline has particularly been associated with convulsions. *Hepatic* and *haematological* reactions may occur and have been particularly associated with mianserin.

Other side-effects of tricyclic and related antidepressants include *drowsiness, dry mouth, blurred vision, constipation,* and *urinary retention* (all attributed to antimuscarinic activity), and sweating. The patient should be encouraged to persist with treatment as some tolerance to these side-effects seems to develop. They are reduced if low doses are given initially and then gradually increased, but this must be balanced against the need to obtain a full therapeutic effect as soon as possible. Gradual introduction of treatment is particularly important in the elderly, who, because of the hypotensive effects of these drugs, are prone to attacks of *dizziness* or even *syncope*. Another side-effect to which the elderly are particularly susceptible is *hyponatraemia* (see CSM advice on p. 187). *Neuroleptic malignant syndrome* (section 4.2.1) may, very rarely, arise in the course of antidepressant treatment.

Limited quantities of tricyclic antidepressants should be prescribed at any one time because they are dangerous in overdosage. For advice on **overdosage** see Emergency Treatment of Poisoning, p. 24.

WITHDRAWAL. If possible tricyclic and related antidepressants should be withdrawn slowly (see also section 4.3).

INTERACTIONS. A tricyclic or related antidepressant (or an SSRI or related antidepressant) should not be started until 2 weeks after stopping an MAOI (3 weeks if starting clomipramine or imipramine). Conversely, an MAOI should not be started until at least 7–14 days after a tricyclic or related antidepressant (3 weeks in the case of clomipramine or imipramine) has been stopped. For guidance relating to the reversible monoamine oxidase inhibitor, moclobemide, see p. 193. For other tricyclic antidepressant **interactions**, see Appendix 1 (antidepressants, tricyclic).

Tricyclic antidepressants

AMITRIPTYLINE HYDROCHLORIDE

Indications: depressive illness, particularly where sedation is required; nocturnal enuresis in children (section 7.4.2)

Cautions: cardiac disease (particularly with arrhythmias, see Contra-indications below), history of epilepsy, pregnancy and breast-feeding (Appendixes 4 and 5), elderly, hepatic impairment (avoid if severe), thyroid disease, phaeochromocytoma, history of mania, psychoses (may aggravate psychotic symptoms), angle-closure glaucoma, history of urinary retention, concurrent electroconvulsive therapy; if possible avoid abrupt withdrawal; anaesthesia (increased risk of arrhythmias and hypotension, see surgery section 15.1); porphyria (section 9.8.2); see section 7.4.2 for additional nocturnal enuresis warnings; **interactions:** Appendix 1 (antidepressants, tricyclic)

DRIVING. Drowsiness may affect performance of skilled tasks (e.g. driving); effects of alcohol enhanced

Contra-indications: recent myocardial infarction, arrhythmias (particularly heart block), not indicated in manic phase, severe liver disease

Side-effects: dry mouth, sedation, blurred vision (disturbance of accommodation, increased intra-ocular pressure), constipation, nausea, difficulty with micturition; cardiovascular side-effects (such as ECG changes, arrhythmias, postural hypotension, tachycardia, syncope, particularly with high doses); sweating, tremor, rashes and hypersensitivity reactions (including urticaria, photosensitivity), behavioural disturbances (particularly children), hypomania or mania, confusion (particularly elderly), interference with sexual function, blood sugar changes; increased appetite and weight gain (occasionally weight loss); endocrine side-effects such as testicular enlargement, gynaecomastia, galactorrhoea; also convulsions (see also Cautions), movement disorders and dyskinesias, fever, agranulocytosis, leucopenia, eosinophilia, purpura, thrombocytopenia, hyponatraemia (may be due to inappropriate antidiuretic hormone secretion) see CSM advice, p. 187, abnormal liver function tests (jaundice); for a general outline of side-effects see also notes above; **overdosage:** see Emergency Treatment of Poisoning, p. 24

Dose: depression, initially 75 mg (elderly and adolescents 30–75 mg) daily in divided doses *or* as a single dose at bedtime increased gradually as necessary to 150–200 mg; CHILD under 16 years not recommended for depression

Nocturnal enuresis, CHILD 7–10 years 10–20 mg, 11–16 years 25–50 mg at night; max. period of treatment (including gradual withdrawal) 3 months—full physical examination before further course

Amitriptyline (Non-proprietary) PoM
Tablets, coated, amitriptyline hydrochloride 10 mg, net price 20 = 56p; 25 mg, 20 = 58p; 50 mg, 20 = 86p. Label: 2
Available from Alpharma, APS, DDSA (*Elavil*®)

Oral solution, amitriptyline (as hydrochloride) 25 mg/5 mL, net price 200 mL = £10.73; 50 mg/5 mL, 200 mL = £18.00. Label: 2
Available from Rosemont (sugar-free)

■ Compound preparations

Triptafen® (Goldshield) PoM ▣▬
Tablets, pink, s/c, amitriptyline hydrochloride 25 mg, perphenazine 2 mg. Net price 20 = £4.25. Label: 2

Triptafen-M® (Goldshield) PoM ▣▬
Tablets, pink, s/c, amitriptyline hydrochloride 10 mg, perphenazine 2 mg. Net price 20 = £3.80. Label: 2

AMOXAPINE

Indications: depressive illness
Cautions: see under Amitriptyline Hydrochloride
Contra-indications: see under Amitriptyline Hydrochloride
Side-effects: see under Amitriptyline Hydrochloride; tardive dyskinesia reported; menstrual irregularities, breast enlargement, and galactorrhoea reported in women
Dose: initially 100–150 mg daily in divided doses *or* as a single dose at bedtime increased as necessary to max. 300 mg daily; ELDERLY initially 25 mg twice daily increased as necessary after 5–7 days to max. 50 mg 3 times daily; CHILD under 16 years not recommended

Asendis® (Goldshield) PoM
Tablets, amoxapine 50 mg (orange, scored), net price 84-tab pack = £16.78; 100 mg (blue, scored), 56-tab pack = £18.65. Label: 2

CLOMIPRAMINE HYDROCHLORIDE

Indications: depressive illness, phobic and obsessional states; adjunctive treatment of cataplexy associated with narcolepsy
Cautions: see under Amitriptyline Hydrochloride
Contra-indications: see under Amitriptyline Hydrochloride
Side-effects: see under Amitriptyline Hydrochloride
Dose: initially 10 mg daily, increased gradually as necessary to 30–150 mg daily in divided doses *or* as a single dose at bedtime; max. 250 mg daily; ELDERLY initially 10 mg daily increased carefully over approx. 10 days to 30–75 mg daily; CHILD not recommended

Phobic and obsessional states, initially 25 mg daily (ELDERLY 10 mg daily) increased over 2 weeks to 100–150 mg daily; CHILD not recommended

Adjunctive treatment of cataplexy associated with narcolepsy, initially 10 mg daily gradually increased until satisfactory response (range 10–75 mg daily)

Clomipramine (Non-proprietary) PoM
Capsules, clomipramine hydrochloride 10 mg, net price 28-cap pack = £1.21; 25 mg, 28-cap pack = £1.29; 50 mg, 28-cap pack = £2.42. Label: 2
Available from Alpharma, APS, Generics, Hillcross, IVAX

Anafranil® (Cephalon) PoM
Capsules, clomipramine hydrochloride 10 mg (yellow/caramel), net price 84-cap pack = £3.23; 25 mg (orange/caramel), 84-cap pack = £6.35; 50 mg (grey/caramel), 56-cap pack=£8.06. Label: 2

of choice are **phenelzine** or **isocarboxazid** which are less stimulant and therefore safer.

Phobic patients and depressed patients with atypical, hypochondriacal, or hysterical features are said to respond best to MAOIs. However, MAOIs should be tried in any patients who are refractory to treatment with other antidepressants as there is occasionally a dramatic response. Response to treatment may be delayed for 3 weeks or more and may take an additional 1 or 2 weeks to become maximal.

WITHDRAWAL. If possible MAOIs should be withdrawn slowly (see also section 4.3).

INTERACTIONS. MAOIs inhibit monoamine oxidase, thereby causing an accumulation of amine neurotransmitters. The metabolism of some amine drugs such as *indirect-acting sympathomimetics* (present in many cough and decongestant preparations, see section 3.10) is also inhibited and their pressor action may be potentiated; the pressor effect of tyramine (in some foods, such as mature cheese, pickled herring, broad bean pods, and *Bovril*®, *Oxo*®, *Marmite*® or any similar meat or yeast extract or fermented soya bean extract) may also be dangerously potentiated. These interactions may cause a dangerous rise in blood pressure. An early warning symptom may be a throbbing headache. Patients should be advised to eat only fresh foods and avoid food that is suspected of being stale or 'going off'. This is especially important with meat, fish, poultry or offal; game should be avoided. The danger of interaction persists for up to 2 weeks after treatment with MAOIs is discontinued. Patients should also avoid alcoholic drinks or de-alcoholised (low alcohol) drinks.

Other antidepressants should **not** be started for 2 weeks after treatment with MAOIs has been stopped (3 weeks if starting clomipramine or imipramine). Some psychiatrists use selected tricyclics in conjunction with MAOIs but this is hazardous, indeed potentially lethal, except in experienced hands and there is no evidence that the combination is more effective than when either constituent is used alone. The combination of tranylcypromine with clomipramine is particularly **dangerous**.

Conversely, an MAOI should not be started until at least 7–14 days after a tricyclic or related antidepressant (3 weeks in the case of clomipramine or imipramine) has been stopped.

In addition, an MAOI should not be started for at least 2 weeks after a previous MAOI has been stopped (then started at a reduced dose).

For other interactions with MAOIs including those with opioid analgesics (notably pethidine), see Appendix 1 (MAOIs). For guidance on interactions relating to the reversible monoamine oxidase inhibitor, moclobemide, see p. 193; for guidance on interactions relating to SSRIs, see p. 193.

PHENELZINE ◢

Indications: depressive illness

Cautions: diabetes mellitus, cardiovascular disease, epilepsy, blood disorders, concurrent electroconvulsive therapy; elderly (great caution); monitor blood pressure (risk of postural hypotension and hypertensive responses—discontinue if palpitations or frequent headaches); if possible avoid abrupt withdrawal; severe hypertensive reactions to certain drugs and foods; avoid in agitated patients; porphyria (section 9.8.2); pregnancy and breast-feeding; surgery (section 15.1); **interactions:** Appendix 1 (MAOIs)

DRIVING. Drowsiness may affect performance of skilled tasks (e.g. driving)

Contra-indications: hepatic impairment or abnormal liver function tests (Appendix 2), cerebrovascular disease, phaeochromocytoma; not indicated in manic phase

Side-effects: commonly postural hypotension (especially in elderly) and dizziness; less common side-effects include drowsiness, insomnia, headache, weakness and fatigue, dry mouth, constipation and other gastro-intestinal disturbances, oedema, myoclonic movement, hyperreflexia, elevated liver enzymes; agitation and tremors, nervousness, euphoria, arrhythmias, blurred vision, nystagmus, difficulty in micturition, sweating, convulsions, rashes, purpura, leucopenia, sexual disturbances, and weight gain with inappropriate appetite may also occur; psychotic episodes with hypomanic behaviour, confusion, and hallucinations may be induced in susceptible persons; jaundice has been reported and, on rare occasions, fatal progressive hepatocellular necrosis; paraesthesia, peripheral neuritis, peripheral neuropathy may be due to pyridoxine deficiency; for CSM advice on possible hyponatraemia, see p. 187

Dose: 15 mg 3 times daily, increased if necessary to 4 times daily after 2 weeks (hospital patients, max. 30 mg 3 times daily), then reduced gradually to lowest possible maintenance dose (15 mg on alternate days may be adequate); CHILD not recommended

Nardil® (Hansam) PoM ◢
Tablets, orange, f/c, phenelzine (as sulphate) 15 mg, net price 20 = £3.99. Label: 3, 10, patient information leaflet

ISOCARBOXAZID ◢

Indications: depressive illness
Cautions: see under Phenelzine
Contra-indications: see under Phenelzine
Side-effects: see under Phenelzine
Dose: initially 30 mg daily in single or divided doses until improvement occurs (increased after 4 weeks if necessary to max. 60 mg daily for 4–6 weeks under close supervision), then reduced to usual maintenance dose 10–20 mg daily (but up to 40 mg daily may be required); ELDERLY 5–10 mg daily; CHILD not recommended

Isocarboxazid (Non-proprietary) PoM ◢
Tablets, pink, scored, isocarboxazid 10 mg. Net price 50 = £26.71. Label: 3, 10, patient information leaflet
Available from Cambridge

TRANYLCYPROMINE ◢

Indications: depressive illness
Cautions: see under Phenelzine
Contra-indications: see under Phenelzine; hyperthyroidism
Side-effects: see under Phenelzine; insomnia if given in evening; hypertensive crises with throbbing headache requiring discontinuation of treatment more frequent than with other MAOIs; liver damage less frequent than with phenelzine